Prevention and Treatment of
RUNNING INJURIES

SECOND EDITION

Editors: Robert D D'Ambrosia, MD
David Drez Jr, MD

1989

SLACK Incorporated, 6900 Grove Road, Thorofare, New Jersey 08086

SLACK International Book Distributors

In Europe, the Middle East and Africa:
John Wiley & Sons Limited
Baffins Lane
Chichester, West Sussex P019 1UD
England

In Canada:
McAinsh and Company
2760 Old Leslie Street
Willowdale, Ontario M2K 2X5

In Australia and New Zealand:
MacLennan & Petty Pty Limited
P.O. Box 425
Artarmon, N.S.W. 2064
Australia

In Japan:
Central Foreign Books Limited
1-13 Jimbocho-Kanda
Tokyo, Japan

In Asia and India:
PG Publishing Pte Limited.
36 West Coast Road, #02-02
Singapore 0512

Foreign Translation Agent:
John Scott & Company
International Publishers' Agency
417-A Pickering Road
Phoenixville, PA 19460

Publisher: Harry C. Benson
Managing Editor: Lynn Borders
Editor: Cheryl D. Willoughby
Designer: Susan Hermansen
Production Manager: David Murphy

RD
560
,P73x
1989

Printed in the United States of America

Library of Congress Catalog Card Number: 86-428639

ISBN: 0-943432-99-5

Published by: SLACK Incorporated
6900 Grove Rd.
Thorofare, NJ 08086

Last digit is print number: 10   9   8   7   6   5   4   3   2   1

Dedication

BARBARA

Lisa
Chris
Matt
Peter

Acknowledgements

Editing a multiauthored text can be a time-consuming project not only for the editors, but also for the many authors on whom the editor depends for contributions. The authors who wrote this text did outstanding jobs with their individual chapters, and their efforts combined to make this book what it is.

The final product was largely made possible through the efforts of Marie Grassi, our research associate who guided and directed this second edition. Her dedication and perseverance is deeply appreciated.

We also acknowledge the help of the secretarial staff of the LSU Department of Orthopedic Surgery under the guidance of Phyllis Casey and Clythia Anderson.

Special appreciation must go to David Drez for his help in putting together the first edition of this text.

Contents

Preface to the Second Edition

No sport has captured the imagination of such a large segment of our population as running. The enthusiasm generated for this activity has approached overwhelming proportions—it has become not only a sport, but a philosophy of life. This over-zealousness has pushed runners to try to make their bodies reach new physical limints. Understandably, many running injuries have resulted.

As physicians who have enjoyed the avocation of running since high school track, we recognize the fact that runners naturally seek physicians who have some empathy for their running problem. Eleven years ago, because of the increase in running injuries presented to us, we decided to establish a running clinic to accommodate the needs of our running population. We found that the team approach was essential for the best care for our runners. Our team consists of orthopedists, a physical therapist, and an orthotist. This approach has proved to be exceedingly beneficial in helping runners with musculoskeletal problems; we have also gained much knowledge about running problems; and especially about how best to prevent such injuries from occurring.

Similar clinics have been set up in diverse areas of the United States, and the sharing of our various experiences has been valuable. This book evolved from our contact with other running-oriented physicians, physical therapists, orthotists, and nutritional experts throughout the United States and Canada. Great care was taken to seek out authorities for the different subject areas of the text in an attempt to amass the most current knowledge currently available on ways to prevent and treat running injuries.

In this second edition we have not only updated our previous text but have attempted to broaden the scope of the text and have added clinical sections on foot injuries, eccentric exercise, and chronic tendonitis, plus added depth to the biomechanics of motion and for the first time have shown the importance of agonist and antagonist muscle and the role of muscle synergism.

Editor

Robert D. D'Ambrosia, MD
Professor and Chairman
Department of Orthopaedics
Louisiana State University School of Medicine
New Orleans, Louisiana

Associate Editor

David Drez, Jr., MD
Clinical Professor of Orthopaedics
Louisiana State University School of Medicine
New Orleans, Louisiana

Contributors

William G. Clancy, Jr., MD
Professor and Head, Section of Sports
    Medicine
Division of Orthopaedic Surgery
University of Wisconsin
Madison, Wisconsin

Sandra Curwin, Ph.D.
Assistant Professor
School of Physiotherapy
Dalhousie University
Halifax, Nova Scotia

Virginia B. Davis, M.A., P.T.
President
Cresent City Physical Therapy
    and Sports Rehabilitation
    Services, Inc.
New Orleans, Louisiana

Roy Douglas
Certified Prosthetist
Associate Professor
Department of Orthopaedics
Louisiana State University School of
    Medicine
New Orleans, Louisiana

Peter G. Hanson, MD
Professor of Medicine
Director, Rehabilitation Program
University of Wisconsin
Madison, Wisconsin

Diane M. Huse, R.D., M.S.
Assistant Professor of Nutrition
Mayo Medical School
Nutritionist, Mayo Clinic
Rochester, Minnesota

Douglas W. Jackson, MD
Director, Southern California
    Center for Sports Medicine
Medical Director, Memorial Bone and
    Tissue Bank
Long Beach, California

Robert E. Leach, MD
Chairman and Professor
Department of Orthopaedics
Boston University Medical Center
Boston, Massachusetts

Roger A. Mann, MD
Private Orthopaedic Practice
Oakland, California
Associate Clinical Professor of
    Orthopaedic Surgery
University of California School
    of Medicine
San Francisco, California

Angus McBryde, Jr., MD
Charolotte Orthopaedic
Clinical Assistant Professor
    of Surgery
Duke University Medical Center
Durham, North Carolina

Lyle Micheli, MD
Director of Sports Medicine
Children's Hospital
    Medical Center
Boston, Massachusetts

Scott J. Mubarak, MD
Associate Clinical of
    Orthopaedic Surgery
University of California San Diego
Pediatric Orthopaedic Surgeon
Children's Hospital
San Diego, California

G. Richard Paul, MD
Associate Professor
    of Orthopaedics
Vice Chairman
Department of Orthopaedics
Boston University School
    of Medicine
Boston, Massachusetts

G. James Sammarco, MD
Center for Orthopaedic Care
Cincinnati, Ohio

Moshe Solomonow, Ph.D.
Director, Bioengineering Laboratory
Department of Orthopaedics
Louisiana State University School of
    Medicine
New Orleans, Louisiana

William D. Standish, MD
Associate Professor of Surgery
Dalhousie University
Halifax, Nova Scotia

CHAPTER 1

Biomechanics
of Running

Roger A. Mann, M.D.

Introduction

The biomechanics of running are somewhat difficult to discuss because of the great variability of the activity, ie, from the slow recreational jogger to the world class sprinter. In the biomechanical studies of "normal" human walking, subject variability is minimal and the speed of gait is constant, as are the range of motion of the joints of the lower extremity, phasic muscle activity, and forces. In running, there is a broad spectrum of speed resulting in extreme variability in the range of motion of the joints, phasic muscle activity, and ground reactions. To fully appreciate the biomechanical aspects of running, I believe we should compare it with an established standard. Because walking has been carefully studied, it will be used as the standard to which various speeds of running will be compared. All the data will be for steady-state walking and running. The acceleration or deceleration of gait will not be discussed.

All unreferenced data presented have been obtained from work carried out at the Gait Analysis Laboratory at Shriner's Hospital for Crippled Children in San Francisco, California.

Gait Cycle

The gait cycle is a useful framework by which the various events that occur during human locomotion can be expressed. The gait cycle begins and ends with heel strike of the same foot. That sequence also constitutes a stride, which consists of two steps. In the case of a person running on his toes, the gait cycle will obviously be from the time of initial ground contact until the same extremity

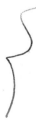

once again comes into contact with the ground. The cycle is further divided into a stance phase and a swing phase. During walking the stance phase occupies about 60% of the gait cycle and the swing phase 40%. Two periods of double-limb support occur during the first 12% and the last 12% of the stance phase, and a period of single-limb support occupies about 35% of the walking cycle. During walking there is no period in which both feet are off the ground (Figure 1-1).

As the speed of gait increases, the period of stance phase decreases and swing phase increases (Figure 1-2). As the speed of gait continues to increase, there is a period, termed the non-support or float phase, in which both feet are off the ground. So as the speed of running increases, the stance phase decreases, swing phase increases, and float phase increases (Figure 1-3).

Angular Rotation of the Lower Extremity

During normal locomotion, motion occurs in the lower extremities in the transverse, sagittal, and frontal planes. In walking, this motion has been well documented and has been measured by many laboratories.[1,2] The results of the measurements basically agree with one another. When a person starts to run, however, the measurement of the rotation in the transverse plane becomes much more difficult and as a result, no reliable quantitative measurement of the transverse plane rotation have been made yet (Figure 1-4). The sagittal-plane motion, however, has been well documented;[3] the sagittal-plane rotation of the hip, knee, and ankle, during walking, jogging, and running, is presented (Figure 1-5). Frontal-plane motion of the hip joint, namely hip abduction and adduction, is also presented (Figure 1-6).

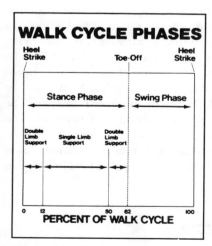

Figure 1-1. Phases of the walking cycle.

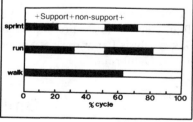

Figure 1-2. The support or stance phase is in black and the non-support or swing phase is in white. Note: As the speed of gait increases, the period of support decreases and the period of non-support increases.

Forceplate Analysis of Gait

During locomotion, forces are exerted against the ground. These forces are measured by use of a forceplate. The forces that are measured consist of the vertical, fore and aft shear, medial and lateral shear, and torque. The force data for walking are presented here (Figure 1-7). The forceplate analysis for running and jogging demonstrates much more variability from step to step, as compared with walking. The vertical, fore and aft shear, and medial and lateral shear for jogging and running are also presented here (Figure 1-8).

A comparison of the force data for walking and running readily demonstrates the marked increase in the ground reaction of running. The magnitude of the vertical force in walking at a cadence of 120 steps per minutes (60 strides) rarely exceeds 115% to 120% of body weight. The inclination and magnitude of the initial spike on a vertical force curve are much greater for running than for walking. In walking, the initial spike is about 70% of body weight, whereas jogging barefooted increases the spike to almost 200% of body weight. Also, interestingly, the two peaks that are normally seen in the vertical force curve for walking are no longer present during running, probably because only one extremity is on the ground at a time during the stance phase of running, whereas the stance phase of walking includes two periods of double-limb support.

The fore and aft shear pattern demonstrates the same basic configuration for walking, jogging, and running; however, the magnitude is increased about 50% for running. The medial and lateral shear curves for walking, jogging, and running also demonstrate the same general pattern, although again magnitude is increased in running.

The torque measurement during walking demonstrates an initial internal torque followed by an external torque against the ground. This sequence correlates well with the transverse rotation curve of the lower extremity, in that internal rotation occurs in the lower extremity at the same time that an internal

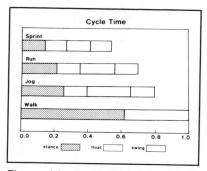

Figure 1-3. As the speed of gait increases, there is a period of time in which both feet are off the ground. This period is known as the float phase. As the speed of gait increases, the length of the stance phase decreases and the period of float phase increases.

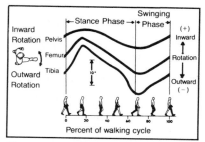

Figure 1-4. Transverse plane rotation of the pelvis, femur, and tibia. Note that maximum internal rotation is achieved by approximately 15% of the walking cycle and maximum external rotation at the time of toe-off.

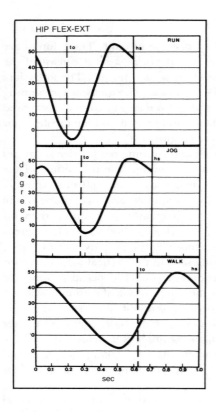

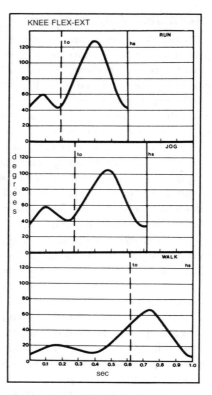

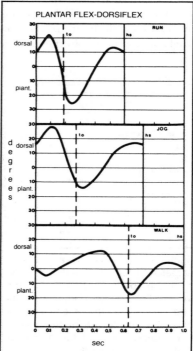

Figure 1-5. Sagittal plane motion of the lower extremity during walking, jogging, and running.

torque occurs against the ground, and conversely, external rotation occurs in the lower extremity, associated with an external torque against the ground. Because torque has been adequately measured only for walking, no data are presented for jogging and running.

Electromyography of the Lower Extremities

The phasic activity of the muscles of the lower extremities during walking is shown (Figure 1-9). The phasic activity has been presented by muscle groups such as the hip flexors and extensors, knee flexors and extensors, and ankle dorsiflexors and plantar flexors, because these muscles are essentially functioning as a unit, rather than as individual muscles. The muscles of the lower extremities do not have a fine neurologic and cerebral representation, as do the muscles of the upper extremities. The overall muscle function is much more gross in the lower extremity than in the upper extremity, and as the speed of gait increases, it has been found that the phasic activity of the various muscles function even more as a group than during walking. Electromyographic activity of the muscles of the lower extremity for walking, jogging, running, and sprinting is presented (Figure 1-10).

Biomechanical Principles

Several basic principles should be kept firmly in mind when evaluating the changes in the biomechanics of the lower extremities as the speed of gait increases. The transverse rotation that occurs in the lower extremity during the walking gait has been documented both quantitatively and qualitatively, but quantitative data of running have been difficult to obtain. Qualitative data obtained from high-speed movies show that the same basic type of rotation

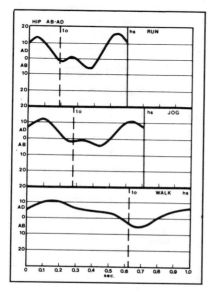

Figure 1-6. Frontal–plane motion of the hip joint, namely, hip abduction and adduction during walking, jogging, and running.

occurs during running, and the rotation seems to be of somewhat greater magnitude than that observed during walking. The transverse rotation, which occurs in the lower extremity at the time of initial ground contact, is transmitted across the ankle joint to the subtalar joint. The subtalar joint is an oblique hinge that is aligned at about 45° to the horizontal plane and deviates 16° from medial to lateral in relation to the foot (Figure 1-11). The subtalar joint, acting as an oblique hinge, translates the transverse rotation of the lower extremity into inversion and eversion of the calcaneus.[4,5,6]

Internal rotation of the lower extremity everts the calcaneus, and conversely, external rotation of the lower extremity inverts the calcaneus (Figure 1-12). The motion in the subtalar joint essentially controls the subsequent stability of the forefoot through its control of the transverse tarsal joint, and therefore controls the stability of the longitudinal arch of the foot. The function of the transverse tarsal joint, which is composed of the talonavicular and calcaneocuboid joints, is

Figure 1-7. Forceplate analysis of walking.

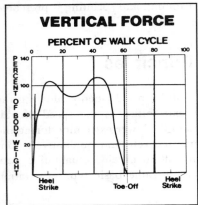

a. Vertical force

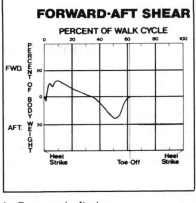

b. Fore and aft shear

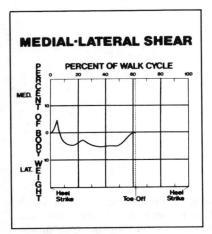

c. Medial lateral shear

d. Torque

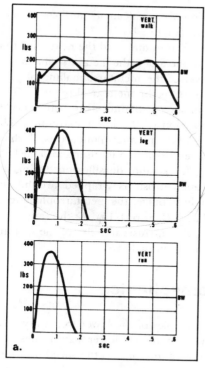

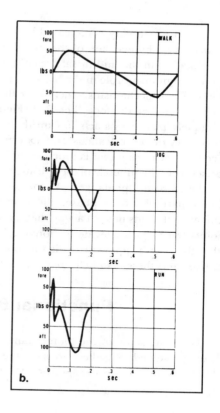

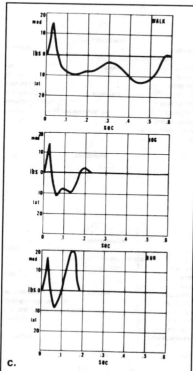

Figure 1-8. Comparison of the force-plate analysis for walking, running, and jogging.

such that its stability is increased by inversion of the calcaneus, and conversely, is decreased by eversion of the subtalar joint (Figure 1-13).

Rotation in the mid-tarsal area of the foot is minimal, and the next joint that plays a significant role in the biomechanics of the foot is the metatarsophalangeal joint. Two mechanisms function at the level of the metatarsophalangeal joint help to stabilize the foot. The first (Figure 1-14) is the metatarsal break.[8,9] This obliquely placed axis acts to cam the foot in such a manner as to help produce inversion of the calcaneus and external rotation of the lower extremity. The second mechanism that is functioning is that of the plantar aponeurosis,[10] which arises from the tubercle of the calcaneus, passes forward, and inserts into the base of the proximal phalanges. As the toes are forced into dorsiflexion during the latter part of stance phase, the plantar aponeurosis is wrapped around the metatarsal heads in such a way that it not only stabilizes the metatarsophalangeal joints but helps to elevate the longitudinal arch (Figure 1-15). At the same time that the plantar aponeurosis is functioning, the intrinsic muscles of the foot are active, and these also help to stabilize the longitudinal arch.

Functional Biomechanics

Thus far, some of the biomechanical principles of the lower extremity have been presented. Needless to say, the function of the lower extremities is a dynamic one, and as the speed of gait increases, not only is the speed by which

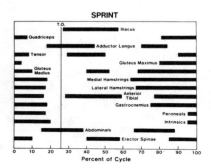
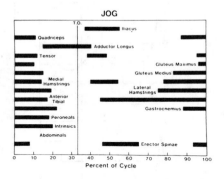
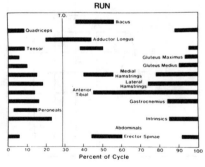

Figure 1-9. Electromyographic activity of the muscle groups of the lower extremity during walking, jogging, running, and sprinting.

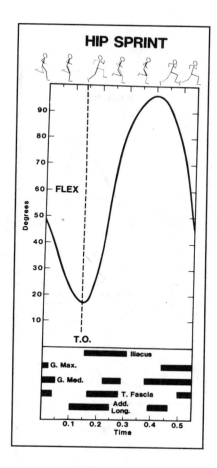

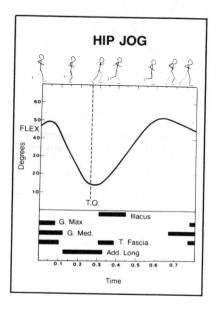

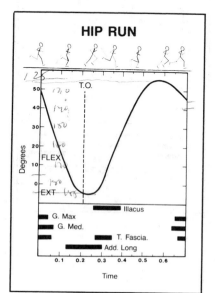

Figure 1-10. Electromyographic activity of the muscle of the lower extremity during walking, jogging, running and sprinting, in relationship to the range of motion of the joint.

10A. Hip joint

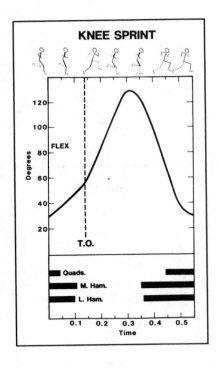

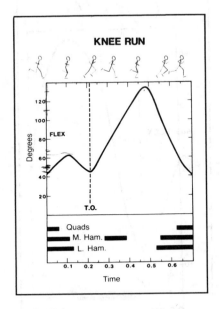

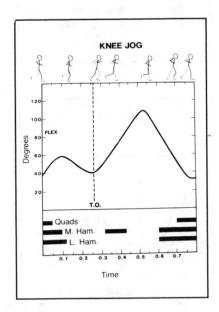

10B. Knee joint.

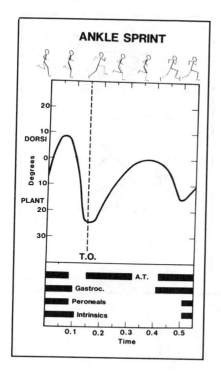

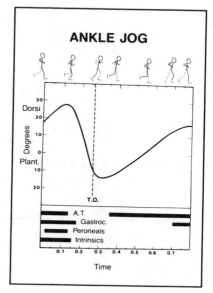

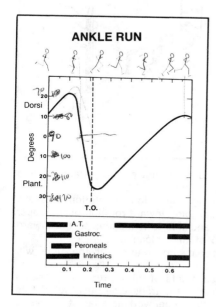

10C. Ankle joint.

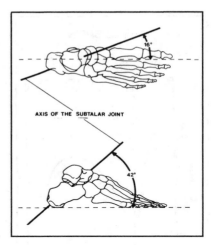

Figure 1-11. Axis of the subtalar joint.

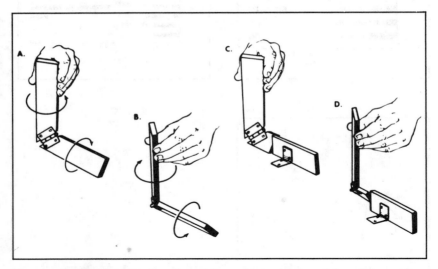

Figure 1-12. Model of the function of the subtalar joint as it translates motion from the tibia above into the calcaneus below.

A. Action of a mitered hinge demonstrating translation of rotation across a 45° hinge. This is analogous to the subtalar joint. Inward rotation of the upper stick causes rotation of the lower stick, and this is analogous to the inward rotation of the tibia, producing eversion of the calcaneus.

B. Conversely, it is demonstrated that outward rotation of the tibia will produce inward rotation of the calcaneus.

C. The addition of a pivot between two segments of the mechanism presents the analogy as above, but with the addition of the transverse tarsal joint. This is depicted by the pivot point beyond the 45° hinge, working against the distal segment, which is fixed on the ground. This distal segment represents the forefoot that is firmly planted on the ground. The inward rotation of the tibia, which produces eversion of the calcaneus, will obviously have an effect on the transverse tarsal joint.

D. See Figure 1-12C.

each of these mechanisms occurs increased but, the magnitude of the force involved increases greatly.

At the time of initial ground contact, internal rotation occurs in the lower extremity, and as the foot is loaded, concomitant eversion occurs in the calcaneus. The eversion of the calcaneus starts a series of movements that results in pronation of the longitudinal arch. The eversion of the calcaneus results in a flexible transverse tarsal joint, which permits a certain degree of collapse of the longitudinal arch as the foot is applied to the ground. This mechanism of eversion of the calcaneus, along with flexibility of the longitudinal arch, is purely passive and is not under any muscle control, per se. The factors limiting the degree of collapse of the longitudinal arch after initial ground contact appear to be only those provided by the axis of the motions of the joints of the foot, shape of the bones of the foot, and their connecting ligaments. Pronation is a normal occurrence in the foot at the time of initial ground contact (Figure 1-16).

Once the foot is firmly on the ground, progressive external rotation occurs in the lower extremity. This external rotation passes across the ankle joint to the

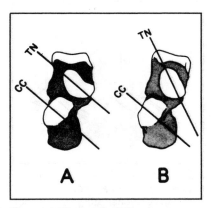

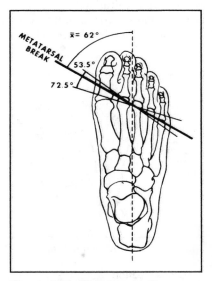

Figure 1-13. Axes of the transverse tarsal joint (TN = talonavicular and CC = calcaneocuboid joint).
A. When the calcaneus is in eversion, the conjoint axes between the talonavicular and calcaneocuboid joints are parallel to one another, so that there is increased motion in the transverse tarsal joint.
B. When the calcaneus is in inversion, the conjoint axes between the talonavicular and calcaneocuboid joints are not parallel to one another, so that there is decreased motion in the transverse tarsal joint.

Figure 1-14. Variation in the angulation of the metatarsal break.

subtalar joint. In response to this external rotation, the subtalar joint brings about inversion of the calcaneus, which in turn stabilizes the transverse tarsal joint, and helps to create a rigid longitudinal arch. As the weight–bearing progresses along the foot to the metatarsal head area, bringing about dorsiflexion of the metatarsophalangeal joints, the oblique metatarsal break further helps to bring about inversion by increasing external rotation of the tibia. Stability of the foot is further enhanced by the action of the plantar aponeurosis and intrinsic muscles of the foot.

The actions that have just been described are active mechanisms, as opposed to the passive mechanism of pronation. The external rotation of the stance limb is initiated by the forward motion of the swing leg, which helps to bring the swing leg side of the pelvis forward. As this occurs, the stance leg femur, which is fixed to the pelvis by the electrically active adductor muscles of the thigh, is externally rotated. The external rotation of the femur passes across the knee joint, which is stabilized by its ligaments, as well as by the popliteus muscle. This external rotation force passes through the tibia and across the ankle joint to the subtalar joint, which through its control of the calcaneus and transverse tarsal joint then stabilizes the longitudinal arch, creating a rigid lever of the foot.

The motion occurring in the sagittal plane at the hip, the knee, and the ankle demonstrates some interesting changes as the speed of gait increases. Generally

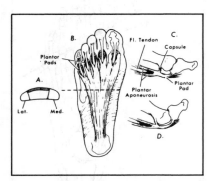

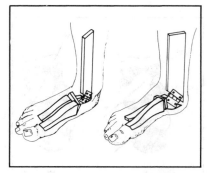

Figure 1-15. The plantar aponeurosis.
A. Cross section
B. The plantar aponeurosis divides as it proceeds distally to allow the flexor tendons to pass through the aponeurosis.
C. The plantar aponeurosis combines with the joint capsule to form the plantar pad of the metatarsophalangeal joint.
D. Dorsiflexion of the toes forces the metatarsal head into plantar flexion and brings the plantar pad over the head of the metatarsal.

Figure 1-16. A model of the linkage between the tibia, hindfoot, and forefoot, demonstrating the effect on the longitudinal arch.
A. Internal rotation of the tibia produces eversion of the calcaneus, which in turn produces a flexible transverse tarsal joint and flattens the longitudinal arch, bringing about pronation of the foot. This occurs at the time of initial ground contact.
B. External rotation of the tibia brings about inversion of the heel, stability of the transverse tarsal joint with elevation of the longitudinal arch, giving rise to a supinated firm forefoot.

speaking, the total range of motion increases in each of these joints during jogging and running (Figure 1-5). At the time of initial ground contact, there is an increased amount of flexion at the hip joint, rapid flexion at the knee joint, and dorsiflexion at the ankle joint. This increased joint motion functions mainly to help the body absorb the sharply increased impact of initial ground contact. The most significant change is at the ankle joint, where at the time of initial ground contact, plantar flexion occurs during walking; but during running, rapid dorsiflexion occurs.

Our laboratory has obtained high-speed movies of many long-distance runners, and with few exceptions, initial ground contact is either heel first or foot flat. Even a sprinter's foot, which lands in plantar flexion, undergoes a certain degree of dorsiflexion after initial ground contact, although the degree of dorsiflexion is not sufficient to permit the sprinter's heel to strike the ground. During the mid-stance phase, progressive extension occurs at the hip joint and continues until after toe-off. The knee joint, after undergoing rapid flexion during the first half of stance, rapidly extends during the remainder of the stance, until toe-off. The ankle joint, after rapid dorsiflexion, which peaks at mid-stance, undergoes rapid plantar flexion. This continues until after toe-off. In contrast to the runner, the few sprinters we have studied had gradual extension of the hip joint after initial ground contact and progressive flexion of the knee joint, but the same type of rapid dorsiflexion of the ankle joint until mid-stance, when rapid plantar flexion began.

The frontal–plane motion of the hip joint demonstrates adduction at the time of initial ground contact, which increases in magnitude with increased speed of gait (Figure 1-6). This adduction of the hip joint accounts for the initial medial force spike noted in the forceplate data (Figure 1-8). We then see progressive abduction of the hip, which reaches its peak after toe-off, and this is what accounts for the lateral force curve noted throughout the remainder of stance phase.

Electromyography

The electromyographic data of the phasic activities of the muscle in the lower extremities also change as the speed of gait increases. Generally speaking, by percentage, the muscles have a longer period of stance phase activity than that normally seen in walking. As an example, it is rare to see a muscle group active for more than 50% of the stance phase during walking, but in jogging, running and sprinting, there is activity during 70% to 80% of the stance phase (Figure 1-9). The muscle function about the hip joint demonstrates that, during walking, the gluteus maximus is active from the end of the swing phase until the foot is flat on the ground (Figure 1-10). It is probably functioning to help decelerate the swinging thigh and to provide stability at the hip joint at the time of initial ground contact.

During the running gaits, the gluteus maximus likewise has terminal swing phase activity, but remains active during the first 40% of the stance phase in jogging. During that period, rapid hip extension occurs, and the gluteus maximus appears to help bring this about. The hip adductors function during terminal swing and throughout the first 50% of the stance phase during walking, jogging, running, and sprinting. The adductors function to stabilize the stance leg side of the pelvis at the time of initial ground contact, which helps prevent excessive sagging of the swing leg side of the pelvis.[11] The period of activity in the hip adductors definitely changes as the speed of gait increases. During walking, the hip adductors are active during the last third of the stance phase, whereas during jogging, running, and sprinting, they demonstrate similar stance–phase activity, and the activity continues into the swing phase. Data about the activity of the hip adductor muscles have always been difficult to collect and are highly variable. A larger series of runners should be studied to further our knowledge regarding phasic activity.

The quadriceps group of muscles about the knee joint appears to perform the same functions during both walking and running (Figure 1-10B). At the end of swing phase they bring about terminal knee extension, and stabilize the knee after initial ground contact, through the period of initial knee flexion. These muscles, however, remain active during about 30% to 40% of the stance phase in running, as compared with only 25% during walking. The period of swing phase activity during running and sprinting increases considerably, probably to help bring about the rapid knee extension that is required as the speed of gait increases. During walking, knee extension is a fairly passive mechanism. The hamstring muscles are active during the end of swing and into mid-stance phase, until the foot is flat on the ground, which is about 10% of the walking cycle. As the speed of gait increases, the hamstrings become active during the last third of swing phase, at which time the hip and knee joints become extended. Because this is a two-joint muscle, it probably helps to initiate extension of the hip joint, which occurs simultaneously. Once stance begins, the hamstrings remain active for about 60% of the stance phase, during which time rapid extension continues, whereas the knee rapidly flexes.

A significant change occurs about the ankle joint in the phasic activity and the function of the anterior and posterior calf muscles. During walking, the anterior compartment is active from late stance through the first 50% of stance phase. The anterior compartment still initially undergoes a concentric contraction at the time of toe-off, and the concentric contraction continues after initial ground contact until maximum dorsiflexion is reached, at about 50% of stance phase. During walking, the anterior compartment functions to restrain plantar flexion of the foot after initial ground contact, but during running, the anterior compartment appears to be accelerating the tibia over the fixed foot. This may be one of the mechanisms by which the body maintains, and possibly increases, its velocity of gait. Further study of the function of the anterior compartment is needed to elucidate this possibility.

During walking, the posterior calf muscles restrain the forward movement of the tibia over the fixed foot. The posterior calf muscles are active from about 25% of the stance phase until 50% of the stance phase and, for the most part, undergo an eccentric type of contraction (Figure 1-10C). It is only during the last 25% of its activity that this muscle group starts to undergo a concentric contraction that initiates active plantar flexion. This muscle group, by functioning to restrain the forward movement of the tibia, permits the body to lean forward and to take a longer stride.[12,13] Active plantar flexion, causing push-off or forward propulsion of the body during walking, does not seem to occur.

During jogging, running, and sprinting, the posterior calf becomes functional at the end of swing phase and undergoes a rapid eccentric contraction at the time of initial ground contact, as rapid dorsiflexion of the ankle joint occurs. The posterior calf then continues its activity for about 60% of the stance phase. Activity ceases, however, after about half of the plantar flexion of the ankle joint has occurred. The posterior calf probably functions initially to help stabilize the ankle joint at the time of initial ground contact, by controlling the forward movement of the tibia. In the latter part of the stance phase, the posterior calf probably provides some degree of propulsion, but how much it provides remains to be determined.

The posterior calf does perform push-off during the acceleration phase of running, as well as during sports that require rapid starting, such as squash, racquetball, or tennis; but in steady-state running, push-off appears to be minimal.

Pronation

As pointed out previously, pronation is a normal function of the foot at the time of initial ground contact. Pronation itself is a passive event brought about by the weight of the body against the lower extremity and the subsequent loading of the subtalar joint, which will normally collapse into an everted position at ground contact, due to the configuration of the joint. The constraints of pronation are the shape of the joints of the subtalar joint complex, along with their ligamentous support, and, to a lesser degree, the muscle support. As pronation occurs, the tibia rotates internally, which, again, is secondary to the eversion movement of the subtalar joint. Hypothetically, if one were to place the calcaneus in a device that would not permit eversion, and then load the extremity, there would be little or no internal rotation of the tibia; conversely, if the calcaneus were to be held into extreme eversion, there would be extreme flattening of the longitudinal arch, along with an increased internal rotation of the lower extremity.

This sequence of events is observed clinically in a person who has a flat foot or a cavus foot. In a person with a flat foot, at the time of initial ground contact, eversion of the subtalar joint increases, which results in an increase in the degree of internal rotation of the lower extremity, as well as increased flattening of the longitudinal arch. In the cavus foot, the opposite occurs; ie, the motion of the subtalar joint decreases and as a result, internal rotation of the subtalar joint and flattening of the longitudinal arch are both minimal. The flat foot represents an increase in the absorption of the impact, in which we observed increased motion in the lower extremity with repetitive stress; this situation may cause various clinical problems in some persons. In the cavus foot, the absorption of the impact actually decreases, which results in increased stresses being placed on the lower extremity. Just because someone has this type of foot configuration, however, does not necessarily mean the foot will be symptomatic.

Runners develop problems mainly because of the repetitive stress imparted to the lower extremity. An average 150-lb man who is walking with a step length of 2½ feet and taking about 2,110 steps to walk a mile will absorb at initial ground contact, considering an impact of 80% of the body weight, a total of 253,440 lbs.

(127 tons) or 63½ tons per foot. If the same person were running a mile, taking a step of 3½ feet and taking about 1,175 steps, he would absorb at initial ground contact, considering an impact of 250% of body weight, a total of 440,625 lbs. (220 tons) or 110 tons per foot.

The other factor that must be taken into account when considering pronation is the time interval in which the pronation occurs. In walking, pronation is completed by about 15% of the walking cycle or 25% of the stance phase. The internal rotation of the lower extremity usually reaches its peak at the same time, according to the torque measurements of the forceplate. In real time, for a person walking at a normal pace of 120 steps per minute, full pronation occurs within about 150 milliseconds (total stance time of about 600 milliseconds), whereas for a person who is running at a six-minute-mile pace, maximum pronation occurs within 30 milliseconds (total stance time about 200 milliseconds). Therefore, the pronation that occurs during running takes place in about one fifth of the time as that observed during walking. In a study by Cavanagh et al,[14] an estimate was made of the angular velocity of the pronation, and they noted that although the maximum degree of pronation occurs by 30 milliseconds, the actual angular velocity of subtalar joint reaches its maximum at 15 milliseconds. High-speed movies in our laboratory have shown that, as the foot strikes the ground, the heel is in a slightly inverted position so that, on initial ground contact, the calcaneus is rapidly brought out of this slightly inverted position and, as it is loaded with about 2½ times the body weight, it rapidly passes into eversion. The remainder of the weight acceptance and associated pronation is carried out at a slightly slower rate, possibly because of the impact–absorption mechanism of the limb, namely the rapid dorsiflexion of the ankle joint and flexion of the knee joint. An interesting correlation in data of Cavanagh et al was that the medial shear reached its peak after about 10 milliseconds, and is probably accounted for in part by the inverted position of the subtalar joint at initial ground contact, after which the direction of the force changes to that of a lateral shear, which reaches its peak by 30 milliseconds, probably because maximum pronation has occurred.

Effect of Orthotic Devices on Hindfoot Motion

In a small percentage of runners, an overuse syndrome can occur as a result of the repetitive stress of running. Such persons generally tend to have a more pronated foot than the average population, but a few may also have a cavus type of foot. Other malalignment problems, such as genuvarum and valgum, and toeing–in and toeing–out, can also lead to clinical problems secondary to the stress of running. Various types of orthotic devices have been used by runners, and the question that always arises is: what, if anything, does an orthosis do, from a biomechanical point of view? One of the problems in making such a determination is the actual measurement of tibial and subtalar joint rotation during running. Unfortunately, no reliable method is available at this time, but a fairly good estimate of subtalar joint motion can be obtained by placing a series of dots along the posterior aspect of the calf, the heel, and the shoe. By a photometric method of analysis, a general quantitation of the motion of the subtalar joint has been obtained.

In a review of several of the studies, in most cases, the overall configuration of the curve of pronation of the hindfoot seemed to follow along the same general was obtained for walking. The use of some type of a support along the medial side of the foot will bring about a decrease in the amount of eversion of the calcaneus, and subsequent pronation of the longitudinal arch. The thicker the material, the greater the decrease in eversion of the calcaneus. The study by Cavanagh et al, in which increasing thicknesses of felt were selectively placed along the medial border of the foot (eventually equivalent to 9.5 mm), showed a decrease in the degree of pronation and a sharp decrease in the angular velocity of the pronation. They further studied the subject, using a forceplate, and the only significant change was in the medial and lateral shear, in which the medial shear was decreased considerably, in the subject using the medial support.

By careful laboratory study of high-speed motion pictures of runners, we have been able to demonstrate a qualitative decrease in pronation, as well as medial deviation of the inner border of the foot and ankle, with increased support along the medial side of the foot.

An orthosis providing a medial arch support, therefore, appears to play a role in the control of the foot, by decreasing the total number of degrees, as well as the rate of pronation of the foot. This type of device would be of clinical benefit in a certain select group of symptomatic runners.

REFERENCES

1. Levens, AS, Inman, VT, Blosser, JA: Transverse rotation of the segments of the lower extremity in locomotion. J Bone Joint Surg 30A:859-11948.
2. University of California (Berkeley), Prosthetic Devices Research Project, Subcontractor's Final Report to the Committee on Artificial Limbs National Research Council; Fundamental studies of human locomotion and other information relating to design of artificial limbs, 1947. Two volumes.
3. Sutherland DH, Hagy JL: Measurement of gait movements from motion picture films. J Bone Joint Surg 54A:787- 797, 1972.
4. Wright DG, Desai ME, Henderson BS: Action of the subtalar and ankle-joint complex during the stance phase of walking. J Bone Joint Surg 46A:361, 1964.
5. Close JR, Inman VT: The action of the subtalar joint. Univ. Calif Prosthet Devices Res Rep Ser 11, Issue 24, May 1953.
6. Manter JT: Movements of the subtalar and transverse tarsal joints. Anat Rec 80:397, 1941.
7. Elftman H: The transverse tarsal joint and its control. Clin Orthop 16:41, 1960.
8. Inman VT: The Joints of the Ankle. Baltimore, Waverly Press, 1976.
9. Isman RE, Inman VT: Anthropometric studies of the human foot and ankle. Bull Prosthet Res 10-11:97, 1976.
10. Hicks JH: The mechanics of the foot, II. The plantar aponeurosis and the arch. J Anat 88:25, 1954.
11. Inman VT: Functional aspects of the abductor muscles of the hip. J Bone Joint Surg 29:607, 1947.

12. Simon SR, Mann RA, Hagy JL, Larsen LJ: Role of the posterior calf muscles in the normal gait. J Bone Joint Surg 29:607, 1947.

13. Sutherland DH: An electromyographic study of the plantar flexor of the ankle in normal walking on the level. J Bone Joint Surg 48A:66-71, 1966.

14. Cavanagh PR, Clarke T, Williams K, Kalenak A: An evaluation of the effect of orthotics on force distribution and rearfoot movement during running. Presented at the Am Orthop Soc Sports Med Meeting, Lake Placid, NY, June 1978.

CHAPTER 2

Muscle Synergism and the Biomechanics of Joint Motion in Running

M.Solomonow, PhD.
Robert D'Ambrosia, M.D.

Introduction

Coordinated movement of an athlete during a specific sports activity is the grand total of many joints acting in synergy with each other. During running, for example, it seems that the joints of the lower extremities (ie, ankle, knee, hip, etc.) interact in a highly coordinated fashion to provide the necessary gait pattern, including stride length, speed and push-off force while maintaining balance and stability. Such sports activity, however, is not limited to the synchronous activity of the lower extremities alone, but is substantially assisted by coordination from the joints of the upper limbs and the spine. With this overall picture in mind, it is rather simple to conclude that single joint motion is the elementary building block of any given sports activity.

Focusing on the joint itself, one can immediately observe, just from its anatomy, that a multi-component system composed of two bones, agonist/antagonist muscle groups, ligaments, sensory receptors, reflex arcs, and various connective tissues, are involved. While the visible outcome of a joint is the angular displacement of its two bones relative to each other, or the generation of torque about their axis of rotation (or a combination thereof), the activity of all of the joint's components is responsible for such functional outcome.

The interactive relationship of the various joint components responsible for its complex functions is the focus of our interest. The understanding of such interactive functions of the components during joint motion will allow us an in-depth appreciation of the various injuries that may occur to the musculoskeletal system, and may assist us in developing some thoughts relative to the prevention and treatment of fractures, ligament tears, dislocations, over-stretched muscles/tendons, etc., as they pertain to running.

The Muscles

Joint motion is a synergistic affair in which two muscle groups act simultaneously, in such a manner that the intended function is achieved while maintaining balance and stability. The fact that both agonist and antagonist muscles of a given joint are active during the movement performance is established in the physiological literature, even if we consider only the reciprocal innervation of their receptors - muscle spindles and Golgi tendon organs.[1] From the bio-engineering standpoint, such agonist/antagonist activity is not surprising, because it may easily serve one or more of the following functions: dynamic braking of the joint before the movement stops, torque or position regulation, increased motion accuracy, compensating for external disturbances and possibly internal disturbances, among others.[2,3]

At this point, based on our intuitive notions, it may be appropriate to ask the following questions: "What is the detailed relationship between the agonist/antagonist muscles of a joint?" and "What is the functional purpose of such a relationship?" We attempt to provide clearly defined answers to the above questions with the data obtained from the following series of experiments.

Agonist/Antagonist Force Interaction About the Joint

Twelve adult subjects, ages 18-42, were each seated in a chair as depicted in Figure 2-1. Each subject grasped the handle on a metal rod connected to a force transducer firmly attached to the rigid frame. The subjects performed a series of isometric elbow flexion and extension tests at various levels of effort

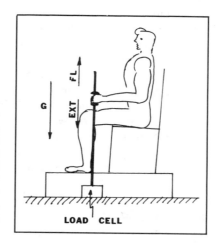

Figure 2-1. The experimental conditions in which a subject generates isometric contraction of the elbow flexors and extensors against a metal rod connected to a load cell attached to the floor. Note the gravity vector and its direction which opposes elbow flexion (ie, acts on the forearm mass and its length to produce extension forces).

from 20% and up to 100% maximal effort. The elbow angles tested were 45°, 90°, and 135° of flexion. To assess the activity of each muscle group – flexors (biceps and brachialis) and extensors (triceps) – we monitored the surface EMG throughout the test. The EMG was full-wave rectified and smoothed with a 120m/sec time constant, yielding its mean absolute value (MAV).

Figure 2-2 shows the level of activity of the joint force vs the EMG of the agonist and antagonist. Both force and MAV were normalized with respect to their maximal value of each elbow angle.

Several important conclusions could be drawn from Figure 2-2. The first is based on the relatively constant slope of the MAV vs force curves corresponding to the agonist in each test configuration. It remained at about 1.16 throughout the joint angle changes, indicating that the agonist muscle group responsible for generating most of the joint's force is concerned exclusively with doing just that, regardless of the joint position.

The second conclusion is that the muscle serving as antagonist at any given joint angle and loading level is always active to some degree, although at a substantially lower level than its agonist muscle. Furthermore, as the force

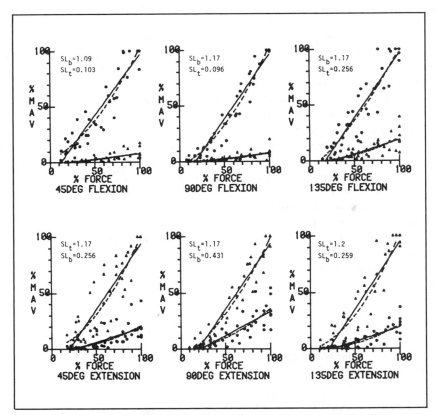

Figure 2-2. The normalized force vs normalized EMG (MAV) of the agonist and antagonist during elbow flexion and extension at three different joint angles. Note that the agonist slope is nearly constant at about 1.17, but the antagonist slope varies with the joint angle, reflecting the effect of gravity on the forearm mass and its length.

generated by the agonist increases, so does the force generated by the antagonist muscle, but at a different rate of increase (ie, slope).

Finally, the MAV vs force slopes of the antagonist vary widely as the joint angle changes. Figure 2-3 shows the slopes of the EMG- force slope as a function of joint angle.

The interpretation of the data is rather straightforward. Each time the joint is required to generate torque, the agonist muscle group is charged with the mission of producing the force necessary to yield that torque level (considering the moment arm formed from the muscle's line of action and the center of rotation, which is discussed later in detail).

The antagonist muscle is also active, as is evident from its myoelectric activity, but at a much lower level than the agonist muscle. Although the agonist muscle response is consistent regardless of the joint's angle, the antagonist's response varies and depends on the angle. Considering the variable effect of the gravity vector on the forearm's weight and effective length (which changes with the elbow angle, and therefore has a variable lever arm), the changes in the antagonist level of activity are not surprising. During flexion, when the torque generated by the flexors (biceps and brachialis) is opposed by the gravity, the extensors (triceps) reduce their activity at a joint angle of 90°, at which the total length of the forearm is the effective lever arm subjected to gravity, and thereby compensates for that gravitational effect. At angles of 45° and 135°, when the effective length of the forearm subjected to gravity forces is reduced, the extensors (triceps) increase their level of activity in order to balance the torques and force about the joint, since the effect of gravity is reduced. Similarly, the situation is reversed during attempted extension, showing that the flexors (antagonists in this case) deal with the gravitational effects.

The major conclusion from these observations is that the antagonist muscle is very important in regulating the joint torque by dealing effectively with disturbances that are external to the anatomy —gravity, in this case.[4] The agonist muscle, having consistent response at all elbow angles, is not concerned with compensation for any disturbances.

Considering the established important role of the antagonist muscles in regulating the joint's activity, one may ask if they are active during movement in the horizontal plane, when gravity is not affecting the joint in its direction of motion. Proceeding to answer this question, we arranged the experimental set-up shown in Figure 2-4. The arm was resting on a horizontal rigid tray, eliminating

Figure 2-3. The antagonist EMG vs force slope is shown as a function of elbow angle. Note the largest increase of the flexors antagonist slope at 90° during extension(along the gravity vector), and the largest decrease of the extensors antagonist slope during flexion at the same angle when the contraction is in an opposing direction to the gravity vector.

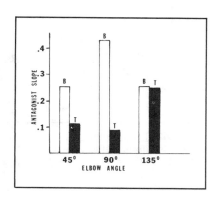

any reaction to gravitational forces while the same flexion-extension tests as described in the previous test were repeated at joint angles of 45°, 90°, and 135°.

Figure 2-5 presents the EMG-force curves from the agonist/antagonist muscles during the various trials. Observing the slopes of the agonists at all six configurations, we receive solid confirmation of our previous conclusion that the agonist's response, being of a steady slope of about 1.16, is consistent, regardless of joint angle. The antagonist's slope, again, varies widely from one configuration to the other, and the explanation is not easily forthcoming, especially with only three data points for each antagonist group at 45°, 90°, and 135° of the joint angle.

To obtain more data points, we repeated the experiment on the Cybex II dynamometer with the subject's arm resting on the crank and the EMG recorded

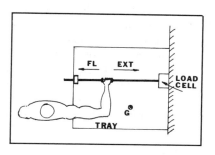

Figure 2-4. Top view of the experimental conditions when isometric contractions are performed when the shoulder is elevated laterally 90° and rested on a wooden tray to eliminate the affect of gravity.

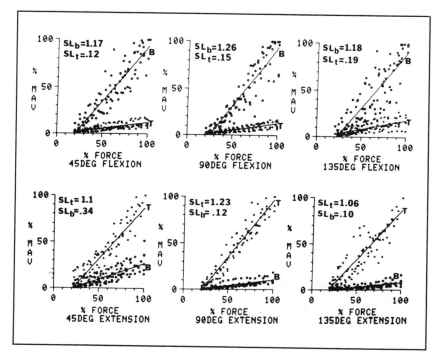

Figure 2-5. The normalized EMG (MAV) vs force of the flexors and extensors at various elbow angles showing the variability of the antagonist slope, which is probably due to changes in its moment arm, as will be shown later.

from flexors and extensors, simultaneously. The crank speed was set at 15°/sec
to simulate the quasi-isometric condition throughout the joint range of motion of
DE-140° in flexion and extension. Similar to the static test, the EMG of the
flexors and extensors acting as antagonists were normalized with respect to the
EMG value of the same muscle when acting as agonist in maximal effort at each
angle throughout the complete range of motion.

Figure 2-6(A,D) shows the normalized antagonist EMG of the elbow flexors
and extensors as a function of joint angle. Figure 2- 7(A,D), presented just below
Figure 2-6, shows the variations of the same muscle's moment arm (distance from
the muscle's line of action to the joint's center of rotation) as a function of joint
angle.[5-12] Surprisingly enough, the antagonist's EMG is inversely related to its
instant moment arm over the joint's range of motion.

Similar experiments, with the quadriceps and hamstrings EMG recorded
during slow–isokinetic maximal–effort flexion-extension of the knee of the
horizontal plane, yielded identical results, indicating that each muscle, when
acting as antagonist in the plane normal to the gravity, compensates for the
variations in its moment arm, with the appropriate increase or decrease in its
level of activity.

Assuming that the EMG represents the muscle force,[13] the antagonist's
normalized torque could be calculated using the moment arm data of Figure 2-7.
Figure 2-8 shows the antagonist's normalized torque. It is evident from the figure

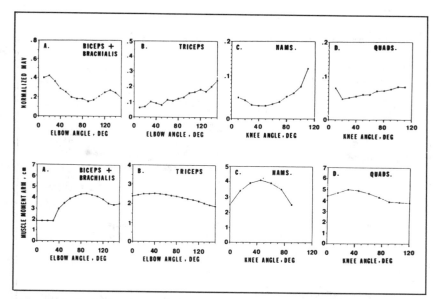

Figure 2-6. Pattern as a function of the joint angle for the elbow flexors (A)
and extensors (B) and knee flexors (C) and extensors (D) during maximal effort
isokinetic motion at 15°/sec.

Figure 2-7. The muscle moment–arm variations, as a function of joint angle,
are shown for the elbow flexors (A) and extensors (B), and for the knee flexors
(C) and extensors (D). Note that the moment arm vs angle pattern of each
muscle is inversely related to its antagonist EMG discharge pattern shown in
the corresponding Figure 2-6.

that nearly constant opposing torque is applied to the joint by the antagonist throughout the full range of motion.

We can now add to our knowledge that the antagonist also regulates for internal disturbances, in this case, the variations in its own moment arm.

Why would the antagonist be active at all? What are the advantages of providing constant opposing force? These are two very important questions, indeed.

The answers to the above questions are rather straightforward if figures 2-9A,B,C,and D are considered. If only the agonist muscle (flexors in flexion and extensor in extension) were active, the articular surface of the joint would be subject to force applied only to its anterior (or posterior) aspects. This, in turn, would cause the most anterior (or posterior) areas of the articular surface to serve as the contact point about which the two bones rotate relative to each other, while the remaining area of the articulation would not be in contact as the figure depicts. A direct corollary of the limited contact area is that the articular surface pressure distribution is disrupted, creating a focal stress point with high pressure on the area in contact only.[14]

Obviously, such high pressures cause accelerated use and deterioration of a specific point of the articular surface, leading to various early symptoms of joint diseases. Arthritis, in particular, may develop in any of the three compartments of the knee which are at risk. Chondromalacia in the posterior femoral compartment or medial compartment arthritis are most common forms, but no area of the knee is immune from the wear and tear.

It is therefore easy to understand why the antagonist muscle applies low levels of opposing torques to the joint. This opposing antagonist torque assures total articular surface contact as well as more favorable articular pressure distribution; even, smooth movement of the joint is accomplished along the complete contact surface of its articulation.

Are athletes subjected to any unfavorable conditions compared with normal, nonathletic persons from whom the above data was derived?

This could be determined by subjecting specific athletes to the same test

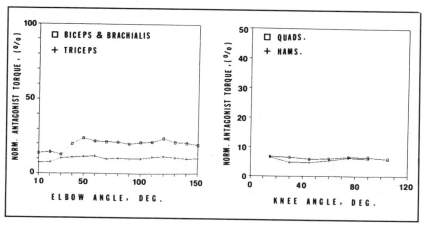

Figure 2-8. The normalized opposing antagonist muscle torque vs joint angle is shown for the flexors and extensors of the elbow and knee.

described above. Figure 2-10 shows the antagonist coactivation pattern of a large group of joggers, basketball players, and volleyball players using the same slow isokinetic test. One should keep in mind that athletes in the above categories use their quadriceps under more strenuous conditions than in other sports (the impact applied to the foot in heel strike during landing is 3-6 times body weight, and is partly absorbed by the anti-gravity muscles, ie, quadriceps, leading to their hypertrophy). This quadriceps hyperactivity is emphasized in a jogger running down hills (or steps) while more activity is seen in the hamstrings in runners on level surfaces due to the need to clear the calf and foot over the surface during the swing phase.

As is immediately evident from Figure 2-10B, the hamstrings antagonist coactivation is grossly inhibited compared with that of normals (See Figure 2-6D). Athletes active in sports that require various types of "jumping" and sustained anti-gravity control against high impact forces do not receive the benefit of hamstring coactivation during extension and may be subject to high risk of early joint damage of various types. One should also consider the excessive loading of the anterior cruciate ligament, having to perform as the sole anterior restraint mechanism of the knee with an inhibited hamstring that does not provide its usual posteriorly directed pull to the tibia, as described in the following section.

The Ligament-Muscle Synergy

During knee extension, the anterior cruciate ligament applies substantial posterior pull to the head of the tibia in the last 50° before full extension.[15] With

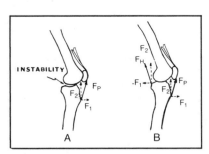

Figure 2-9A. Shows the articular surface of the knee when only the quadriceps force and its components are considered. Note the F2 component tends to concentrate the articular surface contact pressure at a single point, see (B), while F2 tends to pull the tibia anteriorly. Both effects are adverse to the joint from its stability standpoint.

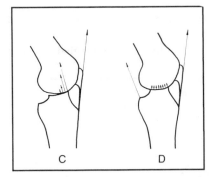

Figure 2-9C. Shows the balanced joint when the force components generated by the antagonist (hamstrings) are considered. The horizontal components oppose each other, preventing any possible excursion of the tibia, while the F2 components are applied at both sides of the articular surface allowing a more favorable pressure distribution as shown in (D).

our knowledge of the antagonist opposing force and torque applied by the hamstrings during extension, it may be important to identify any interesting correlation between the two organs (ACL and hamstrings).

Selecting a group of 12 patients with a midsubstance tear of the ACL, verified by arthroscopy, we performed the same standard maximal-effort isokinetic knee flexion and extension test, using the Cybex.

Figure 2-11 shows a typical torque, joint angle as well as hamstrings and quadriceps EMG of one such patient. The patient reported an episode of subluxation in the mid-range of the motion, which was verified by the data with several distinct features. First, the dramatic torque failure at about 42° was evident, indicating the temporary inability of the quadriceps to generate force because of the pain and discomfort of subluxation. This is well-supported by the sharp decrease in quadriceps EMG. A striking, but almost anticipated, feature is the sharp rise in the hamstrings antagonist EMG, indicating that it provided a fast increase in posterior pull to the head of the tibia, substituting for the lost ACL functional properties.

The joint angle demonstrates a continuous, undisrupted time progression, as well as completion of the function within the specified time, indicating that quadriceps inhibition and the increased temporary excitation of the hamstrings all occurred in a fast, reflexive manner, and were probably based in spinal sensory motor arcs rather than central perceptual-motor loops that require substantially longer time for execution.[16]

The conclusion is, however, that hamstring antagonist activity is also necessary and required for knee joint stability. If we can further generalize this observation, we could conclude that part of the antagonist coactivation serves the purpose of maintaining joint stability secondary to the ligaments, the primary restraints.[17-19,20-22]

The above conclusion causes a natural distress when one reconsiders the inhibited hamstrings antagonist coactivation in athletes engaged in anti-gravity functions, reemphasizing their vulnerability to ACL injuries.

Can something be done to improve athletes' antagonist coactivation with the objective of increasing the contribution of the musculature to joint stability?

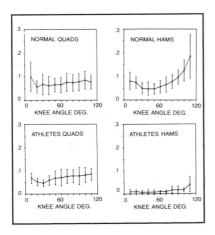

Figure 2-10A. Shows the antagonist EMG (MAV) vs knee angle for the quadriceps and hamstrings of normals. Figure 2-10B. Shows the same recordings from a group of high performance athletes with hypertrophied quads and without hamstrings exercise. Note that while the EMG (MAV) vs angle pattern of the quadriceps is nearly identical in both subject groups, the hamstring pattern of the athletes is substantially depressed. This may place such individuals at high risk of all injuries.

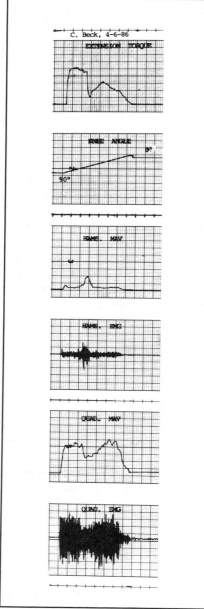

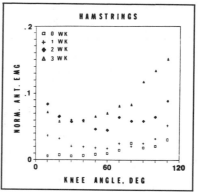

Figure 2-11. A recording of (from top to bottom) extension torque, knee angle, hamstrings MAV, hamstrings EMG, quadriceps MAV, and quadriceps EMG from an ACL deficient patient whose knee became unstable, triggering short increase discharge in the hamstrings and temporary inhibition in quadriceps EMG. (From Solomonow et al., Am. J. Sports Med. 15:207-213, 1987.)

Figure 2-12. Hamstrings antagonist EMG vs knee angle from an athlete with depressed hamstrings activity. The recording shows weekly increase in activity during three weeks of daily strength exercise of the hamstrings.

The Effect of Strength Training on Antagonist Coactivation

Two athletes who demonstrated inhibited antagonist coactivation in their hamstrings were selected for this study. Each subject performed a typical strength exercise of his/her hamstring on a daily basis for three weeks. The exercise consisted of performing knee flexion (curls) with 80% of maximal load. Three sets, each consisting of 12 repetitions, were done daily. The subjects were tested at the end of each week with the standard maximal-effort isokinetic test, while their quadricep and hamstring EMG were monitored.

Figure 2-12 shows a typical performance of the hamstring antagonist coactivation of one subject. It is easily confirmed that the hamstring's strength exercise improved its antagonist coactivation dramatically. Large improvements for knee angle range of 0°-50° flexion were observed within one week, and a normal antagonist coactivation pattern was evident by the end of the third week. A similar response was obtained in the other subject.

The direct conclusion drawn from this study is that athletes whose muscles, due to their sports specialization, underwent modifications inhibiting antagonist coactivation could (and should) engage themselves in an augmentative exercise of the antagonists in order to maintain normal supportive, stabilizing contribution from the musculature to the joint. Failure to maintain such augmentative exercise places the athlete in the high-risk category as far as ACL injuries are concerned, as well as other damages to the joint.[23,24]

Conclusion

To appreciate some of the interesting highlights from the series of experiments described above, one should recognize that "running" is not limited to joggers, but to many other sports in which short or long bursts of running and jumping are required, as in basketball, football, volleyball, and tennis. In fact, some of the above activities are the background of more risky and taxing running conditions, requiring rapid initiation and breaking of running, or fast and unpredictable changes in direction and coordination of balance and posture of the trunk, and upper and lower extremities. Jumping by itself can produce landing impact of several times body weight, most of which is absorbed by the viscoelastic properties of the muscles and ligaments.[25,26] A substantial component of such impact is also transmitted via the long bones and articular surfaces of the joints and spine, hence the importance of the musculature and ligaments in regulating joint motion in a stable, safe manner.

The regulatory role of the musculature, and especially of the antagonist muscles during a specific function, was shown to be multidimensional. The antagonist muscles provided regulation in the face of the effect of gravity on the limb mass and its distance from the joint's center of rotation. This, of course, is an external disturbance applied by the environment.

The regulatory role of the muscle antagonist was further extended to negotiate with internal disturbance imposed by the anatomy, namely, the variations of its own moment arm as the joint angle, muscle line of action, and instant center of rotation are changing. Further evidence of synergistic coordination with the joints and ligaments was also presented, indicating that joint stability is also influenced by the musculature.

Finally, high-performance athletes who obtain high efficiency in some specialized movements due to the nature of a specific sport tend to inhibit the antagonist discharge. This inhibition places such athletes at risk for various joint and ligament injuries, but such injuries could be easily prevented if augmentative exercise of the antagonist is done.

As the musculature is maintained in a balanced, well-conditioned state, various loads, forces, and impacts are properly dissipated in their viscoelastic, shock-absorbing components, and is not fully transferred to the long bones, ligaments, and joint articular surfaces, where they might cause substantial damages, especially when the compounded effect of continuous, repetitive activity under unbalanced conditions is imminent.

REFERENCES

1. Mountcastle, V.: Medical Physiology, Vol. 1, Part V. CV Mosby Co., St. Louis, 1974.
2. Basmajian, J., and DeLuca, C.: Muscles Alive, 5th Edition. Williams and Wilkins, Baltimore, 1985.
3. Sherington, C.: Reciprocal Innervation of Antagonist Muscles, 14th Note on Double Reciprocal Innervation. Proc. Royal Society (Lond.), Ser. B., 91:244-268, 1909.
4. Solomonow, M., Guzzi, A., Baratta, R., Shoji, H., and D'Ambrosia, R.: The EMG-Force Model of The Elbow's Antagonistic Muscle Pair: Effect of Gravity, Joint Position and Recruitment. Am. J. Physical Med., 65:223-244, 1986.
5. Smidt, G.: Biomechanical Analysis of Knee Flexion and Extension, J. Biomech., 6:79-92, 1973.
6. Amis, A., Dowson, D., and Wright, V.: Muscle Strength and Musculoskeletal Geometry of the Upper Limb, Engineering in Medicine and Biology, 8:41-48, 1979.
7. Messier, R., Duffy, Litchman, H., et al.: The Electromyogram as a Measure of Tension in the Human Biceps and Triceps Muscles, J. Mech. Sci., 13:585-588, 1971.
8. Braune, W., and Fischer, O.: Die Rotationsmomente der Beugemusckeln an Ellen Bogengelenk des Menschen, abh. d. Doniglesach. Ges. Wiss. Mateh. Phv., KI. 15, 1980.
9. Wilkie, D.: The Relation Between Force and Velocity in Human Muscle, J. Physiol., (Lond.), 110:249-280, 1949.
10. Haxton, H.: A Comparison of the Action of Extension of the Knee and Elbow Joints in Man, Anat. Rec., 94:279-286, 1945.
11. Kaufer, H.: Mechanical Function of the Patella, J. Bone Joint Surg., 53A:1551-1560, 1971.
12. Haxton, H.: The Function of the Patella and the Effects of Its Excision, Surg. Gynecol. Obstet., 80:389-395, 1945.
13. Solomonow, M., Baratta, R., Zhou, B. H., Shoji, H., and D'Ambrosia, R.: The EMG-Force Model of Electrically Stimulated Muscle: Dependence on

Control Strategy and Predominant Fiber Type. IEEE Trans. Biomed. Eng., 34:692-703,1987.

14. Himeno, S., An, A., Tsumura, H., et al.: Pressure Distribution on Articular Surface, Proc. N. Am. Congress on Biomechanics, P:97-98, Montreal, Canada, 1986.

15. Renstrom, P.,Arms, S., Stanwyck, T., et al.: Strain Within the ACL During Hamstring and Quadriceps Activity, Am. J. Sports Med., 14:83-87, 1987.

16. Solomonow, M., Baratta, R., Zhou, B. H., Shoji, H., Bose, W., Beck, C., and D'Ambrosia, R.: The Synergistic Action of the ACL and Thigh Muscles in Maintaining Joint Stability, Am. J. Sports Med., 15:207-213, 1987.

17. Louie, J., and Mote, C.: Contribution of the Musculature to Rotary Laxity and Torsional Stiffness at the Knee, J. Biomech., 20:281-300, 1987.

18. Pope, M., Johnson, R., Brown, D., and Tighe, C.: The Role of the Musculature in Injuries to the Medial Collateral Ligament, J. Bone Joint Surg., 61A:398, 1979.

19. Shoemaker, S., and Markolf, K.: In Vivo Rotary Knee Stability: Ligamentous and Muscular Contributions, J. Bone Joint Surg., 64A:208-216, 1982.

20. Walla, D., Albright, J., McAuley, E., et al.: Hamstring Control and the Unstable Anterior Cruciate Ligament- Deficient Knee, Am. J. Sports Med., 13:3439, 1985.

21. McDaniels, W., and Dameron, T.: Untreated Anterior Cruciate Ligament Rupture, Clin. Orthop., 172:158-163, 1983.

22. Giove, T., Miller, J., Kent, B., et al.: Non-Operative Treatment of the Torn ACL, J. Bone Joint Surg., 65A:184-192, 1983.

23. Steiner, M., Grana, W., Chilag, K., et al.: The Effect of Exercise on Anterior-Posterior Knee Laxity, Am. J. Sports Med., 14:24-28, 1986.

24. Skinner, H., Wyatt, M., Stone, M., et al.: Exercise Related Knee Joint Laxity, Am. J. Sports Med., 14:30-34, 1986.

25. Solomonow, M., and D'Ambrosia, R.: Biomechanics of Muscle Overuse Injuries, Clinics in Sports Medicine, 6:241-257, 1987.

26. Proske, V., and Morgan, D.: Tendon Stiffness: Methods of Measurements and Significance for the Control of Movement, J. Biomech., 20:75-82, 1987.

CHAPTER 3

Examination of the Lower Extremity in Runners

David Drez, Jr., M.D.

Introduction

As should be evident from the previous chapter on biomechanics, doing a detailed examination of the lower extremity in the runner is a necessity. Such an examination permits one to recognize anatomic abnormalities that could cause the runner problems. Even subtle anatomic deviations can produce injury, because of the large forces that the lower extremity is subjected to during running and jogging. This chapter discusses possible sites of injury in the lower extremity.

General Principles

The lower extremity should be examined while the runner is sitting, reclining, and standing, while walking, and in some cases while running. Dynamic evaluation is important because some abnormalities that are accentuated under cetain conditions might otherwise be overlooked. In addition, the runner should be scrutinized from the front, the back, the side, close, and at a distance. The examining room surface should be hard, rather than soft or carpeted, to avoid observing certain alterations in the foot. In addition to the lower extremity, the entire torso should be examined.

Examination of the Erect Patient

Standing

Spinal alignment is observed while the patient is erect, and with forward flexion. The spine must also be viewed laterally. Spinal mobility and hamstring tightness can be ascertained by forward flexion, with the arms extended to touch the toes.

Leg length discrepancies can be detected by palpating and marking the iliac crests or anterior superior spines and noting any differences in height of the marking on one side compared with the other.

Extremity alignment is observed next. The area of the knee is of prime importance. Any genu varum or genu valgum is measured with a goniometer. Some degree of genu valgum in women is not uncommon, but in my opinion should not exceed 5°. Genu varum in men is likewise not uncommon. Five degrees again probably represents the upper limits of normal. Flexion contractures or recurvatum at the knee are noted as, well. Patellar position is observed and the Q angle is measured.

Walking

While the patient walks back and forth, the examiner looks for asymmetrical arm motion, excessive pelvic tilt, and any other deviations in the gait pattern. Femoral rotation, patellar position, patellar tracking, and knee alignment are noted. The entire foot is again evaluated. Dynamic gastroc-soleus tightness, not seen at rest, may become more pronounced during walking; the heel may never touch the floor. Heel and toe walking should be done.

Running

Observing the patient running or jogging is helpful in some cases, although it demands a degree of dedication that time constraints make difficult in the usual practice situation. In cases that are difficult to diagnose, however, this examination is recommended.

Examination of the Sitting Patient

Leg lengths are checked again by having the runner sit with the back against the wall and knees extended. Hamstring tightness and sciatic nerve irritation can be evaluated by the examiner's passively extending each of the seated patient's legs. Full extension should be possible without undue lumbar extension or discomfort. The deep tendon reflexes should be checked also.

Patellar position and patellar tracking are observed on flexion and extension. The anterior aspect of the knee is palpated as it is flexed and extended. Extension of the knee against resistance may provide information regarding patellofemoral pathology.

Areas about the knee–in particular, the patella, the patellar tendon, the tibial tubercle, the lateral femoral epicondyle, and pes anserinus tendon area–should be palpated. The degree of tibial torsion is also observed.

Examination of the Reclining Patient

Supine

Leg lengths are again determined by measuring from the anterior superior iliac crest to the medial malleolar area. Strength of the abdominal muscles is evaluated by having the patient do sit-ups with the knees flexed.

Range of motion of the hips and knees is checked. A thorough examination of the knee is mandatory.

The amount of hip flexion with the knee extended allows assessment of hamstring flexibility. In my opinion, at least 60° of hip flexion should be possible in the runner.

(Hamstring stretchability should be measured as outlined in Chapter 13, Figures 13-7 and 13-8).

With the patient in the supine position, have him flex the hip to 90° with the knee also flexed. The patient should maintain 90° of hip flexion throughout the test, by placing both hands around his thigh. Extend the flexed knee as far as possible and measure the angle at the knee to determine hamstring flexibility/tightness (Figure 11-8A). The long axes of the fibula and the femur should have an angle of 0°. Hamstring tightness is present if the angle is greater than 0°.

Ankle dorsiflexion with the leg extended is measured; I believe at least 10° should be possible in the runner.

Peripheral pulses are palpated, and muscle strength in the lower extremity is grossly evaluated. Palpation of major muscle masses, such as the quadriceps, to ascertain any differences in muscle tone, is important. A sensory examination can be rapidly and easily done.

Prone

With the patient prone, the knees are flexed and the amount of hip rotation is measured. External rotation and internal rotation of the hip, in most cases, are equal; a difference of 30° in one side compared with the other is significant.[1,2]

The amount of ankle dorsiflexion is again checked with the foot in slight eversion. It should be at least 10°.

The amount of inversion and eversion of the subtalar joint is measured. Normally, inversion is around 30°, and eversion, 10°.[3,4]

The neutral position of the subtalar joints should be determined by the following technique.[5,6,7] With the patient prone, the foot is grasped, over the fourth and fifth metatarsal heads, with the index finger and thumb. The other index finger and thumb are used to palpate the talar head (Figure 3-1). The foot

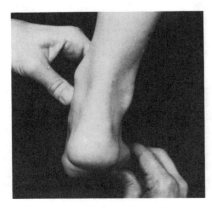

Figure 3-1. With patient prone, the foot is held at the fourth and fifth metatarsal heads with the thumb and index fingers of one hand while the other index finger and thumb palpate the talar head.

is maximally just anterior to and below the medial malleolous (Figures 3-2 to 3-4).

The foot is now maximally inverted and the talar head is felt to bulge just lateral to the midline, and just anterior to the lateral malleolus (Figures 3-5 and 3-6). The subtalar joint is then placed in a position in which no bulge is felt medially or laterally (Figure 3-7). The subtalar joint is now said to be in a neutral position and congruently aligned with the tarsal navicular (Figure 3-8).

After the neutral position has been achieved, observations are made for abnormalities of alignment. The first measurement is that of the leg-heel alignment. A line drawn to bisect the lower third of the leg just before the gastrocnemius muscle belly should fall directly over or parallel to a line that bisects the bony outline of the calcaneus (Figure 3-9). Some 2°-3° of varus of the heel is normal. Next, heel-forefoot alignment is determined. A line bisecting the bony outline of the os calcis should be perpendicular to the plane of the first through the fifth metatarsal heads (Figure 3-10).

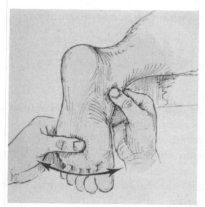

Figure 3-2. Subtalar joint is being everted and inverted.

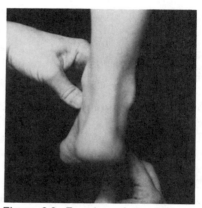

Figure 3-3. Eversion of the foot.

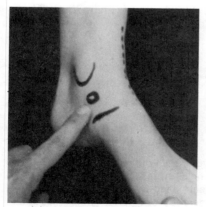

Figure 3-4. Area where talar head is palpated when foot is everted.

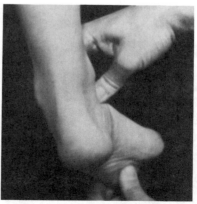

Figure 3-5. Foot maximally inverted.

Abnormalities or deviations of the leg-heel alignment are present if the heel is in a varus or valgus position to the line bisecting the lower third of the leg (Figure 3-11). These deviations are measured with a goniometer and are recorded as degrees of heel valgus or heel varus.

Deviations of heel-forefront alignment exist when the forefoot is either in a valgus or varus relationship to the normal perpendicular arrangement between the heel and forefoot valgus or forefoot varus (Figure 3-12).

Mobility of the mid tarsal joints and first ray are noted. Dorsiflexion and plantar flexion should be free and nonpainful. Motion of the first metatarsophalangeal joint should be free and without pain. Note should be made of excessive

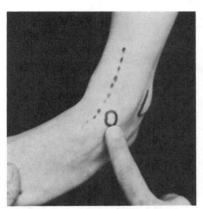

Figure 3-6. Area where talar head is palpated when foot is inverted.

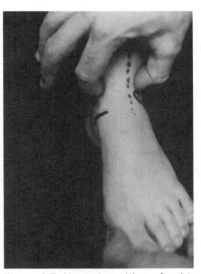

Figure 3-7. Neutral position of subtalar joint, no bulge of talus medialy or laterally.

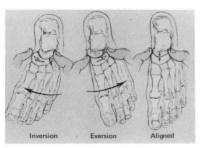

Inversion   Eversion   Aligned

Figure 3-8. Neutral position of subtalar joint.

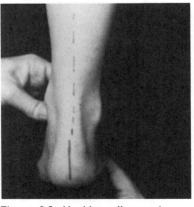

Figure 3-9. Heel-leg alignment.

callus formation on the plantar aspect of the foot and toes or on the dorsum of the foot and toes.

Certain areas in the foot and ankle deserve special attention. The peroneal tendons, as they course behind the lateral malleolus, should be examined. Tenderness or synovitis in this area can be secondary to subluxation or dislocation of these tendons. Eversion of the foot against resistance will allow one to demonstrate subluxation or dislocation of the peroneal tendons. The area around the anterior or posterior tibial tendons is evaluated for tenderness, as well. Lateral ligamentous instability of the ankle is checked by the anterior drawer and inversion stress test. Palpation of the interdigital space, especially the third and fourth, may indicate the presence of an interdigital neuroma. The Achilles tendon should be palpated along its entire course, from its insertion to the musculotendinous junction. Tenderness and thickening may indicate abnormalities. The inner border of the mid and distal tibia should be palpated. Enlargement or tenderness in this area may be present and indicative of a stress reaction. The undersurface of the foot should be palpated. Tenderness over the

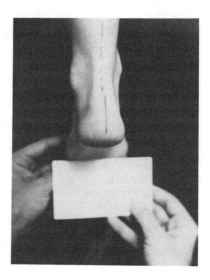

Figure 3-10. Heel-forefoot alignment.

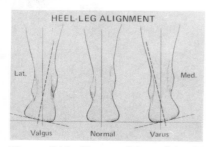

Figure 3-11. Abnormalities of heel-leg alignment.

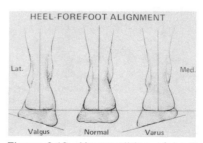

Figure 3-12. Abnormalities of heel-forefoot alignment.

metatarsal heads, the plantar fascia and anterior aspect of the os calcis should be sought.

Summary

The examination of the lower extremity outlined above emphasizes the importance of detecting minor anatomic abnormalities in runners. Such abnormalities may produce significant symptoms because of the tremendous loads imposed on the runner's musculoskeletal system.

REFERENCES

1. Mann RA, et al: Running symposium. Foot and Ankle 1:199, 1981.
2. James SL: Examination of Runners, videotape. American Academy of Orthopedic Surgeons, 1981.
3. Inman CT: The Joints of the Ankle, Baltimore, Williams and Wilkins Co., 1976.
4. James SL, et al: Injuries to runners, Sports Med 6:43, 1978.
5. Langer S: A Practical Manual for a Basic Approach to Biomechanics, Vol 1, Deer Park, NY Langer Acrylic Lab, 1972.
6. James L, et al: Injuries to runners, Sports Med 5:40-42, 1978.
7. Drez, D: Running footwear. Am J Sports 8:141, 1980.

CHAPTER 4

Stress Fracture in Runners

Angus McBryde Jr.,M.D.

Introduction

The stress fracture is a repetitive stress injury of soft tissue and bone. It was first described in 1855 by Breithaupt and has since been identified by numerous appellations, including March fracture, fatigue fracture, overload fracture, exhaustion fracture, and runner's fracture.

During World War II, numerous reports detailed stress fracture of pelvic and lower extremity bones. These reports documented a broad clinical experience. The running-based military training activities provided experience pertinent to the modern-day runner, [1-3] but with definite clinical differences between the military stress fracture and those occurring in the athletic population. [4,5]

There is substantial running literature with information about the stress fracture, [6,7,8] and numerous more specific articles. [9,10] There are two older more general, but excellent monographs on stress fractures. [11,12] The Morris and Blickenstaff publication is based primarily on a military population, but with selected examples of runner's stress fracture. Devas' book, not military-based, serves as an excellent reference work, and offers theory in certain areas.

Definition

Stress fracture is defined as a partial or complete fracture of bone due to its inability to withstand nonviolent stress that is applied in a rythmic, repeated, subthreshold manner. A distinct series of events-a process and not an occurrence-leads to stress fracture. Wolff's law, stating that "every change in the form and function of a bone, or in its function alone, is followed by a certain definite change in its external conformation," is constantly operative. As an end stage of this series of events, stress fracture is a fascinating, well recognized, and common problem seen in the athletic population in general and in the running population in particular. It occurs both in novice recreational and experienced competitive runners. In running any weight–bearing bone (spine and lower extremities) can have stress fracture, including, the proximal fibula[13] and patella[14] cuboid and sesamoid (Figure 4-1A-C).

Stress fracture in runners has no single etiology. Skeletal malsymmetry, malalignment or leg-length discrepancy,[15] as well as poor condition, variations of gait, hard or canted surface running, prior injury, and other body and performance factors, can all predispose to stress fracture.[16,17] These running characteristics underscore that the concept of "margin of error" for stress fracture and, in fact, any repetitive stress injury, is an individual variable. It is difficult for a runner to understand that he or she may have an "at risk" status compared to a running companion. This lack of understanding can lead to injury.

Running is the common denominator for most sports. The fibula ("Runner's Fracture"), along with the metatarsal and tibia, are most commonly involved (Table 4-1A and B).[18-21] The prototype fracture, the fibula, occurs three to five centimeters proximal to the level of the ankle joint. Typically, symptoms occur with running and subside with rest. At two weeks, there is specific clinical point localization to the distal fibula. Complete cessation of running is not necessary during healing, (Figure 4-2) but running must be reduced below the level at which symptoms occur, to permit successful remodeling and union of the fibular stress fracture.

Table 4-1A STRESS FRACTURES IN RUNNERS		
Tibia		34%
Upper metaphysis	7%	
Upper shaft	12%	
Mid shaft	4%	
Lower tibia	11%	
Fibula		24%
Metatarsals		18%
Second	11%	
Third	7%	
Femur		14%
Neck	7%	
Upper shaft	5%	
Distal shaft	2%	
Pelvis		6%
Others		4%
Metatarsals 4 & 5		
Pars, sesamoid		
Navicular, talus		

Cause and Pathology

Older military reports[22] and more recent reports[23] suggest the cause of stress fracture to be repetitive stress due to the increased load after fatiguing of the supporting structures. Other reports[24-26] cite the muscle forces acting across and on the bone, which cause repetitive summation forces exceeding the stress bearing capacity of that bone. In either case, progressive microfractures occur and function as a pathophysiologic precursor, terminating in a clinical fracture a series of events analogous to what may occur in the femoral head.[27]

A simple hypothetical diagram explains the basic relationship between load repetition and bone injury[28] (Figure 4-3). Time, and other unrelated and more general factors, such as the runner's pain threshold, are important.

In metatarsal fractures specifically, a local temperature factor with reactive

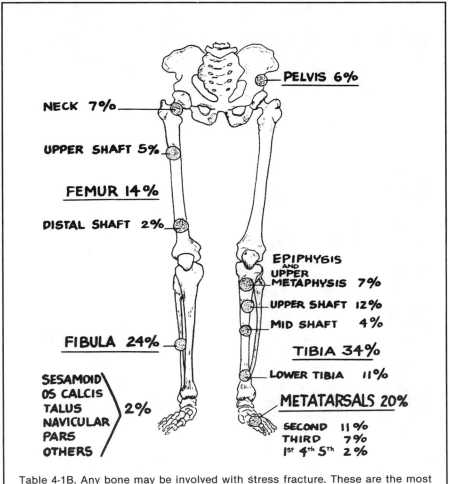

Table 4-1B. Any bone may be involved with stress fracture. These are the most common, based on the author's experience with more than 1000 stress fractures in runners.

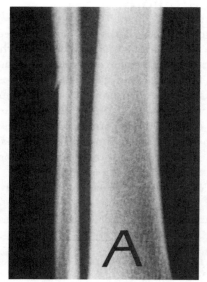

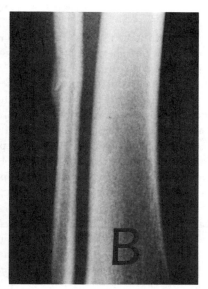

Figure 4-1. FW, a 15-year old female distance runner, showing the six-week evolution of a fibula stress fracture.
A. Two weeks after presentation.

B. Three weeks after diagnosis.

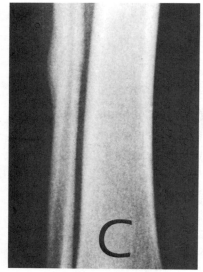

C. After having run track season competitively.

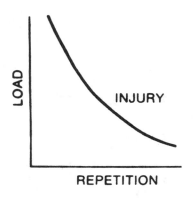

Figure 4-2. Stress fractures lie along this hypothetical fatigue curve. When the repititions reach a certain point, injury can occur even with small loads. From Frankel, Am J Sports Med 6: 396, 1978.

hyperemia occurs and can be measured with thermography.[29] The piezoelectric phenomenon is operative especially in long bones and is an integral basic electrical mechanism affecting cellular and structural activity in a stress fracture.[30]

What is this procession or continuum by which repetitive stress eventually causes a stress fracture (Figure 4-4)?[31,32] That cancellous bone as well as cortical bone has shock-absorption properties has long been hypothesized.[33] These and other properties mesh with the natural process of non-fracture-related osteo-clastic and osteoblastic remodeling, which is ongoing and is increased with stress. The normal remodeling response to what becomes an abnormal stimulus with continued repetitive stress concentration in a certain osseous and juxta osseous area leads to trabecular microfractures. At this point, electron microscopy (EM) can show collagenous fragmentation with obliterated and narrowed canaliculi.[30] As is well known, mechanical properties of bone and its histological structure are correlated. Osteonal anatomy has been correlated with fracture from repetitive stress.[30] Cortical holes representing osteoclastic resorption occur rapidly at sites of accelerated normal cortical bone remodeling. This weakened cortex, including microfractures, leads to periosteal reinforcement[35] until a refilling process has caught up and solidified the cortex.[36] So if the new bone (callous) at the site of these microfractures does not become functional and able to accept further stress, if the trabecular increase in the cancellous bone is not prompt enough, if the numbers and alignment of the osteonal systems of cortical bone are not established quickly enough, and if the osteoclastic activity weakens the bone sufficiently, a certain threshold is exceeded. The result is a peak bone loss occurring at 21 days.[37] It is at that point that clinical stress fracture can occur. (Fatigue infraction, defined as the "incomplete stress fracture," is not a useful concept.)[38] Stress syndrome of bone and stress reaction of bone are more inclusive concepts.[39]

An important clinical corollary to the discussion is that many of the conditions now diagnosed as contusions, strains, medial tibial stress syndrome, shin splints, or periostitis, would, if the inciting activity (running) were allowed to continue, progress to a clinical and roentgenographic stress fracture. Pain, however, causes most runners automatically to adjust their running schedule, thus preventing the end-stage bony structural changes which can be identified as stress fracture.

Incidence and Correlating Factors

The lower extremities account for 95% of all stress fractures in athletes. That fact, of course, reflects running and the primary use of the lower extremity in sports. Of the common runner's injuries, stress fracture constitutes roughly 6% to 10%.[40,41] Earlier reports[42] suggest a lower incidence. With increased awareness by runners and the general public of the preventive methods for more common soft-tissue running injuries, stress fracture can be expected to comprise a larger percentage. Table 4-2 reflects my own experience with an overall stress fracture incidence of 9.6%.

The number of stress fractures quoted in studies does not reflect subclinical and subroentgenographic stress reaction to bone-only those with roentgenographic and clinical evidence of stress fracture (Figure 4-5A and B). The relative incidence

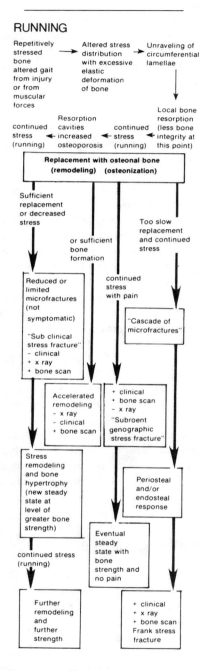

RUNNING

Repetitively stressed bone altered gait from injury or from muscular forces → Altered stress distribution with excessive elastic deformation of bone → Unraveling of circumferential lamellae

Local bone resorption (less bone integrity at this point) ← continued stress (running) ← Resorption cavities increased osteoporosis ← continued stress (running)

Replacement with osteonal bone (remodeling) (osteonization)

Sufficient replacement or decreased stress

Too slow replacement and continued stress

or sufficient bone formation

Reduced or limited microfractures (not symptomatic)

"Sub clinical stress fracture"
– clinical
+ x ray
+ bone scan

continued stress with pain

"Cascade of microfractures"

Accelerated remodeling
– x ray
– clinical
+ bone scan

+ clinical
+ bone scan
– x ray
"Subroent genographic stress fracture"

Stress remodeling and bone hypertrophy (new steady state at level of greater bone strength)

Periosteal and/or endosteal response

continued stress (running)

Eventual steady state with bone strength and no pain

Further remodeling and further strength

+ clinical
+ x ray
+ bone scan
Frank stress fracture

Figure 4-3. A theoretical flow pattern of stress syndromes of bone (stress fracture) seen from the clinician's point of view. (Preparation aided by James A. McAlister, MD)

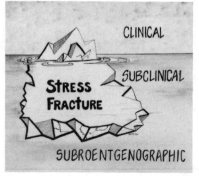

Figure 4-4. Many stress fractures do not become diagnosed clinical entities.

will also vary with the age and type of patient population (eg, university or retirement community, competitiveness, strength of running organization, etc.

Women seem more susceptible to stress fractures,[43] as well as to patellofemoral tracking problems (runner's knee). Their susceptibility may be because of the inherited sociocultural pattern that requires slower conditioning programs for women than for men. The known decreased bone density is a true anatomical difference, as is the width of the woman's child-bearing pelvis. The latter tends to produce a slightly different foot-plant in running gait. These differences alone are decreasing in importance as contributing factors to bony stress syndromes. The distribution of stress fractures and injury patterns in women parallel those in men. Stress fractures can be multiple and bilateral (Figure 4-6), although they are usually single and unilateral. With bilateral fractures, the more symptomatic side usually keeps the running below the level that would cause pain contralaterally, thereby effectively masking the contralateral symptoms.

Stress fractures in Navy and Marine recruits vary in location because of the differing repetitive mechanical high-use activities (Navy/metatarsals vs Marines/os calcis).[44] Though the relationship is not delineated, the toe/heel, heel/toe and other gait variations must similarly play a part in the tendency for anatomical predisposition to certain stress fractures.

Stress fracture occurs primarily in humans, race horses, and racing greyhounds[45-47] those animals who train for maximum performance, with pain (Figure 4-7A-C). Children, whose tibias and fibulas are primarily involved, are no exceptions to this.[48]

In 1935, Dr. Dudley Morton wrote *The Human Foot,* in which he described the "Morton's Foot."[49] Morton's foot is a term abused by lay personnel, runners, and physicians. This condition (short first metatarsal, long second metatarsal, hypermobility of first metatarsal, posteriorly displaced sesamoids) has been linked with many runners' leg and foot problems in general, and with stress fracture of the metatarsals in particular. It is also described as aggravating pronation and predisposing to degenerative changes at the junction of the first and second metatarsal bases.[50] Drez[51] found no statistical difference in relative roentgenographic first and second metatarsal length as it related to metatarsal

Table 4-2 1000 RUNNING INJURIES			
	Male %	Female %	Total %
Knee	32.6	30.8	32.1
Foot	18.3	14.3	17.2
Ankle	13.9	11.5	13.2
Hip	9.1	8.0	8.8
Stress fx	8.0	13.6	9.6
Back	7.1	8.0	7.4
PTSS	6.0	8.0	6.6
Hamstring	3.2	1.8	2.8
CMPT SYN	0.4	1.4	0.7
Misc	1.3	2.4	1.6

stress fractures and to a controlled group. He has defined a short first metatarsal as less than 73% of the length of the second metatarsal. Other studies[52] have not found a positive correlation with specific foot anatomy.

Stress fracture involving the navicular, the anterior tibial cortex, and the proximal fifth metatarsal shaft, occur in relative hypovascular areas. This hypovascularity could predispose these and other areas to union problems and recurrent stress fracture (or stress refracture).

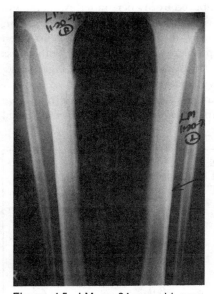

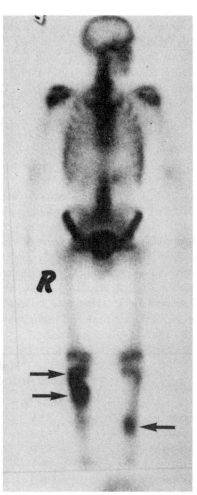

Figure 4-5. LM, a 34-year-old man training at 50 miles per week, premarathon with persistent bilateral tibial symptoms.
A. Anteroposterior roentgenogram, right and left tibia.

B. Corresponding bone scan with right upper tibia and left mid tibial fractures. Biking, as a substitute sport for six weeks, allowed a gradual return to full training, with no further problems.

Diagnosis

Stress fracture diagnosis can be difficult clinically and radiographically. The index of suspicion must be high. On physical examination, local warmth, swelling, and tenderness of juxta osseous soft tissue may be present in superficial bones. Deep bony stress fractures cause diffuse pain and tenderness. Ultrasound

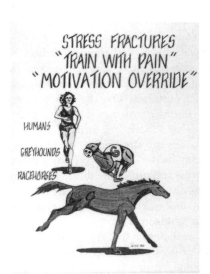

Figure 4-6. That stress fractures are related in normal bone to training and high repetitive stress is underscored by its occurrence in only three athletic animals: race dogs, race horses, and humans.

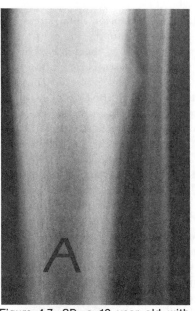

Figure 4-7. SD, a 19 year old with running-related upper tibia lesion.
A. Preoperative lateral view showing periosteal new bone and cortico-cancellous condensation of bone.

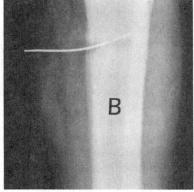

B. Open biopsy and localization.

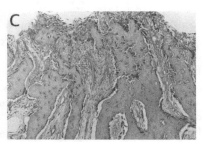

C. Fracture callous and new bone. Cellularity can cause confusion.

treatment may aggravate stress fracture symptoms.[53,54] Further findings of periosteal thickening in subcutaneous bony areas may indicate stress fracture.

Stress fracture of the proximal femur and other deeper bony parts may provide few positive findings on physical examination. The increase of occurrence of pain with active range of motion, but with appropriate painless passive range of motion in addition to relatively painless weight–bearing, implies that the stress reaction has not involved bone.

The clinical differential diagnoses includes shin splints[55] (medial tibial stress syndrome, posterior tibial stress syndrome), tendinitis (musculotendinous inflammation), muscle strain (musculotendinous tear), bursitis (especially pes anserine bursa at the knee), chronic compartment syndrome, fascial hernia, sprained interosseous membrane, and muscle insertional tears.

The term shin splints is a broad non-specific term and should be discarded entirely. Medial tibial stress syndrome[56] or posterior tibial stress, syndrome is a more accurate diagnosis for the entity along the posterior medial tibial border which can culminate in stress fracture if stress continues. The variable bone scan uptake points out the difficulty in diagnosis. The more linear uptake[57,58] present in the early stages can become more localized with continued stress and eventually become a frank stress fracture. Likewise, decreasing stress tends to diffuse the uptake. Any individual runner may have the same predisposition to medial tibial stress syndrome as they do to stress fracture. The fluidity of change with clinical symptoms, scintigraphic findings and physical findings do not make it less important to differentiate stress fracture and medial tibial stress syndrome. Fasciotomy does not help medial tibial stress syndrome.[59]

Clement[60] suggests de-emphasis of the radiologic findings and increased emphasis on early detection, treatment and rehabilitation. This more balanced clinical approach can keep the runner functional, injury at a grade I or II level, and will usually abort a full clinical and roentgenographic stress fracture. Traditional roentgenograms, of necessary high quality, continue to provide the proper tool for diagnosis, differential diagnosis, and follow-up. No other technique is as readily available in a physician's office.

Differential diagnosis roentgenographically includes malignancy, usually osteogenic sarcoma (Figure 4-8A-C), osteomyelitis, and osteoid osteoma. Ill-advised biopsies, and even amputations, have been done for stress fracture. An occasional biopsy in an atypical or questionable lesion should be considered.[13] Seven documented stress fractures or stress syndromes of bone underwent biopsy at the Orthopaedic Hospital of Charlotte during 1978-1979. All of these problems were misdiagnosed preoperatively and corrected retrospectively with appropriate histopathology and a more detailed history. On the other hand, with the increased number of stress fractures seen, the physician should not become complacent with the diagnosis.

Radionuclide (technetium 99M-labelled Medronate sodium) bone scanning, though inherently non-specific, usually can provide the diagnosis as early as two to eight days after the onset of symptoms.[61-65] In this two-to-three week period before roentgenographic visualization, the bone scan can become positive. The early diagnosis may prevent a full clinical and radiological syndrome.[66] Early diagnosis, early recognition of at–risk stress fractures, and more confident

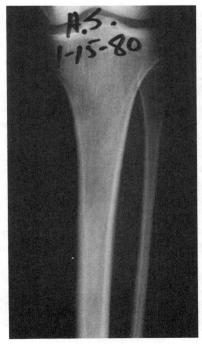

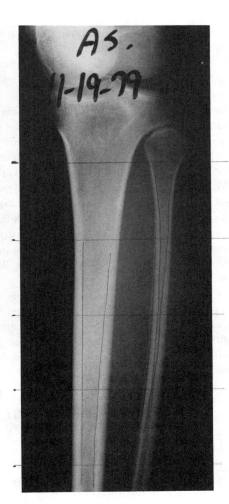

Figure 4-8. AS, a 38 year old woman with left upper tibial pain for two months. months.

A. and B. Negative findings on x-ray film over a six-week period, and no relief with local therapy, aspirin, and reduced mileage.

B.

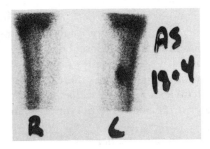

C. Positive bone scan indicating a subroentgenographic stress fracture. Substitute activity allowed her symptoms to subside.

treatment of stress syndromes of soft tissue[67-69] make scanning appropriate in selected and questionable cases.

Scintigraphic characteristics may assume more importance in the future. Mid and distal third tibial stress syndromes tend to involve the posterior medial cortex and be longitudinally oriented, whereas the proximal tibial fractures exhibit a transverse pattern or imaging.[70,71] Clinical applicability will remain important but nonspecific. Already positive results on scans of continually stressed bones, however, may persist for up to 12 months. Physical repetitive stress alone, even at high levels, will not usually cause abnormal imaging, although there is a 10% to 20% false-positive bone scan result with stress fracture because of accelerated bone remodeling. The false-positive finding indicated high sensitivity and low specificity. False-negative scans are rare and essentially exclude the diagnosis of stress fracture.[67,72] In adolescents, positive imaging occurs at the epiphysis and can cause diagnostic confusion, especially since epiphyseal stress fracture does occur.[73-75] Subroentgenographic stress fracture is a true stress fracture and is (Figure 4-9A-E) responsible for much bone pain in the training athlete.[76]

Tomography, computerized tomography[56,77,78] (Figure 4-10) xeroradiography (Figure 4-11A-C), and thermography[79,80,81] (Figure 4-12A-B) can be of occasional differential help.[82] CT scan and/or tomography in particular can help with osteoid osteoma and nidus identification. Other techniques, such as ultrasonic emission, may be useful in the future. Gallium scan[83] has been used, but is not recommended.

Clinical Considerations

Training mistakes,[84] anatomic or malalignment asymmetries or asynchronies, and sudden changes in shoe type or surface contribute to stress fracture. Frequently, a relatively minor soft-tissue injury is allowed to progress with continuation of training at the same or higher level, and a frank stress fracture results. Similarly, a minor injury can cause a significant change in running gait, initiating mechanisms for stress fracture elsewhere.

Runners incur stress fracture of bony elements in the pelvis, as well as in the lower extremities. The fracture may be proximal or distal in the long bone, or characteristic in the pelvis and tarsal bones, and can involve both cortical and cancellous areas. Numerous classification attempts exist.[85] Trabecular condensation of bone visible on roentgenograms typifies metaphyseal long bone or short bone (tarsal) fractures. Cortical break/periosteal reaction typifies primary cortical bone/stress fractures.[86] Beyond this simple categorization, there is little of practical value. The individual's musculoskeletal anatomy, the skeletal maturity, and the point where stress is or is not stopped are the deciding variables and cannot be classified.

Each bone has its own clinical presentation and tendencies. The pelvis fracture causes symptoms of perineal, groin and adductor pain, and usually occurs in the inferior pubic arch.[87] Stress avulsion[88] can also occur and is common in shorter distance runners at the hamstring attachment to the ischium and at the subacetabular level (Figure 4-13A and B). Tibial tubercle and lower

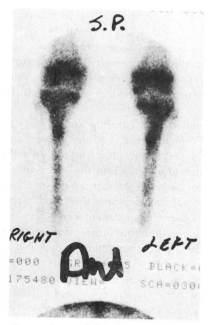

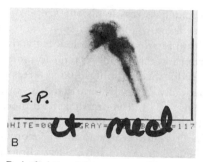

B. Left lateral bone scan. Magnetic resonance imaging confirms the endosteal new bone and cortical response.

Figure 4-9. This 22-year old female cross-country runner had a previously symptomatic left femoral stress fracture, followed by bilateral upper tibial stress fractures.
A. Bone scan, with increased uptake in both tibias.

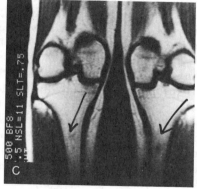

C.

C and D. In these coronal views with Magnetic resonance imaging (MRI), cancellous endosteal new bone is evident.

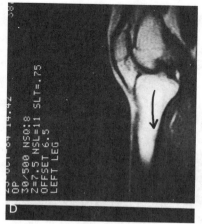

D.

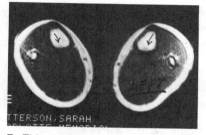

E. This transverse view shows the same endosteal reaction in the upper tibia. Cortical bone changes do not image well.

pole patella stress avulsions are also seen in the skeletally immature runner.[11] Stress fracture of ossified spikes into the patella tendon insertion can occur.

Jumping and more violent leg activities, such as, hurdling, steeplechase, and European cross-country, tend to more proximal lower extremity stress fracture. Long distance running-related stress fractures are more common distally than proximally. Pars interarticularis stress fracture does occur with repetitive loading,[89,90] but is unusual in runners.

Running and/or the stress fractures associated with running are unlikely to play a significant role in the development of osteoarthritis.[91] Many joggers and mid-career runners have early clinical and roentgenographic findings of mild osteoarthritis at the tibiofemoral and patellofemoral joints and the lower spine. Ongoing studies suggest these changes are standard and not increased over those expected in the non-running population.[93] Of course, any displaced stress fracture that causes angulation, torsion, or other malalignment can affect the proximo-distal joints negatively and predispose them to future stress-related problems. Likewise, metaphyseal stress fracture with components extending to the articular surfaces can create permanent problems. Stress fracture of the femoral neck, with displacement, may lead to non-union and/or avascular necrosis of the femoral head. Mechanics of bone hypertrophy and cartilage nutrition and regeneration have not been worked out in regard to repetitive loading in runners.[33,92]

An increasingly important question is the subjection of major weight-bearing joints–the hip, knee and ankle–with known abnormality to the repetitive stresses of running. Postmeniscectomy compartment symptoms and symptoms from old adolescent hip disease (Legg-Perthes or slipped capital femoral epiphysis) commonly occur with running. A general rule for clinicians to follow is that permanently reduced mileage or permanent substitution is indicated if: 1) roentgenographic changes advance more quickly than anticipated;[94] 2) chronic local intra-articular painful symptoms persist; or 3) chronic effusion of synovitis persists.

Treatment

The best treatment is prevention. The principals of prevention of all repetitive stress injuries are emphasized elsewhere in this text.

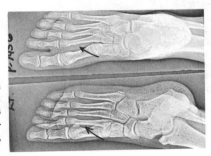

Figure 4-10. Xeroradiography of a metatarsal stress fracture is shown. Heplful cancellous trabecular clarity is present in many occult stress fractures. (Courtesy of David Humphries, M.D., Charlotte, North Carolina).

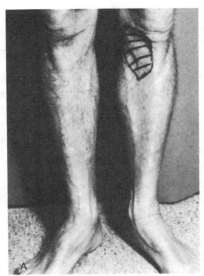

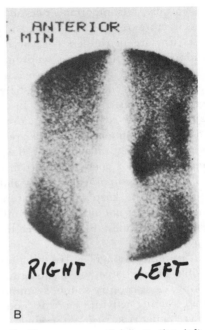

Figure 4-11. Thermography is an ancillary tool in the diagnosis of stress fracture.

A. This runner had pain and tenderness at the lower medial tibial plateau, beneath the pes anserinus bursa.

B. Bone scan uptake at the left medial tibial plateau.

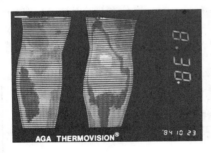

C. Thermography response corresponds to the area of injury. Thermography can detect stress changes in bone easily and within hours of clinical symptoms (Courtesy of James Maultsby, M.D., Greensboro, North Carolina.)

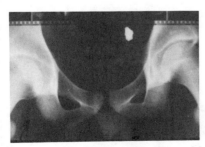

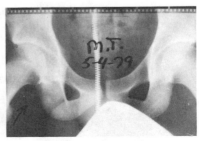

Figure 4-12. MT, an 18 year old 440-yard dash competitor with:

A. Partial avulsion of the hamstrings (semitendinosus).

B. Irregularity of involved area one year later.

Clinically, it is important, relevant and practical to emphasize and categorize stress fracture treatment patterns, and not simply the roentgenographic patterns. Stress fracture in runners has varying clinical significance depending on the location, nature of the stress syndrome, and duration of symptoms (Table 4-3). A clearly visible lucent fracture line traversing the femoral neck indicating predisplacement, demands immediate internal fixation[95] to prevent displacement and serious complications. In this situation and, to a lesser extent in all major long-bone stress fractures, close follow-up is indicated. Though general and specific treatment algorithms are variable,[96,97] a guide is that if a pain does not subside with unloading of the injured part within a few days, total immobilization or operative internal fixation is indicated.

The time of temporary disability and morbidity can be decreased by observing the principle of, "keep the level of running below that which causes pain." The principle implies not only reduced running mileage, but substitution and/or total abstinence at times. Bracing or casting is rarely necessary if this principle is followed.

If "running through" or "running around" the stress fracture symptoms is not possible or advisable, then substitute sports are necessary. Walking or race walking, cross-country skiing, swimming, biking, and selective strengthening or circuit training activities serve as good substitutes. With those fractures of bones that are not at risk, such as the fibula, techniques to permit painless running can be used. Calf sleeves, ice massage, anti-inflammatory drugs (usually aspirin), and gentler training should be tried.

The role of orthoses in stress fracture treatment, or the role of any customized sports applicants built into or within running shoes to better distribute weight to all parts of the foot, is an important one. Orthoses can reroute stress proximally, distally, medially or laterally. Its mechanical and treatment benefits are dis-

Table 4-3
STRESS FRACTURES – RELATIVE IMPORTANCE IN CLINICAL TREATMENT

"At Risk" or Critical

Femoral neck
Upper tibia
Mid Tibia anterior cortex
Navicular

Less Critical

Femoral shaft

Noncritical

Metatarsal
Fibula
Os calcis
Pelvis

cussed elsewhere. Standard prevention and treatment require modification of training, isometric rehabilitation,[60] and gradual, monitored return to running. Electrical stimulation currently has no routine therapeutic role in treating stress fracture, with the possible exception of the anterior tibial cortex.

Specific Stress Fractures

Sesamoids

Both medial (tibia) and lateral (fibula) sesamoids can be involved (Figure 4-13A-G). The differential diagnosis includes sesamoiditis, multipartite bones and osteochondritis/osteochrondrosis. Treatment may require special orthoses and even bone grafting (preferred) or excision.

Metatarsals

Metatarsal stress fracture is common (Table 4-4). All metatarsals can be involved. The second and third are involved most often, and the fourth, first, and fifth, less often (Figure 4-14 A-C). The proximal shaft is involved 5% of the time. Significant displacement or comminution of the metatarsal fracture is rare. Stress fracture can occur at the base of the fifth metatarsal, distal to the tuberosity. This "no man's land" in the area of the described acute Jones fracture tends to delayed/non-union with both acute fracture and stress fracture injuries[98-99]. Treatment with intra-medullary nailing is indicated in selected circumstances.[100]

Stress fracture may seem to be acute due to sudden overload of repetitively stressed bones. Figure 4-15A and B shows consecutive metatarsal fractures from an intra-marathon injury. Before acute injury, this runner probably had a sub-clinical stress fracture.

Table 4-4 STRESS FRACTURES OF THE FOOT & ANKLE IN RUNNERS		
Metatarsals		55%
First	3%	
Second	25%	
Third	19%	
Fourth	2%	
Fifth	6%	
Lateral malleolus		30%
Medial malleolus		9%
Os calcis		4%
Talus		
Navicular		2%
Sesamoid		

Tarsal Bone

Tarsal stress fracture is most common in the os calcis. Condensation of bone roughly parallel to the subtalar joint in the os calcis (Figure 4-16) and parallel to the talonavicular joint in the talus is the usual finding on roentgenogram. In 1944, os calcis stress fractures, usually bilateral, were frequently noted in military training after cross-country runs consisting of the two-mile intermittent walk/run period.[101] With close clinical examination, Achilles tendinitis and retrocalcaneal bursitis can be easily differentiated from stress fracture. Plantar fasciitis can create confusion. Medial lateral compression pain and positive roentgenographic findings at three weeks confirm os calcis stress fracture. Treatment is not critical and symptoms usually permit resumption of a full running schedule at three weeks. Stress symptoms at the os calcis apophysis can occur and are similar to those that occur at the tibial tubercle.

The tarsal navicular stress fracture is now recognized as more common than previously thought.[102] It is a difficult stress fracture to diagnosis, and with high morbidity if diagnosis is unduly delayed (Figure 4-17A-D). Delay is due to a low index of suspicion and false negative x-rays.[103] Anatomic bone scanning and anatomic AP tomograms are necessary for diagnosis.[104] Vague arch pain, increased pain in the midfoot with agility moves, and limited dorsiflexion and/or subtalar motion suggest the diagnosis. The relative avascular middle third of the navicular may predispose that portion to fatigue fracture.[105]

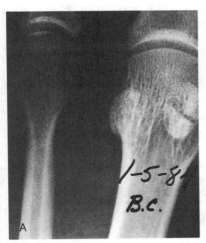
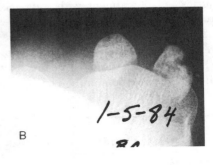
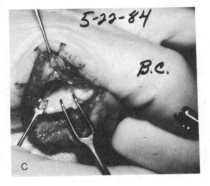

Figure 4-13. The sesamoid stress fracture unites with difficulty. This 32-year old woman, running at a level of 25 miles a week, did not respond to casting and time. A Bone graft for nonunion was performed, and a running program was re-established.
A and B. Anteroposterior and sesamoid views 6 months after injury (January 5, 1984).
C. Exposure of this sesamoid with transverse fracture line (May 22, 1984).

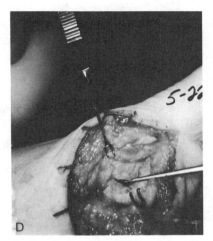

D. Curettement for bone grafting.

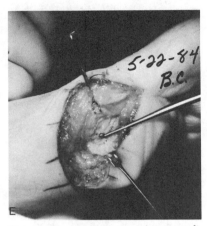

E. Impacting autogenous bone graft from adjacent first metatarsal. The patient had a postoperative plaster cast and a wooden shoe for 6 weeks.

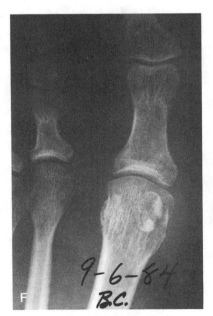

F and G. Anteroposterior and sesamoid views show the healed sesamoid stress fracture with some residual rediolucence. There were no symptoms at this point (September 6, 1984).

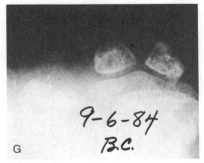

G.

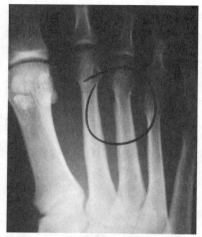

Figure 4-14. CS, a 49 year old marathoner training at 70 miles weekly.
A. Presenting 10 days after pain onset with stress fracture involving the distal diaphysis of the third metatarsal.

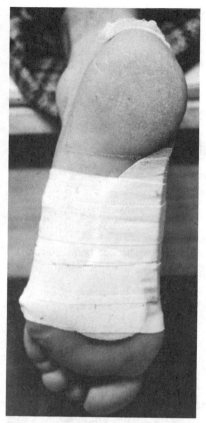

B. Low dye strapping with return to running three weeks after injury.

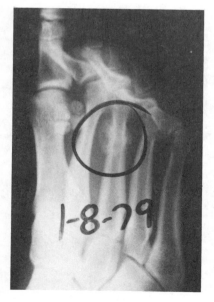

C. Proliferative callous and a limited running program.

Fibula

Fibular stress fracture (Figure 4-18A and B) causes lateral leg and ankle pain and is common in both runners and other athletes.[106] It is not an "at risk" fracture. Its limited weight-bearing function[92] effectively allows "running through" the injury by simply reducing mileage. Drilling[107] is not recommended. Many persons with fibula stress fracture fail to be examined roentgenographically. Proximal fibular stress fracture is uncommon.

Tibia

Tibial stress fracture is common. At-risk potential varies. It is roentgenographically difficult to diagnose a tibial stress fracture. Multiple oblique and marked injury site views may be necessary for accurate identification.

Though medial tibial plateau stress fracture is reportedly benign,[108] complications can occur. Intra-articular extension and displacement can be a particular

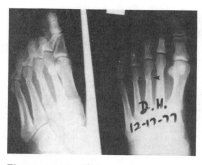

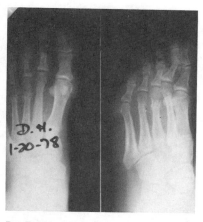

Figure 4-15. DH, a 35 year old marathoner without premarathon foot symptoms. Acute pain at the 15th and 18th miles of the marathon. He finished the marathon.
A. Fractures of necks of third and fourth metatarsals on the day of injury.

B. Early union four weeks later. Short-leg walking cast used for one week, with biking for three weeks. He ran the Boston Marathon successfully four months later.

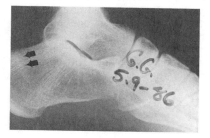

Figure 4-16. The os calsis fracture shown here in the 32-year-old runner is typical. Many os calsis stress fractures cover a longer area and extend more distally in the os calcis.

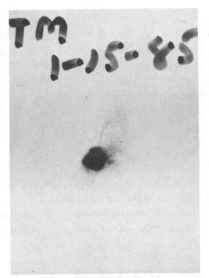

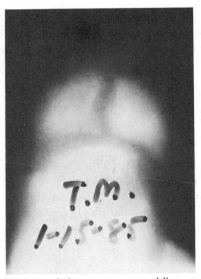

Figure 4-17. A 20 year old runner and soccer player with a one year history of increasing midfoot pain, in retrospect caused by a navicular stress fracture.
A. Initial anatomic AP tomogram one year after symptoms.

B. Lateral bone scan providing a "hot" navicular, including the talonavicular joint.

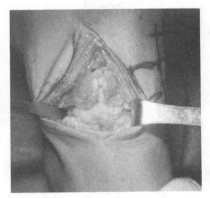

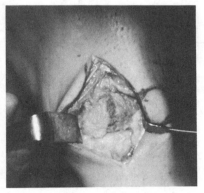

C. The frank pseudoarthrosis present on exploration. Moderate navicular joint change present.

D. The fracture sight was bone grafted from the illiac crest. By the 1986-87 school year, one year after bone graft and union, he had returned to recreational athletics and soccer kicking with minimal discomfort.

problem (Figure 4-19A-D). These proximal subplateau stress fractures frequently appear to be pes anserine bursitis, medial strain or patellofemoral problems. Minor condensation of bone can easily be missed, especially in the younger, but skeletally mature, runner with bony changes of recently closed physes. The proximity of the tibial collateral ligament attachment may be a significant factor.[109]

Often the patient seeks medical aid several weeks after forced mileage reduction, which allows union with minimal symptoms in spite of continued, but lessened, stress. It is rare for a tibial-shaft stress fracture to completely displace, but persistent high mileage or running with pain can cause problems. (Figure 4-20A-E).

The atypical fracture may occur in any athlete[110] or runner. Although not common in runners, the atypical anterior tibial cortical stress fracture is difficult to treat in the running–and–jumping based athlete (Figure 4-21A-D).[111] The tendency to more balanced training and multi-sport competition may increase the incidence in running. An early and more aggressive approach with a total training change and/or non-operative electrical stimulation[112] or early operative excision and grafting[113] may be indicated. This more aggressive treatment, with its follow–up, plus more cases and more basic biomechanical and vascular studies,

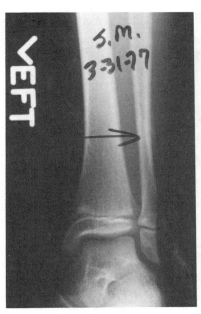

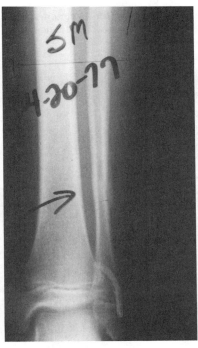

Figure 4-18. SM, a 13 year old boy with an inversion-associated painful ankle for two weeks, from running. A. Periosteal reaction and typical "runner's fracture."

B. Adequate union three weeks later. Minimal interruption of running program.

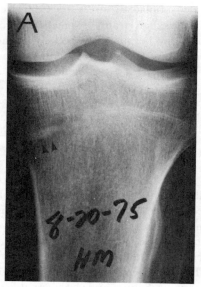

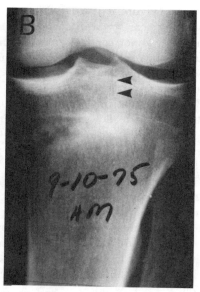

Figure 4-19. HM, a 51–year–old sedentary printer began jogging with a quick mileage increase from five to 15 miles.
A. One week after symptoms appeared. Limits of bony change are hard to define.

B. Limited weight–bearing, but extension to the interspinous articular surface effectively completing the medial tibial plateau fracture.

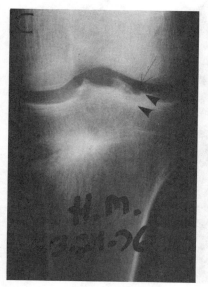

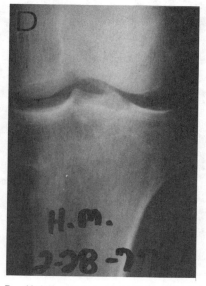

C. Union, but with clinical mild varus of the upper tibia.

D. Union and remodeling. More permanent problems would have occurred if the intra-articular components had violated the medial or lateral compartment.

will clarify which of these fractures will unite and heal. Continued clinical symptoms, diagnostic findings, and a persistent anterior tibial cortical defect at four months require surgical consideration. Distal tibial fracture is less common and is metaphyseal (Figure 4-22A and B).

With tibial stress fractures, it is generally necessary to stop running completely for a four-to-eight-week period, with substitute swimming or biking followed by reinstitution of a more gradual training program. The causative factors in the running history, running style or anatomic makeup should be identified and eliminated or corrected.

Femur

Femoral shaft stress fracture is of three types.[115] Proximal–third shaft fracture at the medial subtrochanteric level is the most common and is typical (Figure 4-23A and B).[11] Midshaft cortical fracture is less common in runners. The distal femur fracture is often metaphyseal and involves the condensation of bone (Figure 4-24A-C).

Femoral Neck

In 1966 Morris and Blickenstaff described femoral-neck stress fracture.[116] Though not running-based, the apparently first- reported displaced femoral-neck stress fracture was an 18-year-old Indian youth who was forced to crawl excessively on his elbows and toes.[117]

The so called "transverse" or "compression" stress fracture of the femoral neck[118] does indeed need treatment. The different roentgenographic appearances, however, generally reflect the same pathophysiologic process at different times in the continuum. The variables of continued vs. lessened stress per unit time determine the roentgenographic appearance. Overinterpretation of the

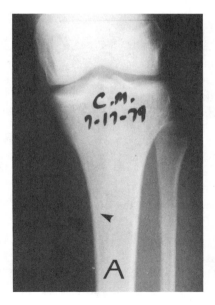

Figure 4-20. CM, a 38 year old man, ran 50 miles per week for two weeks after having been at 30 miles per week for the prior three months.
A. Cortical defect.

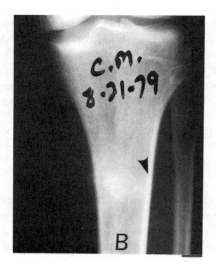

B. Extension of the fracture to the lateral cortex even with decreased stress. Also impressive condensation of bone.

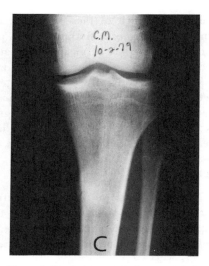

C. and D. Anteroposterior and lateral views still symptomatic three months after onset of symptoms, but running with mild pain against instructions.

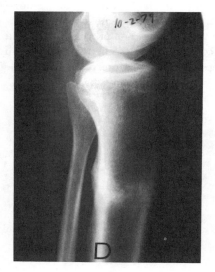

D.

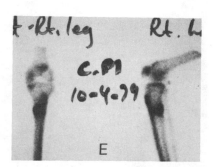

E. Bone scan hotly positive over a wide area. Late remodeling, with minimal varus results.

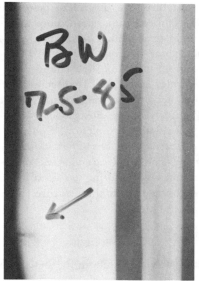

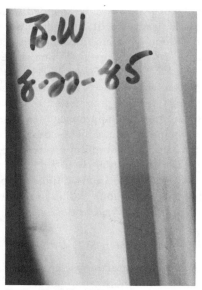

Figure 4-21. 19 year old runner and basketball player with a recalcitrant anterior tibial cortical stress fracture.
A. When initially seen following a basketball season; competed, but with playing time cut in half due to anterior tibial pain.

B. Continued symptoms after strict rest and crutches six weeks later.

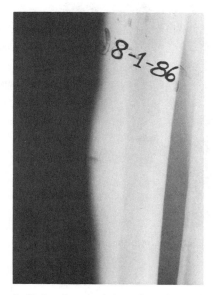

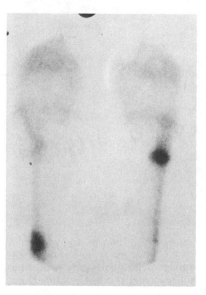

C. Following a winter of moderated activity, continued symptoms in August during summer basketball league, one year after symptoms were presented.

D. Bone scan strongly positive September, 1986, 14 months after symptoms. Note the distal tibial increased uptake on the contralateral side.

roentgenogram must be avoided, but can establish the diagnosis, help judge possible displacement, and verify union. The clinical status, pain, limp, patient cooperation—remain important in determining treatment. Unexplained pelvic, hip, or thigh pain, even with negative radiographic findings, should be watched closely.[119,120] In the femoral neck, roentgenograms may not show changes for up to five or six weeks.[101] Figure 4-25A-F illustrates the typical roentgenographic presentation and progression of the femoral neck stress fracture in a runner resistant to initial appropriate treatment. Figure 4-26A-H illustrates an initially undiagnosed femoral neck stress fracture with acute completion. Subsequent nonunion and complications occurred. *If femoral neck stress fracture does not immediately become pain-free with cessation of running, with or without crutches hip pinning, ie, Knowles pins, is indicated.* Internal fixation and bone grafting are used for late functional nonunion.[121] The immature skeleton can incur this fracture (Figure 4-27A and B) as well as others.[122]

Pelvis

Pelvic stress fracture is seen in the anterior pelvis, usually in the ischiopubic ramus, and is more common in women. The predominant site may depend in

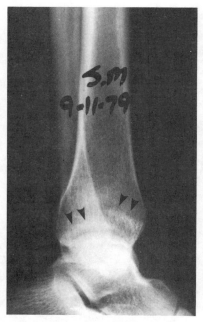

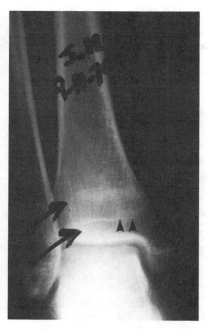

Figure 4-22. SM, a 25 year old woman who, after one month of running at 20 miles per week, had pain involving the ankle joint. Note the dual transverse areas of bone condensation in this metaphyseal fracture.
A. Anteroposterior roentgenogram.

B. Lateral roentgenogram.

part on the differential pull of the adductors medially and the hamstrings laterally.

Parasymphsical stress fracture does occur and must be differentiated from pubic stress symphysitis (osteitis pubis), adductor pulls and tendinitis and rectus insertional problems.

Summary

Stress fractures in runners are common; the incidence is increasing. Causes are similar to those leading to other repetitive stress problems of soft tissue and bone. Treatment varies, but the level of running or nonrunning substitution must be kept below that which causes pain. Treatment of the at-risk fracture demands special attention. The femoral neck fracture can require internal fixation. The navicular, anterior tibial cortex and proximal fifth metatarsal are different management problems in relatively avascular areas. The proximal and distal tibial fracture rarely requires plaster. A high index of suspicion plus good patient understanding and cooperation are extremely important. Without this cooperation, major complications can occur.

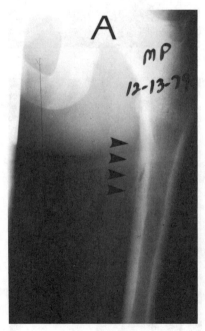 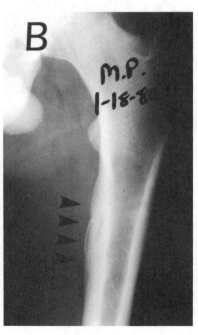

Figure 4-23. MP, an 18-year-old cross-country runner with upper thigh pain one month before being seen. The onset of symptoms was at the last cross-country meet. Abstinence caused loss of symptoms.
A. Roentgenogram taken at first examination.

B. Full activity (basketball guard) without symptoms one month later. Quicker return because of substitute activity.

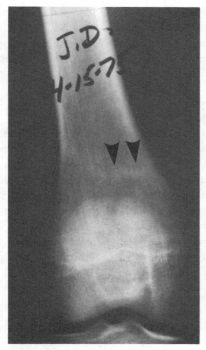

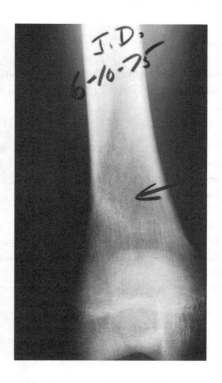

Figure 4-24. JD, a 16 year old distance runner.
A. Two weeks after onset of right knee pain.

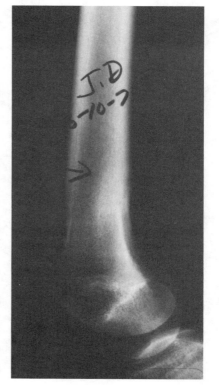

B. and C. Swimming as substitute activity and no symptoms after seven weeks.

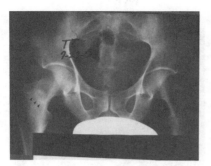

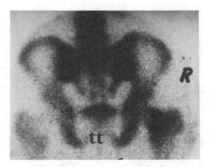

Figure 4-25. TT, a 36 year old marathoner at 50 miles per week with a three-week history of right hip pain worse with running and better with rest.

A. Initial roentgenograms show sclerosis across the distal neck.

B. Bone scan strongly positive.

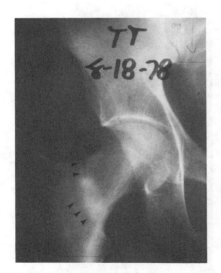

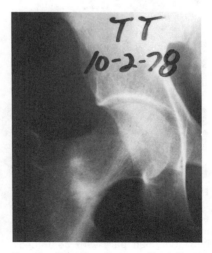

C. More bone condensation. A lucent line to the superior neck is present.

D. Continued stress after three months of symptoms. Surgery not done. Extension of the process is obvious with potential displacement.

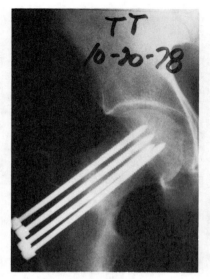

E. Knowles pinning carried out with immediate relief of hip pain.

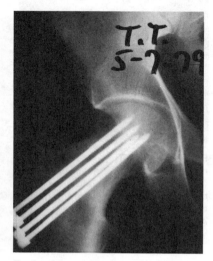

F. Again running at 50 miles per week with a healed femoral neck. The pins will remain unless bursal symptoms develop. He completed a marathon within eighteen months of his fracture.

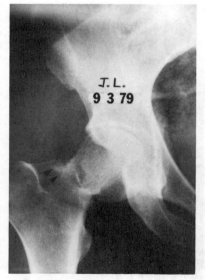

Figure 4-26. JL, a 37 year old with right hip pain four to six weeks after novice jogging. No diagnosis made. Forced to stop jogging but had continued pain with continued activity.

A. Acute hip pain at settling into the water after water skiing. No acute injury. Note sclerosis at the fracture site. Internally fixed.

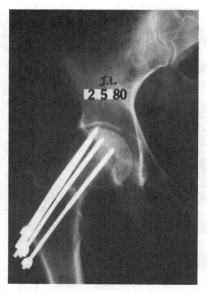

B. Appropriate pinning and position five months postinjury.

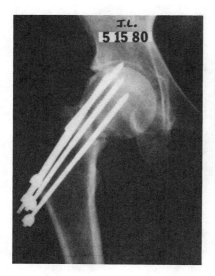

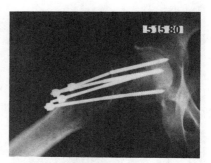

C and D. Eight months postinjury, with non-union, collapse with pin fracture and protrusion. Bone grafting, osteotomy, and internal fixation planned.

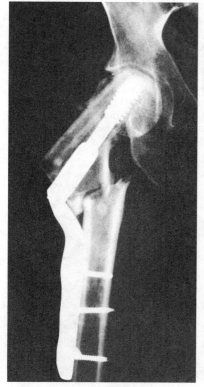

E. Osteotomy with tibial strut bone graft in attempt to salvage the hip.

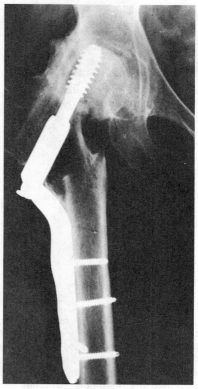

F. Union of osteotomy and incorporation of bone graft, but with upper outer degenerative change, mild subluxation and chronic pain.

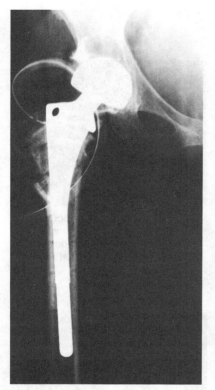

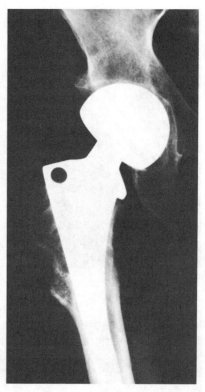

G. Porocoat self centering prosthesis with osteotomy takedown.

H. Competent and relatively asymptomatic total joint replacement. Maximally rehabilitated, but with unfortunate long term result.

Figure 4-27. 12 year old male on an early August running program pre-football with gradually increasing left hip pain. Seen and placed on crutches one month after symptoms with a diagnosis of stress fracture. X-rays confirmed the diagnosis. Crutches and non-weightbearing did not relieve his symptoms.
A. The picture of aggressive sclerosis and bone condensation with a lucent line developed.

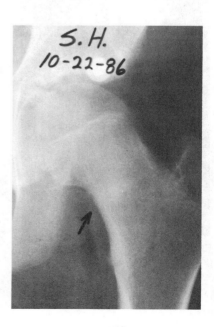

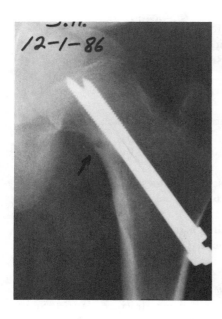

B. Knowles pinning. Note that the pins do not progress across the physis in this immature skeleton.

REFERENCES

1. Wolfe HRI, Robertson JM: Fatigue fracture of femur and Tibia, Lancet 11-13, July, 1945.
2. Mann TP: Fatigue fracture of tibia. Lancet 2:8- 10, 1945.
3. Leveton L: March (Fatigue) Fracture of the long bones of the lower extremity and pelvis. Am J Surg 71:222-232, 1946.
4. McBryde AM: Stress fractures in athletes. J Sports Med 3:212-217, 1975.
5. Greaney RB, Gerber FH, Laughlin RL, Kmet JP, Kilcheski TS, Rao BR, Silverman ED: Distribution and Natural History of Stress Fractures in U.S. Marine Recruits. Radiology 146:339-346, February, 1983.
6. Brody, DM: Running injuries, Ciba Found. Symp., 32:4, 1980.
7. Lutter L, Mann RA, and Baxter D: Running Symposium. Foot Ankle J, 1:190, 1981.
8. Jackson DW, and Strizak AM: Stress fractures in runners excluding the foot. In Mack, RP (ed.): The Foot and Leg in Running Sports. St. Louis, CV Mosby Co., 1982.
9. McBryde, AM: Stress fractures in runners: Clinics in Sports Medicine, Vol. 4, No. 4, 737-752, Oct., 1985.
10. Belkin, SC: Stress fractures in athletes. Orthop. Clin. North Am. 11:735-742, 1980.
11. Morris JM, Blickenstaff LD: Fatigue Fractures: A Clinical Study. Springfield, IL, Charles C. Thomas, 1967.
12. Devas MB: Stress Fractures. Edinburgh, Churchill Livingston, 1975.
13. Newberg, AH, and Kalisher, L: Case report: An unusual stress fracture in a jogger. Trauma, 12:816-817, 1978.
14. Dickson JM, and Fox JM: Fracture of the patella due to overuse syndrome in a child: A case report. Am J Sports Med, 4:248-249, 1982.
15. Frieberg, O: Leg length asymmetry in stress fractures: A clinical and

radiological study. J Sports Med, 22:485-488, 1982.

16. James SL, Brubaker E: Biomechanical and neuromuscular aspects of running. Exercise and Sports Science Reviews. New York, Academic Press 1:189-214, 1973.

17. Corrigan AB, Fitch KD: Complications of jogging. Med J Australia 2:363-368, 1972.

18. Blazine ME, Watanabe RS, et al: Fatigue fractures in track athletes. Calif Med 97:61-63, 1962.

19. Orava PJ, Ala-Ketola L, et al: Stress fractures caused by physical exercise. Acta Orthop Scand 49:19-27, 1978.

20. Devas MB: Stress fractures in athletes. Nurs Times 76:227-232, 1971.

21. McBryde AM, Basset FH: Stress fractures of the fibula, GP 38:120-123, 1968.

22. Bernstein A. Stone JR: March fracture, a report of three hundred and seven cases and new method of treatment. J Bone Joint Surg 26:743-750, 1944.

23. Baker J, Frankel VH, et al: Fatigue fractures: biomechanical considerations, proceedings. J Bone Joint Surg 53.A:1345, 1972.

24. Nickerson SH: March fracture or insufficiency fracture. Am J Surg 62-153.164, 1943.

25. Stanitski CL, et al: On the nature of stress fractures, Am J Sports Med 6:391-396, 1978.

26. Walter NE, Wolf D: Stress fractures in young athletes. Am J Sports Med 5:165-170, 1977.

27. Urovitz EPM, Fornasier VL, et al: Etiological factors in the pathogenesis of femoral trabecular fatigue fractures. Clin Orthop 127:275-280, 1977.

28. Frankel VH: Editorial Comment. Am J Sports Med 6:396, 1978.

29. Brand PW: The cycle of repetitive stress on insensitive feet: Scientific exhibit. Am Acad Ortho Surgeons, March, 1975.

30. Chamay A, Tschantz P: Mechanical influences in bone remodeling. experimental research on Wolff's Law. J Biomechanics 5:170-180, 1972.

31. Scully TJ, and Besterman G: Stress fracture - a preventable training injury. Milit Med 147:285-287, 1982.

32. Skinner HB, and Cook SD: Fatigue failure stress of the femoral neck: A case report. Am J Sports Med 4:245-247, 1982.

33. Radin EL, Parker HG, Pugh JW: Response of joints to impact loading-III. J Biomechanics 6:51-57, 1973.

34. Chamay A, Tschantz P: Mechanical influences in bone remodeling. experimental research on Wolff's Law. J Biomechanics 5:170-180, 1972.

35. Guoping L, Shudong Z, Chen G, Chen H, Wang A: Radiologic and Histologic analyses of stress fracture in rabbit tibias. Amer J Sports Med, 13(5):285-294, 1985.

36. Johnson LK: The kinetics of skeletal remodeling symposia, structural organization of the skeleton, Bergsma, and Milch. Birth Defects. Original Article Series, National Foundation, II:66-142, 1966.

37. Johnson LC, Stratford HT, Geis RW, et al: Histogenesis of stress fractures. J Bone Joint Surg 45A:1542, 1963.

38. Burrows H: Fatigue infraction of the middle of the tibia in ballet dancers. J Bone Joint Surg 38B:83-84, 1956.

39. Marymount JV, Lynch MA, Henning CE: Exercise-related stress of the sarcroiliac joint, an unusual cause of low back pain in athletes. Amer J Sports Med, 14(4):320-323, July- Aug., 1986.

40. James SL, Bates BT, Osternig LR: Injuries to runners. Am J Sports Med, 6:40-50, 1978.

41. Jackson DW, James CM, McBryde AM: Injuries in runners and joggers. In Schneider, RC, et al (eds.): Sports Injuries, Mechanism, Prevention and Treatment. Baltimore, Williams and Wilkins, 1985.

42. Glick JM, Katch VL: Musculoskeletal injuries in jogging. Arch Phys Med 51:123-126, 1970.

43. Micheli LJ: Injuries to female athletes. Surgical Rounds 43.52, May, 1979.

44. lbert RS, Johnson HA: Stress fractures in military recruits. A review of twelve years experiences. Military Med 131:716-621, 1966.

45. Bateman JK: Broken hock in the greyhound: repair methods and the 'plastic scaphiod. Vet Record 70:621-623, 1958.

46. Devas MB: Compression stress fractures in man and the greyhound. J Bone Joint Surg 43B:540-551, 1961.

47. Devas MB: Shin splints or stress fractures in the metacarpal bone in horses and shin soreness or stress fractures of the tibia in man. J Bone Joint Surg 49B: 310-313, 1967.

48. Devas MB: Stress fractures in children. J Bone Joint Surg 45B:528-541, 1963.

49. Morton DJ: The Human Foot: The Evolution, Physiology and Functional Disorders. New York, Columbia Univ Press, 1935, P. 257.

50. Mosley HG: Static disorders of the ankle and foot. Clin Symp 9:85, 1957.

51. Drez D, Young JC, Johnson RD, et al: Metatarsal stress fractures. Am J Sports Med 8:123-125, 1980.

52. Kernodle HB, Jacobs JE: Metatarsal march fracture. Southern Med J 37:579-582, 1944.

53. Goodwin JS: Stress fractures diagnosed by ultrasound. Mediguide Inflammatory Diseases, 4:5, 1983.

54. Devereaux MD, Parr GR, Lachmann SM, et al: Two non- invasive tests allow early diagnosis of stress fractures. J Musculoskeletal Medicine, 49, Nov., 1984.

55. Andrish JT, Bergfeld JA, Walhein J: A prospective study on the management of shin splints. J Bone Joint Surg 56A:1697-1700, 1974.

56. Mubarak SJ, Gould RN, Lee YF, et al: The medial tibial stress syndrome: A cause of shin splints. Am J Sports Med, 4:201-205, 1982.

57. Michael R: The Soleus Syndrome: A Cause of Medial Tibial Stress (shin splints). Presented at The American Orthopaedic Society for Sports Medicine, Anaheim, California, 1984.

58. Lieberman CM, and Hemingway DL: Scintigraphy of shin splints. Clin Nucl Med, 5:31, 1980.

59. Allen JJ, Barnes MR: Exercise pain in the lower leg. J Bone Joint Surg, 68B(5):818-823, Nov. 1986.

60. Clement DB: Tibial Stress syndrome in athletes. Am J Sports Med 2:81-85, 1974.

61. Siddiqui AR: Bone scans for early detection of stress fractures. N Engl J

Med, 198:1033, 2978.

62. Garrick JG: Early Diagnosis of Stress Fractures and Their Precursors. Presented at New Orleans, American Academy of Orthopedic Surgeons, Feb. 2, 1976.

63. Brill DR: Bone imaging for lower extremity pain in athletes. Clin Nucl Med, 8:101-106, 1983.

64. Butler JE, Brown SL, and McConnell BG: Subtrochanteric stress fractures in runners. Am J Sports Med, 10:228-294, 1985.

65. Milgrom C, Chisin M, Giladi M, Chen H, Wang A: Radiographic and histologic analyses of stress fracture in rabbit tibias. Am J Sports Med, 13(5):285-294, 1985.

66. Prather JL, Nusynowitz ML, Snowdy HA, et al: Scintigraphic findings in stress fractures. J Bone Joint Surg 59A:896-874, 1977.

67. Strait JL: Early Diagnosis of Stress Fractures by Bone Scintography. Presented at Sallas, American Academy of Orthopedic Surgeons, Feb 27, 1978.

68. Norfray JF, Schlacter L, Kernahan WT Jr, et al: Early confirmation of stress fractures in joggers. JAMA 243:1647- 1649, 1980.

69. Saunders AJS, Sayed TF, Hilson AJW, et al: Stress lesions of the lower leg and foot. Clin Radiol 30:649-651, 1979.

70. Roub LW, Gumerman LW, Hanley EN Jr, et al: Bone stress: A radionuclide imaging perspective. Radiology 132:431- 438, 1979.

71. Mills GQ, Marymount JH, and Murphy DA: Bone scan utilization in the differential diagnosis of exercise-induced lower extremity pain. Clin Orthop 149:207-210, 1979.

72. Wilcox JR, Moniot AL, et al: Bone scanning in the evaluation of exercise-related stress injuries. Radiology 123:699- 703, 1977.

73. Cahill BR: Stress fracture of the proximal tibial epiphysis: A case report. Am J Sports Med 5:186-187, 1977.

74. Godshall RW, Hansen CA, and Rising DC: Stress fractures through the distal femoral epiphysis in athletes. Am J Sports Med, 2:113.116, 1981.

75. Percy EC and Gamble FO: Case report: An epiphyseal stress fracture of the foot and shin splints in an anamalous calf muscle in a runner. Brit J Sports Med, 14:110-113, 1980.

76. Jackson DW: Shin splints: An update. Phys Sports Med, 51-62, Oct. 1978.

77. Somer K, and Meurman, ROA: Computed tomography of stress fractures. J Comput Assist Tomogr, 6:109-115, 1982.

78. Murcia M, Brennan RE, and Edeiken J: Computed tomography of stress fracture. Skeletal Radiol, 8:193-195, 1982.

79. Harway RA: Thermal imaging and stress fractures. Contemporary Orthopaedics, 13(5):43-45, Nov. 1986.

80. Goodman PH, Heaslet MW, Pagliano JW, Rubin GD: Stress fracture diagnosis by computer-assisted thermography. Phys Sports Med, 13(4):113.132, 1985.

81. Gilstrom, P: Thermography in low back pain and sciatica. Arch Orthop Trauma Surg. 104:31-36, 1985.

82. Berquist TH, Cooper KL, Pritchard DJ: Stress fractures. Imaging of Orthopedic Trauma and Surgery, 755-766, 1986.

83. Marta JB, Williams HJ and Smookler, RA: Gallium 67 Uptake in a stress

fracture. J Nucl Med, 4:271-272, 1981.

84. Graham CE: Stress fractures in joggers. Texas Med 66:68-73, 1970.

85. Kroening PM, Shelton ML: Stress fractures. Am J Roentgen 89:1281-1286, 1963.

86. Savoca CJ: Stress Fractures. Radiology 100:519- 524, 1971.

87. Selakovich W, Love L: Stress Fractures of the pubic ramus. J Bone Joint Surg 36a:573-576, 1954.

88. Mowat AG, and Kay VJ: Case report: Ischial stress fracture. Brit J Sports Med, 2:93.95, 1983.

89. Wiltse LL, Widell EH Jr., Jackson DW: Fatigue fractures: The basic lesion in isthmic spondylolistheses. J Bone Joint Surg 57A:17-22, 1975.

90. Hutton WC, Stott JRR, Cyron BM: Is spondyloysis a fatigue fracture? Spin 2:202-209, 1977.

91. Puranen J, Alaketola L, Peltokallio P, et al: Running and primary osteoarthritis of the hip. Fr Med J 2:423.425, 1975.

92. Lutter, Lowell: Personal Communication. 1987

93. Lambert KL: The weight bearing function of the fibula. J Bone Joint Surg 53A:507-513, 1971.

94. Hunder GG: Harmful effect of jogging. Am Intern Med 71:663.665, 1969.

95. Ernst JR: Stress fractures of the neck femur. J Trauma 4:71-83, 1964.

96. Fullerton LR, and Sowdy HA: Femoral neck stress fracture treatment algorithm. American Academy of Orthopaedic Surgeons Scientific Exhibit, 1984.

97. Harolds JA: Fatigue fractures of the medial tibial plateau. South Med J 5:578-581, 1981.

98. Dameron TB, Jr.: Fractures and anatomical variations of the proximal portion of the fifth metatarsal. J Bone Joint Surg 57-a:788-792, Sept. 1975.

99. Zelko RR, Torg JS, Rachun A: Proximal diaphyseal fractures of the fifth metatarsal - treatment of the fractures and their complications in athletes. Am J Sports Med 7:95-101, 1979.

100. DeLee JC: Stress Fracture of the Base of the Fifth Metatarsal, Distal to the Tuberosity. Presentations AOSSM, July 1986. Sun Valley, Idaho.

101. Hullinger CW: Insufficiency fracture of the calcaneus, similar to march fracture of the metatarsal. J Bone Joint Surg 26:751-757, 1944.

102. Hunter LY: Stress fracture of the tarsal navicular. Am J Sports Med 9(4):217-219, 1981.

103. Goergen TG, Venn-Watson EA, Rossman DL, Resnick D, Gerber KU: Tarsal navicular stress fracture in runners. AJR, 136:201-203, 1981.

104. Pavlov H, Torg JS, Freiberg RH: Tarsal navicular stress fractures : radiologic evaluation. Radiology 148:641-645, Sept., 1983.

105. Torg JS, Pavlov H, Cooley LR, et al: Stress fractures of the tarsal navicular. J Bone Joint Surg, 5:700-712, 1982.

106. Devas BM, Sweeten R: Stress fractures of the fibula. J Bone Joint Surg 38B:818-829, 1956.

107. Wiliams JGP: Recalcitrant stress fractures, a case managed by drilling. Fr J Sports Med 13:83.85, 1979.

108. Engber WD: Stess fractures of the medial tibial plateau. J Bone Joint Surg 59A:767-768, 1977.

109. Protzman RR, Griffis CG: Stress fractures in men and women undergoing

military training. J Bone Joint Surg, 59A:825, 1977.

110. Brahms MA, Fumich RM, et al: Atypical stress fracture of the tibia in a professional athlete. Am J Sports Med 8:131- 132, 1980.

111. Andrish, J: Anterior Tibial Cortical Stress Fractures. Presentation Sports Medicine Meeting, July 1986. Sun Valley, Idaho.

112. Rettig AC, Shelbourne KD, McCarroll JR, Gisesi M, Watts J: The Natural History and Treatment of Delayed-Union Stress Fractures of the Anterior Cortex of the Tibia. Presentation AOSSM, July 1986. Sun Valley, Idaho.

113. Lipscomb B: Stress Fractures. Presentation Sports Medicine Meeting, July 1986. Sun Valley, Idaho.

114. Kimball PR, Savastano AA: Fatigue fractures of the proximal tibia. Clin Orthop 70:170-173, 1970.

115. Provost RA, Morris JM: Fatigue fractures of the femoral shaft. J Bone Joint Surg 51A:487-498, 1969.

116. Blickenstaff LD, Morris JM: Fatigue fracture of the femoral neck. J Bone Joint Surg 48A:1031-1047, 1966.

117. Bingham J: Stress Fracture of femoral neck. Lancet 2:13, July 7, 1945.

118. Devas MB: Stress fractures of the femoral neck. J Bone Joint Surg 47B:728-738, 1965.

119. Bargren JH, Tilson DH, et al: Prevention of displaced fatigue fractures of the femur. J Bone Joint Surg 53A:1115-1117, 1971.

120. Lombardo SJ, and Benson DW: Stress fractures of the femur in runners. Am J Sports Med 4:219-227, 1982.

121. Snyder SJ, Sherman OH, Hattendorf K: Nine-year functional nonunion of a femoral neck stress fracture: Treatment with internal fixation and fibular graft - A case report. Orthopedics 9(11):1553-1557, Nov. 1986.

122. Coldwell D, Gross GW, Boal DK: Stress fracture of the femoral neck in a child (stress fracture). Pediatric Radiology 14:174-176, 1984.

CHAPTER 5

Spine Problems in the Runner

Douglas W. Jackson, M.D.

Introduction

Symptoms related to the spine, restricting running and other strenuous activities, occur most commonly in runners between the ages of 30 and 50. They are often a manifestation of an underlying degenerative process and are similar to those seen in the general population. The onset of the spinal disability may develop in relation to running, or it may develop in an unrelated activity and be accentuated and prolonged by running. Fortunately, most spine problems have a self-limited course, and the runner will be able to resume the desired mileage in time.

Most adults experience a period of low back pain sometime during their lives. The runner may find that running aggravates and prolongs the presence of what otherwise would be mild symptoms. However, disorders associated with more severe pain may result in longer times in which the runner is unable to return to a desired mileage.

A prospective study of 1,000 consecutive adult runners having disabling musculoskeletal complaints showed only 11 (1.1%) related to the spine.[1] The incidence of spinal complaints varies significantly depending on the sampling of a given runner population, the average age of the runner population and the average age of the runners being evaluated. For example, spinal complaints are infrequent in runners under age 25. Determining the exact incidence of spinal problems in the running population is further complicated in that most spinal symptoms are of an aching nature and only intermittently increase in severity to the point that they restrict the runner's mileage. Athletes, or active people, often accept their spinal discomfort and never seek formal medical advice.

Chart # _____

Name _____Age _____ Ht. _____ (in inches) Wt. _____ (in pounds)

Sex   M _____   F _____   Shoe length _____   Width of shoe _____

Dominant hand   Rt. _____ L. _____   Dominant Foot   Rt. _____ L. _____

Symptomatic side   Rt. _____ L. _____ Both _____

　　　　　　　　　　Reinjury   Yes _____ No _____

Body type   Ecto _____   Meso _____   Endo _____

　　　　　　Body frame   S   M   L

Body part involved　　forefoot _____　　midfoot _____　　rear foot _____

　　　　　　　　　　　ankle _____　　fibula _____　　tibia _____

　　　　　　　　　　　femur _____　　knee _____　　hip _____

　　　　　　　　　　　back _____

Severity   Pain only after running _____ Pain before, during and after running,

　　　　　but able to perform workout _____ Workout compromised by pain

　　　　　_____ Unable to work out, or self-imposed rest _____

Activity　　　　　　Distance _____　　Interval _____　　Both _____

Terrain　　　　　　Level　　　　　Hill _____　　　Track _____

　　　　　　　　　Other _____　　If other specify, _____

Surface　　　Paved road _____　Sidewalk _____　　Dirt_____

　　　　　　Grass _____　　　　Soft sand _____　　Packed sand _____

　　　　　　Artifical track _____　Combinations _____ _____ _____

Time of day   Morning _____　　Afternoon _____　Evening _____

Shoe Style   Distance training _____　　Tennis _____

　　　　　Other _____　　　If other, specify _____

Shoe type　　　　　Brooks _____　　Adidas _____　　Etonic _____

　　　　　　　　Nike _____　　New Balance _____Lydlard _____

　　　　　　　　Pony _____　　Puma _____　　Other (write type)

　　　　　　　　　　　　　　　　　　　　　　_____

Socks   Yes _____　　No _____

　　　　If yes, pairs   1 _____   2 _____

Miles per week　　　　　　0-20 _____　　20-40 _____　　40-60_____

　　　　　　　　　　　60-80 _____　　80+ _____

How long have you   less than 3 mos. _____　　less than 6 mos. _____

been running?　　less than 1 yr. _____　　less than 5 yrs. _____

　　　　　　　more than 5 yrs. _____

The farthest mileage   0-2 _____　　　　　3-4 _____

ever run at one time   5-6 _____　　　　　7-10 _____

　　　　　　　10-20 _____　　　　greater than 20 _____

Have you run a　　Yes _____　　　　　No _____

marathon?　　If yes, how may _____

Do you use orthotics?   Yes _____　　　　　No _____

　　　　　　Is yes, rigid _____   or flexible _____

How would you classify your foot structures?   Flat foot_____

　　　　　　　　　　　　　High arch _____ Normal _____

Diagnosis: _____

Figure 5-1. This questionnaire gives the physician a profile of the runner's training and experience. This information can be integrated into the general history obtained for spinal disabilities.

Evaluation of the spinal disability of any runner should be detailed, and a diagnosis established so that a reasonable recommendation and prognosis may be given. The history and additional pertinent questions (Figure 5-1), are of particular interest in the runner, who may also fill out a pain drawing (Figure 5-2), which pictorially represents the pain location and aids the runner in characterizing the nature of the pain.[2,3] It also aids the physician in deciding whether the pain is localized and/or represents referred pain in a dermatomal or sclerotomal distribution. This assessment of the spinal pain and its referred component helps to determine which diagnostic tests are appropriate if conservative treatment measures fail. Runners with referred pain, particularly radicular pain, often require more aggressive restriction than those with more localized musculoskeletal complaints.

The physical examination of the runner with a spinal complaint is similar to an examination for any back problem, and includes documentation of any restriction in the range of motion of the spine and lower extremities, paraspinous muscle spasm, tenderness, reflex changes, sensory changes, motor weakness, and signs of nerve root irritation.

Leg-length discrepancies become more important in distance runners than in the general population. They can be evaluated by many different methods. A film of the pelvis with the patient standing takes into account the entire lower extremity, including the feet bearing weight. Measurements from the anterior-superior iliac crest to the medial malleoli do not take into account foot structure. For example, when one foot is more pronated than the other it contributes to a relative leg-length discrepancy while weightbearing. In the runner complaining of nonspecific spinal discomfort, a discrepancy of greater than one centimeter should be empirically treated in an attempt to see whether such correction will be of some benefit. The question of which leg-length discrepancies are contributing factors is a multi-variable problem to try to evaluate. A lift is an innocuous treatment and can be tried empirically as it does not represent significant cost and seldom aggravates the underlying problem.

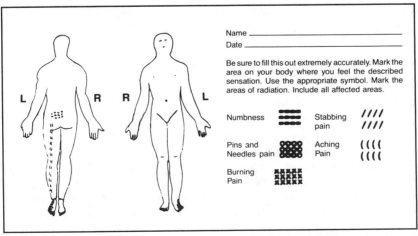

Figure 5-2. The pain drawing is quite helpful in determining if the runner has a dermatomal distribution to pain or if it is localized.

Roentogenographic evaluation of the area of the spine in which the runner is complaining of pain is usually of little help diagnostically in the management or prognosis of the spinal problem. In a series of roentogenograms of the lumbar spine in 90 asymptomatic marathon runners, we found that their incidence of degenerative changes was similar to that of the general population.[4] Many of those with mild roentogenographic changes did not seem to be having any more symptomatic spinal problems than those without changes at the time of their roentogenograms. The presence of changes in the lumbar spine does not preclude a runner from returning to unlimited mileage, and may or may not be associated with the patient's particular pain complex.

Supplemental diagnostic tests beyond the routine roentogenographic survey of the spine in the runner are seldom necessary. The use of electromyogram, myelogram, spinal fluid analysis, venography, bone scan, computerized axial tomography, segmental nerve blocks, Pentothal (thiopental) examinations, and psychometric evaluations are part of the armamentarium directed to those not responding once the initial impression has been made and program started.

Magnetic resonance imaging (MRI) is a revolutionary new scanning method for evaluating the lumbar disc and neural elements. This method has assisted in the early establishment of a specific diagnosis in those runners with refractory symptoms. The absence of ionizing radiation (X-ray) and no need for injecting contrast material (myelogram) has made this test more desired by most runners. There are infrequent instances where the more traditional tests are still indicated. The MRI presently is an expensive test but most runners faced with the restrictions a symptomatic or ruptured disc places upon them have been pleased to have this new technology available.

As a rule, the distance runner does not have the conflicting secondary gain and psychological overlay that interferes with recovery, as often seen in other similarly aged adult patients with spinal complaints. Nevertheless, the psychological aspects of not being able to run cannot be ignored. To advise the runner to give up running as a solution for the spinal discomfort is seldom necessary. Controlled or restricted mileage is often part of the initial treatment program, which should be carefully outlined with the runner. Most runners, however, eventually return to unrestricted running, and telling the patient that fact on the initial evaluation will provide him with a source of relief.

Cervical Spine

The cervical spine infrequently presents symptoms that restrict running programs, but when cervical disc symptoms develop with associated radicular and paracervical pain and muscle spasm, it may curtail running for a significant period of time. The runner who sustains a whiplash injury may prolong the acute phase by continuing to run. Attention to the acute phase of a cervical disc injury, or injury to soft tissue of the cervical spine, may prevent chronic symptoms and headaches. The aggressive restriction of running during the acute phase of a cervical injury is often beneficial. Shoulder movement and motion of the upper extremity, and the muscle interaction with the cervical spine, may increase the pain and lengthen the recovery time. Running in a cervical collar with restricted upper extremity motion is not enjoyable.

The stationary bicycle is an excellent alternative to maintain conditioning and usually will not aggravate the cervical spine during the acute symptoms. Most cervical symptoms will subside with a period of rest, and selected patients may require additional treatment such as cervical traction, immobilization, heat, massage, and other modalities. Acute symptoms may merit a short period of bedrest, with or without cervical traction. A short course of parenteral steroids, or other anti-inflammatory medication, analgesics, and muscle relaxants may be beneficial and could hasten the resolution of nerve root irritation symptoms. These treatments will vary and must be individualized with each case. Surgery usually is not necessary for cervical problems in the runner.

In the older runner, cervical disc disease and associated degenerative boney changes can be associated with neurologic findings in the lower extremities, as well as in the upper extremities. The neurologic status of both the upper and the lower extremities should be thoroughly evaluated in runners who have cervical spine complaints. Careful examination of the long tract signs, including clonus and spasticity, should be evaluated in cervical spine problems.

Occasionally, runners will develop symptoms of an acute "wryneck" in which the runner awakens in the morning with, or gradually develops, stiffness in the neck that is associated with some discomfort. These symptoms usually diminish as the runner warms up related to his running activity, and the cervical discomfort disappears during the workout. The symptoms return after the workout is completed and the runner cools down. This condition is usually a self-limited process unrelated to running and is seen frequently in the general adult population as well as in the runner. It is not associated with a long-term disability and usually the running program is disrupted for only seven to ten days.

In terms of returning the runner to the sport, nearly all cervical spine symptoms resolve readily with conservative measures. Cervical problems in runners are less difficult to manage than those in participants of some other sports in which more head and neck motion is required. Even if surgery is necessary, ie, disc removal and/or fusion, running usually remains an excellent fitness activity after recovery from the surgery.

Thoracic Spine

Pain and disability in the thoracic spine is seldom related exclusively to running. It can be associated with paraspinous muscle spasm, local pain, and radicular pain around the rib cage. The runner who notes an increased sensitivity in the skin in a thoracic dermatomal distribution and who develops radiating pain may be describing the prodromal of shingles, which is something that will become obvious when the skin rash occurs. The amount of pain and irritation that the runner has related to this viral illness varies significantly. The amount of restriction is essentially symptomatic and highly individualized. Occasionally, but rarely, an especially irritating post-therapeutic neuritis can develop.

Persistent localized thoracic pain is rare in the runner. If the tenderness is confined to a spinous process, or is reasonably well-localized, it should raise the suspicion of the possibility of an underlying malignancy or metastic lesion in the middle-aged and older runner. Often careful scrutiny of the anteroposterior and lateral roentogenograms of the thoracic spine, as well as a complete medical examination, will suggest whether further studies are needed. If the pain does not resolve in a reasonable period, a bone scan and tomography of the area may be indicated. Just as metastatic disease and primary tumor involvement in the thoracic spine are infrequent occurrences, and are rare in the runner as well as in the general population, so is unexplained thoracic pain. Suspicion should be aroused. Fortunately such problems are unusual and unrelated to running, but they may develop in the runner and early symptoms should not be neglected.

Spondylitis confined to the thoracic spine also is a remote possibility. Signs and symptoms in other joints should alert the clinician to the appropriate diagnostic studies. Degenerative changes in the thoracic spine and old traumatic compression fractures usually do not restrict the running program, but do need individual assessment.

For those who have irritation with motion of the thoracic spine related to running, once again a stationary bicycle or rollerskating during the recovery period may be an alternative.

Lumbar Spine

The lumbar spine, by far, is the area of greatest disability related directly to running. In all of us, as we grow older, our intravertebral discs alter. Usually this aging process of the disc is not associated with pain and there is gradual and rather uniform narrowing in the disc space. Those who have symptomatic pain with a disc, with or without associated radicular symptoms, may find their running curtailed for a significant period.

In running, as the hind leg trails, it is associated with hyperextension of the lumbar spine.[5] This hyperextension greatly aggravates most causes of lumbar pain and radicular symptoms. The degree of repetitive motion in the lumbar spine during distance running is unparalleled in other sports in the age group between 30 to 50 years. It is primarily the repetitive hyperextension of the lumbar spine that makes running so unique. The low back moves from the flat-backed position as the foot strikes to an extended lordotic position as the trailing leg leaves the ground. Often the more competitive and faster runners will have more extension in the lumbar spine.

The more degenerative arthritic changes seen in the lumbar spine roentogenograms, associated with nerve foramina encroachment and spinal stenosis, may result in actual development of a mild cauda equina syndrome in the older runner. Their presentation may be one of pain and fatigability in the lower extremities with prolonged running. This condition should not be confused with a vascular problem and is related to neural element impingement with manifestations in the lower extremity. This problem is infrequent, as most people with this advanced degree of degenerative lumbar changes have enough associated pain that they are unable to carry out prolonged running.

Spondylolysis, defects of the pars interarticularis, that are present on lumbar films in skeletally mature runners are usually incidental findings (Figure 5-3). The incidence of lumbar pars interarticularis defects among male runners is in the range of 5%, although the percentage may be higher in certain athletic populations.[6-8] Most lumbar pars interarticularis defects develop during childhood or early adolescence and are unrelated to the particular pain pattern in the adult. If localized vertebral instability or associated vertebral slippage is present, however, they may be associated with pain (Figure 5-4A. and B). Often, accelerated disc space narrowing at the level of the instability has been present for some time. Frequently, the symptomatic disc that causes these patients to complain is at the level above the obvious roentgenographic changes and instability.

Pars interarticularis defects in themselves usually will not permanently restrict running. Runners with vertebral slippage often are unaware of their spondylolisthesis until their first x-ray films are obtained in relationship to their new

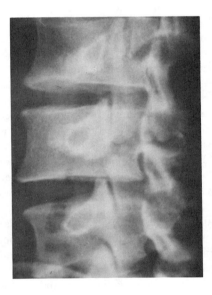

Figure 5-3. This pars interarticularis defect was an incidental finding in a marathon runner. The runner was unaware of its presence and denied spine complications.

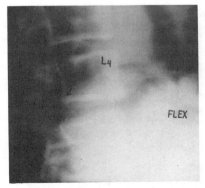 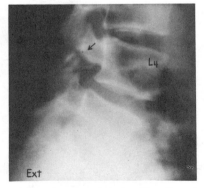

Figure 5-4 A and B. This segmental instability is associated with altered invertebral disc motion between the fourth and fifth vertebrae. This runner complained of persistent discomfort with vigorous running.

lumbar spine complaints (Figure 5-5). They most often will be able to return to running after a conservative treatment program. Spondylolysis and spondylolisthesis are not the result of running, but when increased demands are placed on the lumbar spine, particularly the repetitive extension of the lumbar spine associated with running, the entire area may be more symptomatic and restricting. Although most of those types of low back problems will resolve through a period of rest, some surgical intervention may be necessary, and the possibility that the runners will have some permanent disability related to their running does exist.

Structural changes in the spine, such as scoliosis, thoracic kyphosis and congenital abnormalities, may alter flexibility and restrict range of motion. They may be associated with degenerative changes that become more symptomatic as a result of the aging process, and are aggravated by running. Treatment must be individualized, but most affected patients can return to some type of satisfying fitness program if running is not tolerated. Attention to leg length discrepancies has already been alluded to and is something that needs to be watched for in this group.

Manifestations of inflammatory connective tissue disease in the spine and/or sacroiliac joints may be present in the runner. These seronegative spondyloarthropathies should not be overlooked, particularly in the younger adult age group. The early presentation of spondylitis and its variants should be suspected in young runners complaining of lower spine and sacral discomfort. The tissue typing of HLA-B27 in these runners with unusual low back pain may be particularly worthwhile. A positive HLA-B27 can be obtained in about 7% or more of the normal male population, so it, in itself, is not diagnostic, but when coupled with a dramatic response to an anti-inflammatory medication or a positive bone scan, the diagnosis becomes more apparent.

Pain in the area of the sacroiliac joints in the lower lumbar spine should raise the question of ankylosing spondylitis, as well as variants of Reiter's syndrome. Details related to other joint involvement, arthritis, urethritis, conjunctivitis and mucous membrane lesions, should be obtained appropriately. The bone scan is particularly helpful in those problems involving early sacroiliac joint inflamma-

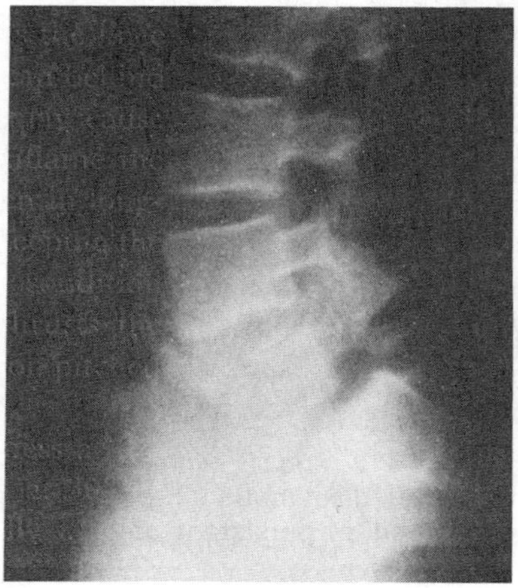

Figure 5-5. Low grade spondylolisthesis is not inconsistent with distance running, and a few internationally known runners have had this entity. They often have intervertebral narrowing at the level of instability.

tory change. The roentogenograms may show no abnormality, and the increased boney activity can often be detected only by increased uptake on the technetium 99 bone scan. If they are part of a self-limited process, these early changes may never be detected on routine roentogenograms, or may develop years later. These processes may be associated with periods of disability that respond to rest and anti-inflammatory medication, and usually the athletes are able to continue with their running, if that is their desire.

Nonspecific urethritis in the runner associated with discomfort in the sacroiliac joints is often associated with a period of disability, and evaluation of this entity may require an extensive rheumatologic or urologic workup.

Treatment of Lumbar Spine Problems

Most conservative programs related to treating acute disc problems associated with radicular pain have, as the basis of their treatment, rest, antilordotic exercises, and positioning. Because runners are subjected to repetitive hyperextension, those interested in the fastest recovery should consider a period of bedrest at the onset of intense acute low back pain. This rest may be associated with traction and analgesics, if necessary. The role of the anti-inflammatory medication and muscle relaxers should be individualized. Runners as a group do not respond favorably to the suggestion of bedrest, although they may pay considerably more attention if they understand its potential role in the ultimate return to their running. Runners tend to be highly activity-oriented people, and often the milder problems can be controlled by limiting their exercise and running program.[9] A period of controlled rest, with restriction in running and other activities, can be tried in the milder cases for a trial period in the treatment program. Abdominal exercises and antilordotic positioning for the lumbar spine should be included, as well as significant reduction in mileage. This rest may be supplemented by the simple use of heat and relaxation techniques, as necessary.

In those runners who have radicular symptoms that persist two to three weeks or longer and do not respond to rest, a lumbar epidural cortisone injection may hasten the resolution of the more chronic symptoms (Figure 5-6). It may significantly reduce the runner's radicular pain and hasten the ability to resume running, after just one injection. The lumbar epidural cortisone injection, coupled with restricted mileage, flexion exercises, and gradual resumption of their running program, has succeeded in about 40% of the athletes on whom we have used it.[10,11] The longer lasting epidural effects of DepoMedrol have been preferred to the shorter-acting water soluable suspensions.

The intradiscal cortisone injection has not been beneficial in any of our runners, and my experience with the lumbar facet injection has been limited. Lumbar facet syndrome is difficult to diagnose. Some runners are believed to have symptoms related to impingement of the facets from repetitive hyperextension of of the lumbar spine during the running gait. If a facet injection is believed to be indicated, localizing the position of the needle in the facet joint usually requires image intensification control, and may even be aided with the use of a facet arthrogram before the injection. It has been reported to be beneficial in some population groups, but has not been reported as a source of success in runners.

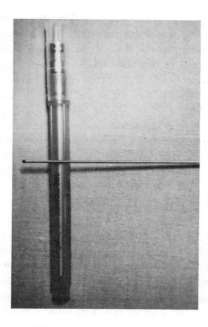

Figure 5-6. The epidural needle facilitates the placement in the epidural space, without penetrating the dura. The short beveled needle helps prevent dural leaks at the time of the epidural injection.

Mobilization (manipulation) of the lumbar spine, both actively and passively, is reasonable in localized lumbar spine problems in distance runners. It can be done by the physician, by a therapist, or by other persons trained in mobilization techniques. Often the runner finds that the treatment relieves symptoms for two to three hours only. On occasion, some treatments may result in dramatic relief. Usually, however, the mobilization techniques are coupled with additional treatments.

The efficiency of transelectrical nerve stimulation (TENS) in the distance runner is limited. It may give temporary noninvasive analgesia while the underlying process proceeds to heal. It should not be used to increase the pain tolerance for prolonged training. Most runners respond to rest with or without TENS.

Corsets and antilordotic braces in the runners are of little value unless used during the acute phase to aid in positioning and restricting activity for a short time. In the milder cases of low back discomfort, wet-suit lumbar binders that increase the local skin temperature may give symptomatic relief while the patient is running.

Some lumbar pain syndromes are aggravated by activities other than running. The running only accounts for a portion of the disability. For example, a person may have a job requiring prolonged sitting, and repeated bending, lifting, and stooping. These activities keep the back aggravated and yet it is during running that the greatest disability is present. Often an effective solution requires altering the entire requirements placed on the back if the runner is to continue running. Time is well spent in reviewing lifting habits, bending techniques, ways of getting into and out of chairs and automobiles, and sleeping positions and surfaces; placing a foot on a short stool if prolonged standing is necessary can be helpful.

The prevention of spinal symptoms in the runner is a goal. Proper stretching, good muscle balance, and proper lifting and posture habits are important in an effective preventive program. To minimize the episodes of difficulty, a runner should stretch regularly, preferably before and after running. Allotting enough time is always difficult, but a runner with a back problem should definitely make a priority of having a stretching program before and after running. Although most runners will spend time stretching the Achilles tendon and the hamstrings, they usually do not specifically work on the spine. A full range of motion of the spine is maintained by stretching. Almost all beneficial stretching avoids hyperextension of the lumbar spine. This factor is particularly important in doing the sit-ups and other calisthenics that some runners do as part of their warm up and cooling down period.

Lumbar surgery in the runner can be highly successful and I am aware of several runners who have returned to marathon running after one level, and multiple level, disc surgery and lumbar spine fusions (Figure 5-7). The ability to run a marathon after lumbar spine surgery remains a possibility, but not in all cases. If recovery is incomplete or the pain is only partially resolved after surgery, and the patient has associated chronic changes related to the neural elements, he may not be able to continue with his running program. For these persons, swimming and bicycling may become substitutes for running. That choice is an individual matter. That someone who has had lumbar spine surgery

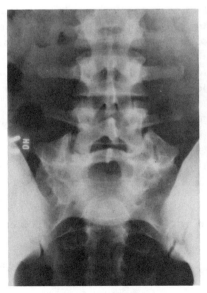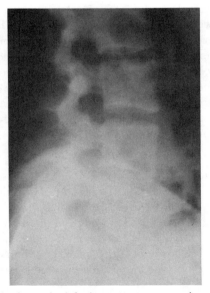

Figure 5-7 A and B. This young runner had a spinal fusion seven years prior to these roentgenograms, for a low grade spondylolisthesis, showing essentially no symptoms associated with running. The spine above the level of the fusion is remarkably free of degenerative changes.

is precluded from future running is a popular misconception.

Lumbar spine surgery for a ruptured or bulging disc in a runner without significant secondary arthritic or boney changes requires limited surgical exposure. New techniques include microsurgery and other percutaneous approaches.[12] In some select cases these may be done as an outpatient procedure. Minimal damage to the overlying paraspinal musculature and boney structures is an important consideration in a runner. The use of chymopapain (an enzyme) to dissolve the center of the disc has pros and cons. Its use is best determined by the treating surgeon. One of its potential advantages remains as a minimally invasive alternative treatment.

As yet there is no conclusive evidence that a postsurgical, pain-free spine more rapidly degenerates with running than does the spine that has never had surgery. The runner who has had a disabling back condition of long duration, with or without surgery, is likely to have recurrent episodes of back disability, whether that person runs or not. Controlled studies have not been done to support positions, for or against running, in patients with lumbar spine problems. My experience is that if the spine can be maintained pain-free, running has not proved to be that detrimental.

Fortunately for the runner, the spine is in an area that does not present a great deal of disability, and usually responds to conservative treatment, enabling the runner to return to unlimited mileage. To minimize spinal problems, each runner should maintain flexibility of the spine, use good lifting habits, and respect warning pains if they should develop. For those few who have a significant problem in spite of their efforts, the prognosis is usually good. Running, with its demands of repetitive range of motion of the lumbar spine, particularly the increasing lordosis related to the trailing leg, may be more than certain spines can tolerate. Tolerance is highly individualized and each patient needs an evaluation and interpretation of his particular case. Many chronic lumbar spine patients do well only in the antilordotic position. It may even mean a certain percentage of runners will need to switch to alternate fitness programs of cycling or swimming. Fortunately, few patients must give up running altogether. Runners should take good care of their spines because the spine is one of the areas in which a chronic disabling condition, if allowed to develop, will significantly limit running.

REFERENCES

1. Jackson DW, Pagliano J: The ultimate study of running injuries. Runners World Nov:42-50, 1980.
2. Palmer H: Pain maps in differential diagnosis of psychosomatic disorders. Med Press May 25, 1960, p 454.
3. Ransford AO, Cairns D, Mooney V: The pain drawing as an aid to psychologic evaluation of the patient with low back pain. Spine 1:127, 1976.
4. Sutker A, Jackson DW: Roentogenographic changes in the lumbar spine in marathon runners. (publication pending)
5. Slocum DB, James SL: Biomechanics of running. JAMA 205:721-728, 1968.

6. Jackson DW, Wiltse LL, Cirincione RJ: Spondylolysis in the female gymnast. Clin Orthop 117:68-73, 1976.

7. Wiltse LL, Widell EH, Jackson W: Fatigue fracture: The basic lesion in isthmic spondylolisthesis. J Bone Joint Surg 57A:17-22, 1975.

8. Jackson DW, Wiltse LL, Dingeman R, Hayes M: Stress reactions involving the pars intaricularis in young athletes. Am J Sports Med 9(5):304-312, 1981.

9. Guten G: Herniated lumbar disc associated with running: A review of 10 cases. Am J Sports Med 9(3):155-159, 1981.

10. Jackson DW, Rettig A, Wiltse LL: Epidural cortisone injections in the young athletic adult. Am J Sports Med 8:239- 243, 1980.

11. Rettig A, Jackson DW, Wiltse LL, Secrist L: The epidural venogram as a diagnosis procedure in the young athlete with symptoms of lumbar disc disease. Am J Sports Med 5:158-162, 1977.

12. Onik G, Helmes C: Percutaneous lumbar discectomy using a new aspirated probe. AJNR 6:290,1985.

CHAPTER 6

Running Injuries of the Knee

Robert E. Leach, M.D.
G. Richard Paul, M.D.

Introduction

When an orthopedic surgeon considers sports injuries of the knee, he usually is primarily concerned with ligamentous instability or meniscal tears. Damage to those structures, however, plays a minor role in running injuries, unless the runner injured them previously and they resurface to cause trouble again. Most problems from running that cause knee pain are due to chronic stress and not to any one single injury.[1,2]

Handling runners with knee pain differs from dealing with other athletes with knee pain. Athletes with a chronically unstable ligament or meniscal tear would be unable to perform in most other sports. Many runners will have problems that produce less disability. The problem may produce pain which, while allowing the runner to run, may keep him from functioning optimally or from running as long as he desires. It may be difficult for a physician not involved with runners to understand why a patient would worry if he can run three miles but not six miles; the tendency is to tell the runner to stop after three miles. This may not be the goal of the runner, nor should it be the goal of the physician. Our aim should be to allow each runner to achieve his own maximum potential and goals, however hard it may prove.

Initial Evaluation

When dealing with knee problems in athletes, physicians usually are concerned with the onset of the acute knee injury and the subsequent disability. Many times runners do not have an acute injury but a series of events on running days in which pain gradually begins. Still, the physician should try to pin the runner down as to the precise time that the pain began. Was there a change in the training pattern, increased mileage, more hill work, or were interval workouts suddenly started? When does the pain occur? Is it present from the start of a run or just near the end? Does the pain persist or increase with running, and what is the pain level the next day? Is this pain present only with running, or is it associated with normal activities? What happens when going up or down the stairs, or up or down ramps or hills? What physical manifestations, such as swelling, has the runner noted? Does the runner detect any noises in the knee with running or climbing, as well as grating or grinding sounds? Finally, the physician must know what treatment the runner has already received. Has there been a shoe change? Orthotics? Medications? Injections? Have rehabilitation exercises been prescribed, and if so, exactly which ones? Have the exercises been performed properly? And what has been their effect?

When evaluating a runner who presents with knee pain, the physician must recognize that the foot, ankle, leg and hip all are interrelated and may contribute to certain knee problems.[3,4] Physical examination of a runner with knee pain includes a look at the runner's standing or weight-bearing position and his gait pattern (Figure 6-1A and 6-1B). Leg lengths (measured from the anterior superior iliac spine to the medial malleoli), femoral anteversion or retroversion, varus or valgus alignment of the knee or of the tibia, and internal or external tibial torsion must be observed. Abnormalities of femoral anteversion/retroversion and tibial torsion may be apparent in the standing position. These findings must be confirmed by examining the patient in the recumbent or seated position, when the true axes of the hip joint, the knee joint, and the ankle joint can be controlled.

In addition to a complete foot and ankle examination, evaluation of the wear pattern of the runner's shoes then must be done, because abnormal foot mechanics may have a direct bearing on a number of knee problems. One must look for varus or valgus alignment of the heel, cavus or planus deformity of the longitudinal arch, and forefoot pronation (Figure 6-2) or supination. A number of seemingly mild abnormalities of the lower extremities combine to form clinical patterns producing knee pain.

After a general examination of the lower extremity has been completed, turn to the knee itself. A systematic examination of the knee includes the usual tests for pathologic menisci and ligamentous instabilities[5] (Figure 6-3). The knee must be evaluated for effusion, joint-line tenderness, meniscal damage, medial or lateral instability on valgus or varus stress, anterior or posterior instability, and rotary instability. The alignment and excursion of the patella also must be assessed. Is there any patellofemoral crepitation on resisted extension of the knee? Is there any angular or rotational malalignment of the patella? Angular alignment of the patella or extensor mechanism is best assesed by the Q angle. This angle is formed by the intersection of a line drawn from the anterosuperior illiac spine to the center of the patella and a line drawn from the tibial tubercle to the center of the patella (Figure 6-4). Normally this angle is 15° or less. An angle greater than 20° is considered abnormal and is frequently associated with patellofemoral pathology.

Particular attention must be paid to the quadriceps and hamstring musculature. Look for atrophy of any of the muscle groups of the thigh, and test for muscle strength. Is there abnormal tightness of the hamstrings, the hip or knee flexors, or the external rotators of the hips? Tightness of any of these muscle groups or of the gastrocnemius-soleus complex may have a bearing on certain knee problems. All painful areas must be carefully assessed; point tenderness will help distinguish referred pain patterns from certain specific syndromes.

Radiographs of the knee should be obtained if intra-articular pathology is suspected. Routine AP, lateral, and intercondylar ("tunnel") projection radiographs should be obtained. A patellar tangential projection of the patellofemoral groove should be obtained in patients with patellar pain or with extensor mechanism malalignment; various techniques for obtaining these views have been described by Hughston[6] (Figure 6-5), by Labelle and Laurin,[7] and by Merchant associates.[8]

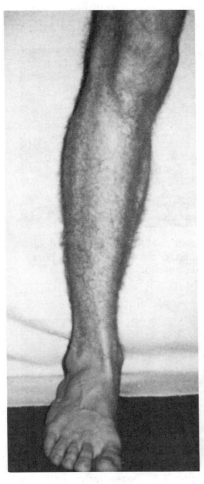

Figure 6-1A. Normal leg.

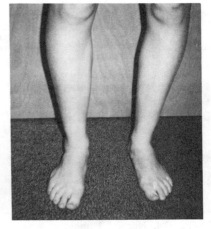

Figure 6-1B. Tibia vara with foot pronation.

Intra-Articular Pathology

Meniscal Injuries

Except for chondromalacia patella, intra-articular pathology is not a common form of disability in runners. Although a runner could tear the medial or lateral meniscus with a misstep, acute meniscal injuries are uncommon. A more common sequence is for the repetitive overloading of running or a misstep while running to aggravate a pre-existing meniscal tear.

The symptoms and findings on physical examination of such a runner will not differ from other athletes with a meniscal tear. There is a history of an acute injury followed by pain. The runner may have felt something giving way within the knee, and swelling usually occurs within the first 12 hours following injury. If the patient's knee recovers from this first episode, then a history of repeated knee clicking or giving way followed by episodes of minor swelling begins. Physical signs usually include a small joint effusion, joint-line tenderness,

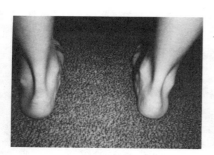

Figure 6-2. Bilateral pronated feet.

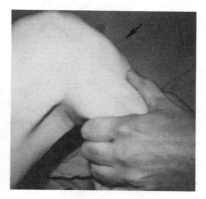

Figure 6-3. Arrow points to tibial tubercle pulled forward in positive anterior drawer sign.

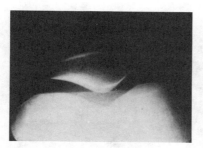

Figure 6-4. Normal Hughston view of the patella.

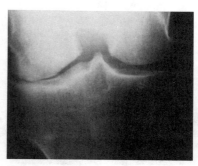

Figure 6-5. Degenerative joint disease on lateral side, secondary to early menisectomy.

localized pain occurring on full knee extension (with the examiner's thumb applying pressure on the affected joint-line), and a positive McMurray test. An arthrogram can be helpful in diagnosis, although we currently prefer arthroscopy. An arthrogram may give a false negative result in 15% of cases;[9] arthroscopy, in contrast, permits one to probe the meniscus to test its patency, as well as to evaluate the articular surfaces, and the anterior cruciate ligament.

If arthroscopy confirms a tear of the meniscus, the offending portion of the meniscus should be removed, unless meniscal repair is possible. All compartments of the knee joint must be examined arthroscopically, because there may be a relatively silent tear on the opposite portion of the joint that is a potential source of future trouble, with a more major tear on the symptomatic side. We believe that arthroscopic partial meniscectomy is the reasonable way to handle certain specific tears.

The postoperative rehabilitation, even if surgery is performed arthroscopically, is important. Many runners have tight hamstrings. While much attention is directed to strengthening the quadriceps muscle, work must also be done to stretch and strengthen the hamstring muscle. To send a runner out onto the road before he has completely rehabilitated the quadriceps and hamstring musculature is asking for recurrent difficulty in the ability of the functionally weakened quadriceps to adequately shock absorb and decelerate in the landing and stance phases of the gait cycle.

Old Trauma

Many runners are more likely to have trouble because of a previous sports injury (Figure 6-6) and resultant intra-articular pathology, rather than because of an acute running injury. Typical of these are people who have played other sports and have had a prior meniscectomy, osteochondritic defect, or ligamentous injury. While the past history is important, and the diagnosis frequently obvious, how well the runner will do depends upon the present integrity of the articular cartilage. With relatively intact articular cartilage, which sometimes can be determined only by arthroscopy, and with a willingness to work to strengthen the quadriceps and hamstring muscles, many patients are able to continue running despite previous knee injuries. They may have to decrease mileage or cut down on certain workouts, such as hill running or interval training. Many people who have had previous injuries, such as an anterior cruciate ligament tear with resultant laxity, are still able to run provided that they do not cut or run on uneven ground. With mild chronic rotary instability, an appropriate brace can be helpful.

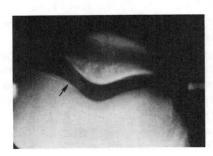

Figure 6-6. Arrow points to osteochondral fragment between patella and femur.

We do not believe it is reasonable to continue running and continuously suppress a synovitis with nonsteroidal anti-inflammatory medication. Short-term use of oral anti-inflammatory agents is excellent, but if the synovitis continues, either the offending pathology must be identified and rectified or the runner should pursue another sport.

Some patients with a history of an old injury and a synovitis produced by running will benefit from nonsteroidal agents, decreasing mileage, and strengthening the thigh musculature. If a runner has synovitis after relatively short runs, he may be unable to continue running and might be better advised to undertake sports such as cycling, swimming, or cross-country skiing. A stationary bike or sliding track (Nordic Track) are two excellent devices that are sparing of the knee and which can be used in all climates and all seasons.

A few patients with long-term symptoms and synovitis may have minor degenerative changes or meniscal tears that can be identified by arthroscopy. If these meniscal changes are minor, partial meniscectomy may cure the problem. We examine arthroscopically such patients who continue to have intermittent synovitis, in order to ascertain the status of the joint and to see whether anything operatively of a relatively minor nature would enable the patient to continue running. The "middle-aged athletic knee" may be helped by arthroscopic debridement and lavage, giving symptomatic relief for many months.

Loose Bodies

Loose bodies constitute an uncommon cause of knee pain in a runner. In most cases, the loose bodies or chondral-osteochondral fragments are the result of previous injury or are fragments of the articular surface of a knee from degenerative arthritis. The usual history is that of occasional catching or giving way of the knee joint. The athlete may state that he can feel something moving with the knee or even feel the loose body. Each episode of pain or transient locking is followed by a brief period of effusion and reduced activity, which gives the knee time to recover.

On physical examination, the examiner may or may not feel the loose body. Radiographs should include intercondylar ("tunnel") and patellar tangential projections. They may show an old osteochondritic defect or, in the younger person, a relatively new defect. Only if the loose body has an ossific portion will it be identified radiographically. With degenerative arthritis, the loose body may represent fragmentation of an osteophyte. If a loose body is suspected, arthroscopy is necessary both for visualization (especially if the loose body is cartilaginous) and for removal of the loose body. If a loose body is causing symptoms, it should be removed, because its continued presence would cause erosion of the articular surface in the future.

One other source of loose bodies is an osteochondral fracture from either the patella or the femur (Figure 6-7) as result of an acute or recurrent dislocation of the patella. The patient will usually be aware of what happened, but in some instances he does not realize the patella has dislocated. A bloody effusion and tenderness on the medial retinaculum of the patella will point to the diagnosis. A small osteochondral or chondral fragment may not be visible on radiographs because there is little bone attached to the articular cartilage. Once again, arthroscopy helps to locate the loose fragment or show the defect in the patellar or femoral articular surface, thereby altering the examiner of the loose fragment, in addition to allowing for removal of the fragment.

Popliteal (Baker's) Cyst

A popliteal cyst, despite its extra-articular location, usually is in continuity with the knee joint and usually occurs as a secondary process in response to an intra-articular problem. Frequently a torn meniscus causes a reactive synovitis and secondary effusion that distends the popliteal cyst. When a patient presents with a popliteal cyst, always look for intra-articular pathology. The cyst usually can be confirmed by either arthrography or ultrasonography.

We do not operate on a popliteal cyst itself, but rather direct our attention toward diagnosis and treatment of the offending intra-articular pathology that has the secondary popliteal cyst. The cyst will then usually receed spontaneously. If a large cyst starts to dissect into the soft tissues of the leg and is causing unremitting pain or swelling, the cyst may need to be removed. One must be careful to differentiate a hypertrophied popliteus muscle belly, which can be easily palpated in a thin runner, from a true popliteal cyst.

Overuse Synovitis

Some runners may have a chronic knee synovitis without apparent intra-articular pathology, and with no history suggesting possible injury, other than that of increased running. One must be certain that no intra-articular pathology is producing the synovitis. In such patients, we usually find a history of increased mileage or more vigorous workouts. In effect, the quadriceps is too weakened functionally at the increased distances to adequately shock absorb and decelerate in the landing phase of the gait cycle.

Nonsteroidal anti-inflammatory medication for several weeks, combined with decreased mileage and less strenuous workouts and ice pack applications to the knee after running, may decrease the synovitis. If the synovitis persists, the

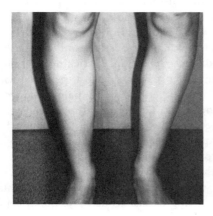

Figure 6-7. Miserable malalignment with tibia vara, pronated feet, and "squinting in" patellae.

runner should stop running until the knee remains free of any synovial effusion for several weeks. Resumption of running on a very graduated basis can then be tried.

Should intra-articular steroid injections be used? We dislike using them because of the deleterious effect on articular cartilage.[10] One must realize that intra-articular steroid causes breakdown of the ground substance and matrix of articular cartilage and thereby contributes to degeneration of the articular cartilage. With this in mind, however, it may still be reasonable on a rare occasion to try an intra-articular steroid injection for synovitis that is secondary to overuse and that has not responded to rest. The runner should not run for the next 14- 21 days, in order to allow both the synovium and the articular cartilage to recover. Running then should be reinstituted on a very graduated basis, in order to allow adequate time for quadriceps and hamstring strengthening.

Intra-Articular Plica

An intra-articular plica as a source of disabling knee pain in runners has become increasingly recognized and diagnosed in recent years, particularly with the advent of arthroscopy.[11] Increased interest in the structure, function, and pathomechanics of these synovial folds of the knee has occurred during this interval. Certain physicians seem to make this diagnosis much more frequently than do others, and in many instances the diagnosis of synovial plica as a common cause of knee pain in runners is over-emphasized.

At one time or another, these once obscure structures have been referred to as plicae, synovial folds, cords, shelves, bands, and alar folds. The plica represents either embryolgic remnants of the septum existing between the superior articular cavity and the suprapatellar bursa or incomplete involution of other embryonic septae. Modern nomenclature has delineated four primary synovial structures now designated as plicae; they are further designated according to their relationship to the patella. The major plicae are the suprapatellar plica, the medial plica, the infrapatellar plica, and the lateral plica. Although plicae were first described in 1918, Iino[12] in 1939 and Mizumachi[13] in 1948, both working in Japan and using early versions of an arthroscope, were the first to implicate the medial plica as a cause of "internal derangement" of the knee.

The medial plica is a fibrotic band originating from the superomedial aspect of the suprapatellar pouch adjacent to the medial pole of the patella and extending distalward to insert on the medial aspect of the infrapatellar fat pad. This tissue is present in most patients but is pathologic in only a few. If it becomes thickened, it can snap over the medial femoral condyle and cause local chondromalacic changes in some patients or cause sensations of clicking or giving way, suggestive of an meniscal tear, in other patients. Most patients will complain of a snapping sensation, whereas others describe pain produced particularly by running inclines or climbing stairs. Tenderness is found over the medial femoral condyle or medial aspect of the patella. Occasionally the examiner can palpate the fibrotic band snapping over the medial femoral condyle on knee motion when a valgus-external rotation stress is applied to the knee.

The diagnosis can be confirmed by arthroscopy, which may demonstrate the plica and identify chondromalacic changes of the femoral condyle. Some patients will respond to conservative measures, including decreased activity, quadriceps strengthening exercises, ice applications after running, and aspirin or anti-inflammatory medications. In others the plica must be resected arthroscopically, particularly if a dense band snapping over the medial femoral condyle has been identified.

From the number of patients whom we have seen who have had a plica previously treated arthroscopically but who continue to have knee pain, we believe the diagnosis of a pathologic synovial plica must be carefully studied before it can be described as a common cause of knee pain in runners.

Patella and Patellar Mechanism Problems

Knee problems were the most common cause of pain in runners in a runner's clinic conducted by James, and the most common causes of knee pain were conditions of the patellofemoral joint.[14] In this section we will attempt to categorize problems of the patella into subdivisions. However, some of these diagnostic entities blend into each other and may represent later stages of the same condition.

First, let us state that we have no idea what the term "runner's knee" precisely describes. To some physicians this means pain occurring on the lateral aspect of the patella. To others, it represents chondromalacia patella or perhaps a nonspecific tendinitis. To runners, it is any pain around the knee joint. In reality it is a meaningless "catch-all" term. As in any other area, physicians dealing with runners should make an accurate diagnosis of the cause of knee pain, thereby enabling more rational treatment.

Lateral Patellar Compression Syndrome

The lateral patellar compression syndrome is characterized by pain on the lateral aspect of the knee along the patellofemoral joint.[15,16] Increased mileage, hard running surfaces, interval workouts, and running hills all may contribute to the problem. Runners describe the pain as being deep and aching, relieved only by rest or reduction in their workouts. Sometimes the runners feel uncomfortable when sitting for a long time, particularly with their knee in flexion, or state that their knees feel tight or creaky as they move about afterwards.

On physical examination, there is no effusion. There may be mild patellofemoral crepitus on resisted extension, and compression of the patella against the underlying lateral femoral condyle may elicit pain. The Q angle is usually normal, with little tendency to lateral subluxation of the patella. If the patella is examined arthroscopically, the articular surface looks normal.

Perhaps the lateral compression syndrome is a precursor of chondromalacia. Perhaps it is not. This pain on the lateral aspect of the knee may be caused by static deformities, such as foot pronation or tibial varum, which causes pressure of the lateral facet of the patella. Some patients have the miserable malalignment syndrome (Figure 6-8) described by James et al[14] and by Kennedy,[15] which includes internal rotation of the hips or femoral anteversion, medial squinting of the patella, varus alignment of the knee or of the tibia, external tibial torsion, and excessive forefoot pronation, all of which cause altered patellofemoral mechanics.

We direct treatment toward proper alignment of the whole lower extremity and a careful review of the runner's training program. During the painful phase, we ask runners to decrease their mileage, run on controlled surfaces, stay off hills, and stop interval workouts. At this time, we try to correct any static foot or lower extremity deformities. For a pronated forefoot, an orthotic to control heel strike in the stance phase of the gait cycle may help. Many of these runners have tight Achilles tendons, and stretching of the gastrocnemius-soleus muscle Achilles tendon complex is mandatory. We demand that the patient strengthen the quadriceps musculature, initially with isometric resistance exercises. After several weeks of these exercises, he progresses to terminal extension isotonic quadriceps strengthening exercises, working from 20° of knee flexion to full extension. In general, runners start with low weights and a high number of repetitions and gradually increase in weight resistance. Adolescent runners may be helped with a patella-stabilizing device. Aspirin is the usual medication we recommend, although nonsteroidal anti-inflammatory agents may be tried. Intra-articular steroid injections should not be used, for reasons outlined in the section on Overuse Synovitis.

Lateral retinacular release may be required for intractable cases of lateral patellar compression syndrome,[16] particularly if lateral tilt of the patella has been demonstrated on patellar tangential projection radiographs. Here, one eliminates the offending retinaculum causing abnormal compression of the lateral facet of the patella.

Chondromalacia Patella

Chondromalacia patella signifies physical damage to the articular surface of the patella (Figure 6-9), and possibly similar damage to the opposing surface of the femoral condyle. It is a common cause of knee pain in runners, and the physical complaints are similar to those of the lateral patellar compression syndrome. With chondromalacia patella, the pain is usually more severe and of longer duration. The runner will frequently complain of a noisy knee, particularly while descending stairs. In many instances, the runner is able to localize the

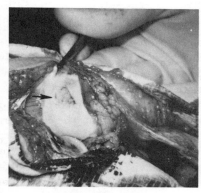

Figure 6-8. Arrow points to severe chondromalacic changes on patella.

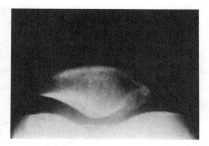

Figure 6-9. Damage to medial facet of patella secondary to dislocation.

pain and crunching sensation to a particular arc of the full range of knee motion. Hill running, especially down hill, increases the pain, and increased mileage may cause swelling of the knee joint as well.

On physical examination, there is audible and palpable patellofemoral crepitation as the knee moves from flexion to extension on resisted extension. The examiner will find tenderness on the undersurface of the patella either medially (Figure 6-10) or laterally, and compressing the patella against the femur causes intense pain. We produce patellofemoral compression by having the knee flexed 20°, stabilizing the patella with the hand. The patient then attempts to extend the knee, which causes intense pain if he has chondromalacia. An effusion indicates synovial irritation and probably severe chondromalacic changes. Some patients will have an increased Q angle (Figure 6-11) and lateral subluxation of the patella. Some will have the same lower extremity findings seen in the lateral compression syndrome, such as excessive foot pronation, tibia varum, external tibial torsion, and femoral anteversion. However, many runners with patellofemoral complaints will have none of these findings.

Treatment of chondromalacia patella is similar to that for lateral patellar compression syndrome, except that it may take longer for successful results, and some patients may not respond to conservative measures. We ask the runners to decrease their mileage, stay off hills, and stop interval workouts. We ask if they have been running on a particular surface that seems to bother them. Sometimes running on a particular track or a pitched road will put stress on one leg and force the foot into pronation or the knee into valgus, which would cause lateral

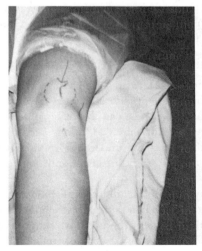

Figure 6-10. Increased Q angle in patellar subluxer.

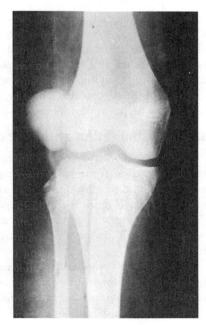

Figure 6-11. Acute patellar dislocation.

tracking of the patella. Static defects of the lower extremity must be corrected. Not all patients with chondromalacia patella need orthotics, but some do and they respond well to them.

Treatment is directed to increasing quadriceps strength and stretching the hamstring muscles. This includes isometric and terminal extension isotonic quadriceps ("short-arc quads") progressive resistance exercises, coupled with an active hamstring stretching program. If the patient has an effusion, we stop his running completely and put him on a regimen of progressive resistance exercises and anti-inflammatory medications or aspirin. During this period, we ask him to keep his cardiorespiratory system in tone by swimming or biking. Cycling allows for lower extremity strengthening in a manner simulating that of running, with the exception that shock absorption in the landing or deceleration phase of the gait cycle is avoided. Cycling, however, does bother some patients with advanced chondromalacia. Once the symptoms and effusion have resolved, the runner may resume running, but the terminal extension isotonic quadriceps strengthening exercise program must be continued.

In those patients with a loose patella, a stabilization device of the patella helps. These devices are commercially available, or they can be readily fabricated by cutting out a horseshoe-shaped piece of felt that is held in position with an elastic wrap or Neoprene knee sleeve. Other devices, such as the patellar alignment control braces devised by Marshall and Palumbo, can be equally helpful. Evaluation and treatment of more significant patellar laxity is described in the subsequent section.

If the runner, after following the conservative measures outlines above, continues to have pain with running, arthroscopy is advised. This procedure gives the physician precise knowledge of the amount and location of damage to the articular surface of the patella, and he can observe any abnormal tracking of the patella on knee motion. With significant damage and pain, surgical realignment of the patella is indicated. A variety of procedures - such as lateral retinacular release and arthroscopic abrasion chondroplasty or shaving, lateral retinacular release alone, soft tissue or bony extensor realignment procedures, and even the tibial tubercle anterior transposition osteotomy of Maquet and Ficat[18]- may help some runners return to their sport.

Patellar Subluxation and Dislocation

Some patients with chondromalacia patella have recurrent patellar subluxation or dislocation. If the runner's complaint is less of pain and more of sudden knee collapse and physical findings show that the patella can be easily subluxed, diagnosis is easy (Figure 6-12). Such patients usually have a Q angle exceeding 20°, valgus alignment of the knee or tibia, and an underdeveloped vastus medialis portion of the quadriceps muscle, as well as findings of chondromalacia patella.

In those patients who have recurrent patellar subluxation or dislocations and major physical findings but who want to continue to run, a trial to strengthen the quadriceps musculature should be undertaken. One of the patellar realignment braces may help in the milder cases. If little or no progress has been made after two months of such a therapeutic trial, particularly in those with poor development of the vastus medialis or in those in whom the vastus medialis ends too proximal to the patella, a realignment procedure of the extensor mechanism should be undertaken.[6,17] A variety of procedures has been described. One must decide initially whether alignment from above or below (ie, proximal or distal to the patella) is required; then one must decide whether soft tissue or osseous realignment, or a combination of both, is required. In those patients having a Q angle less than 20° and no significant valgus of the lower extremity, we perform a release of the lateral patellar retinaculum combined with vastus medialis advancement and imbrication of the medial patellar retinaculum and capsule. If the Q angle is greater than 20° or if there is significant valgus alignment of the knee or lower extremity, we perform either a Trillat medial transposition of the tibial tubercle or a medial transfer of the medial half of the patellar tendon combined with vastus medialis advancement and medial capsular imbrication, as well as lateral retinacular release (Figure 6-13). (Note the apparent discrepancy in functional application of the Q angle: all procedures are designed to correct an excessive Q angle, and yet they further increase the Q angle). The vastus medialis must then be strengthened after all surgical procedures. Fortunately, not all patients subjected to this extensive reconstructive surgery will be able to return to running. Some patients may find they are better off pursuing another sport.

Patellofemoral Arthrosis/Arthritis

In those few patients who have severe patellofemoral arthrosis or arthritis and who cannot be helped by other therapeutic modalities or procedures, osteotomy and anterior transposition of the tibial tuberosity described by Maquet[18] may be beneficial (Figure 6-14). This procedure should be reserved for those patients who do not respond to conservative measures or to other operative procedures. It is unrealistic to tell any runner with severe patellofemoral arthrosis that any surgical procedure can allow him to resume running, but the Maquet procedure offers at least that possibility.

Quadriceps Tendinitis/Tendon Rupture

The quadriceps muscle itself is not a common source of disabling pain, other than when it is directly contused. Some new joggers may start out more strongly

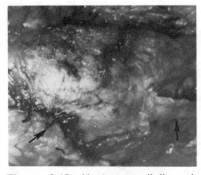

Figure 6-12. Vastus medialis advancement (top arrow) and medial placement (distal arrow) of part of patellar ligament.

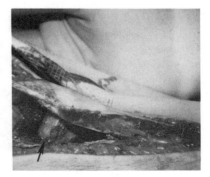

Figure 6-13. Bone graft (arrow) in Maquet tibial tuberosity advancement.

than they should, and muscles will ache afterwards for the first several days. This aching usually passes quickly, once the muscles accommodate to the increased activity.

More common than quadriceps muscle pain is chronic pain from quadriceps tendinitis. The quadriceps tendon has a broad insertion into the upper pole of the patella, and this broad insertion of the quadriceps tendon functions to dissipate the quadriceps muscle power. This area is not inclined to break down as quickly as is the patellar tendon, where it originates from the lower pole of the patella. Quadriceps tendinitis is characterized by pain in the upper pole of the patella, usually more along the lateral aspect of the superior pole than along the medial aspect. Quadriceps tendinitis is increased by more mileage and particularly by running hills.

Most runners can decrease symptoms by lowering their mileage or changing their running course, as well as ice applications to the area after running. If the symptoms are severe, aspirin or nonsteroidal anti-inflammatory agents can be helpful. We have usually found that aspirin and ice applications are enough to control pain. Quadriceps strength must be maintained, and isometric progressive resistance strengthening exercises are mandatory. Pain does not seem to increase if weight resistance is applied with the knee in full extension. We ask runners to increase endurance by increasing repetitions of low weights rather than increasing to high weights. Isokinetic eccentric quadriceps strengthening exercises may be helpful in patients with quadriceps tendinitis.[19] It is also important to be sure that the runners routinely perform their stretching exercises, which include stretching of both the hamstring and the quadriceps

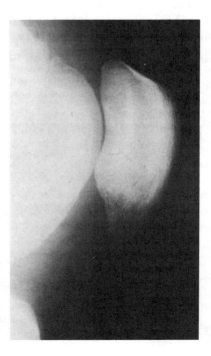

Figure 6-14. Distal patella elongation in patellar tendinitis.

muscle both before and after running. Local steroid injection into the area of tenderness is seldom needed, and it carries the inherent long term risk of destruction of tendon ground substance and matrix.

Ruptures of the quadriceps muscle or tendon are uncommon except in more violent physical activity, such as football, basketball, or pole vaulting, with their inherent greater forceful overloading of the quadriceps mechanism. Quadriceps rupture can occur if a runner going down hill misstepped and regained his balance with sudden violent contracture of the quadriceps. Following this catastrophic event, he either would be unable to extend the knee or would have extreme pain and weakness on attempted knee extension. Localized tenderness and a palpable defect within the quadriceps tendon at its attachment to the superior pole of the patella would be noted. Because this defect may fill shortly with organizing hematoma, the presence of local tenderness is a distinct diagnostic help. Quadriceps rupture can be treated nonoperatively if the defect is minor; operative repair is required if the defect is significant.

Patellar Tendinitis

"Jumper's knee" is the term for the condition characterized by tenderness at the patellar tendon (or patellar ligament, as some anatomists prefer) originating from the lower pole of the patella.[21] It is particularly common in basketball players and certain track athletes, such as high jumpers and hurdlers, but less common in distance runners. The condition results from chronic repetitive stress on the patellar tendon, particularly the sudden impact overloading associated with jumping. Pain is felt below the patella; usually the patient can localize it to the origin of the patellar tendon at the lower pole of the patella. Soft tissue swelling is evident. The pain increases with physical activity and decreases with rest. Many runners have a long history of difficulty, extending over several years (Figure 6-15). Conservative measures include a slow warm-up and ice application after activity. We frequently prescribe oral anti-inflammatory agents, starting with aspirin and progressing to NSAIDs, if the aspirin is ineffective. Sometimes a Neoprene knee sleeve with a patellar opening will help, acting as a counter-force brace. Rest frequently improves the condition, but a return to activity may be accompanied by a recurrence of pain. In our experience, conservative measures have not always worked and some people continue to have pain when they run or jump. It is particularly difficult to treat high-jumpers and hurdlers, because of the force generated by the take-off and landing. Putting an athlete into a cast will cause significant quadriceps atrophy, but we have sometimes used a knee immobilizer for a short interval to decrease pain while the anti-inflammatory agents are being used. The quadriceps must be kept strong, and isometric quadriceps strengthening exercises are necessary. Eccentric resistance quadriceps strengthening exercises also have helped some patients with patellar tendinitis.

On rare occasions we have given a one-time injection of a steroid preparation into the locally tender area, just superficial to the tendon itself. The more acute the tenderness, the more likely the steroid injection will help. Following the injection, the athlete must be restricted from running for a minimum of two weeks. The steroid injection leads to the destruction of the ground substance of the tendon, ultimately weakening the tendon, for which restricted activity is required during the healing phase. Rarely, a patient is unable to continue running and surgery may be needed. An incision is made directly over the tender area and the patellar tendon split longitudinally. There is usually an area of mucinoid degeneration, which may be only a few millimeters in diameter, which must be resected. The base of the patella also is curetted, in an attempt to stimulate vascularization and thereby promote healing of the tendon, and the tendon is reattached to the patella. Do not hasten the athlete's return to action too quickly following surgery. It takes three months before everything heals to allow the athlete a return to normal activity.

Osgood-Schlatter's Disease and Residuals

Osgood-Schlatter's disease as an active process is an osteochondrosis or traction apophysitis confined to young athletes or adolescents, some of whom are runners. Pain presents at the attachment of the patellar tendon to the tibial tuberosity, and the condition is due to chronic stress caused by the quadriceps mechanism. In later years, once the tibial tuberosity apophysitis has fused, one may be left with the residuals of the active adolescent condition - a prominent tibial tuberosity, pain while running or climbing, and a loose ossicle within the patellar tendon - of an earlier neglected case of Osgood-Schlatter's disease.

Osgood-Schlatter's disease is characterized by the prominence and tenderness of the tibial tuberosity, as well as inflammation of the overlying soft tissues. It represents a traction apophysitis of the tuberosity, and the base should be placed at complete rest to prevent the permanent changes previously mentioned. This

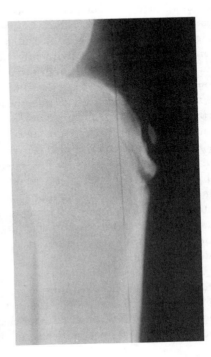

Figure 6-15. Osgood-Schlatter disease with loose ossicle.

frequently requires immobilization and a long leg cyclinder cast for six weeks, so that normal apophyseal remodeling can be restored.

One occasionally sees an older patient with a prominent tibial tuberosity as the residual of Osgood-Schlatter's disease at an earlier age. There may be tenderness at the patellar tendon attachment. At this point, it should be called patellar tendinitis or Osgood-Schlatter's residuals, rather than Osgood- Schlatter's disease. We find it useful to explain to the person what the bump represents. In most instances, conservative measures, such as decreased running and application of ice packs, are enough to allow people to continue sports. If the small bursa deep to the distal patellar tendon is inflamed, a steroid injection can help. In this instance, we inject deep to the patellar tendon just proximal to its insertion into bone rather than into the patellar tendon itself.

If in adult years a loose ossicle is present in the patellar tendon as a residual of earlier Osgood-Schlatter's disease, it can cause pain as the ossicle impacts against the underlying tibial cortex with running, climbing, or kneeling. Surgical removal of the ossicle provides immediate and gratifying relief of the pain.

Ligament Injuries

Sprains or major tears of the ligaments of the knee, such as the medial and lateral collateral and anterior and posterior cruciate ligaments, are uncommon in runners. If, however, the runner slips or has a misstep and puts appropriate stress on the knee, sprains or tears may occur. This type of stress might happen in crosscountry events where the runners are often on uneven surfaces. A runner could land awkwardly on his leg and apply a valgus stress to his knee, causing pain and soft tissue swelling around the medial collateral ligament. In such an instance, the knee would almost always be stable. We treat this type of sprain with a commercially available knee immobilizer for 14 to 21 days; we use removable immobilizers, rather than casts, when the ligament is intact.

Another rare ligamentous injury for a runner occurs if he lands on the extended knee and feels a popping sensation. If this is followed by an effusion (or hemarthrosis), a tear of the anterior cruciate ligament is likely. Aspiration of the knee would reveal gross blood. A careful physical examination may show a positive Lachman test even with a negative anterior drawer sign. A hemarthrosis of the knee is a frequent sign of an anterior cruciate ligament tear and warrants careful follow-up. Arthroscopy and stress examination under anesthesia is the logical next step. Arthroscopic examination should be directed to both the cruciate ligaments and the posterior corners of the menisci to see whether there is a peripheral tear. Although it depends on the surgeon's experience and his philosophy, in most instances we perform a primary augmented repair or reconstruction of an acute tear of the anterior cruciate ligament in a young athlete.

Prior ligament injuries may play a major role for runners when the athlete turns to running as his new sport. Many people with previous ligament injuries are able to run without significant difficulty as long as there is no articular cartilage damage. Running straight ahead is not difficult, but when one starts to pivot or cut, the knee ligament instability syndromes are a problem. In some patients with old ligamentous injuries causing instability, the increased activity causes synovitis. We must be careful to see whether the patient is injuring himself by continuing to run. Major muscle rehabilitation programs of both the quadriceps and hamstrings may allow such a person to run. In other instances, an appropriate brace may help. Some people with instability and articular cartilage damage may be better off undergoing ligament reconstruction or not running at all.

Bursitis/Tendinitis

Running frequently produces inflammatory changes in the tendons about the knee, other than those involving the quadriceps-patellar mechanism. The repetitive motion of running also leads to the development of friction syndromes or inflammation of bursae.

Prepatellar Bursitis

Prepatellar bursitis, while uncommon in runners, is occasionally seen. The runner feels pain in the soft tissues overlying the superficial surface of the patella. It may be induced by chronic stress, such as kneeling in a tile installer, or occasionally from a blow to the knee. Prepatellar bursitis must be differentiated from both patellar and quadriceps tendinitis, as well as from patellofemoral arthritis. The soft-tissue swelling in the prepatellar area is confined to a distinct bursa, and there may be fluid within the bursa.

Application of ice packs several times a day, combined with compression, may be enough to control symptoms. If the bursa is enlarged, we sometimes aspirate the bursa and advise rest and compression while the inflammatory process resolves. If this is not enough, a steroid injection into the bursa may help. On rare occasions, excision of the bursa is needed.

Iliotibial Band Friction Syndrome

The iliotibial tract or band is an important lateral stabilizer of the knee and very important in running. Before and during foot strike, it helps to externally rotate the leg and stabilize it during the early phase of foot strike. As the knee moves from flexion to extension and back, the iliotibial tract passes from behind the lateral femoral epicondyle to in front of it; repeated excursion may cause irritation of the iliotibial tract[22] against the lateral epicondyle and inflame the areolar tissue in this area (Figure 6-16). Characteristically, this is seen in long-distance runners and is particularly painful when running downhill. Keeping the knee relatively straight while walking usually relieves the pain. The condition also is seen when there is a varus deformity of the knee, which thrusts the iliotibial band against the lateral femoral epicondyle, or from running on pitched surfaces, such as a road with a significant side slope.

On physical examination, the only positive finding is local tenderness at the lateral epicondyle where the iliotibial band crosses. Pain is maximal at 30° of flexion, as the iliotibial band goes over the lateral epicondyle, especially when a varus stress is applied to the knee. There may also be some swelling and occasional soft-tissue thickening in this area.

Initial treatment is directed toward decreasing mileage, improving foot strike, and protecting against any excessive wear on the lateral aspect of the heel that might tend to cause foot pronation or knee varus. Decreased mileage, application of ice packs after activity, and oral anti-inflammatory agents will help a number of patients. Some, however, will need a steroid injection into the locally tender area, followed by two weeks of rest. The steroid is injected into the areolar tissue just under the iliotibial tract. Noble[23] has reported doing a surgical partial release of the iliotibial band in a few recalcitrant cases.

Pes Anserinus Bursitis

One interesting condition occurring primarily in runners is characterized by pain on the medial aspect of the knee below the joint line in the area of the pes anserinus bursa (Figure 6-17). In all runners, the hamstring muscles are constantly acting during deceleration and knee flexions, which is controlled by the hamstrings. The medial hamstrings act as knee flexors and internal rotators of the tibia, and must act to counterbalance the external rotation and pronation of the foot, which occurs after heel strike during running. The large pes bursa is located between the medial collateral ligament and the three tendons (forming a duck's foot) overlying the ligament as they cross to attach to the medial aspect of

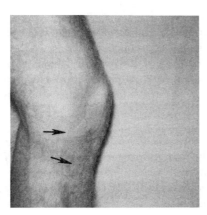

Figure 6-16. The painful area (x) in illiotibial tract syndrome.

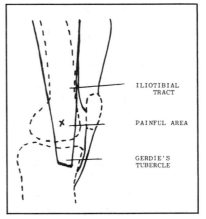

Figure 6-17. Physical examination shows local tenderness within the pes anserinus bursa, together with soft tissue swelling and even local crepitus. If the examination is done with the knee extended, the pain may appear to be near the joint line, but if the knee is flexed the tenderness will be detected within the pes anserinus bursa, a fact which easily distinguishes it from a tear of the medial meniscus.

the tibia. Characteristically, pain occurs in both distance runners and intermediate sprinters, with less trouble for people who run dashes.

Treatment is directed toward decreasing the inflammatory response. If there are static foot abnormalities, shoe orthotics may help in trying to decrease the tendency towards external rotation or pronation of the foot. As with so many knee conditions, decreasing mileage, limiting interval workouts, and applying ice after running is helpful. Some runners have found that wrapping the upper leg with an elastic bandage or Neoprene sleeve is helpful. Oral anti-inflammatory agents are especially effective. If pain persists and the runner is unable to continue, we believe that a local injection of a steroid will not harm the runner. After receiving the injection, the runner should rest for at least 14 days.

Pes anserinus bursitis is a condition seen particularly in runners on indoor tracks with tight or heavily banked corners. As they round the curve, they must drive off hard on the outside foot, causing a tendency for the muscles on the inner aspect of the leg to contract tightly. It is difficult to have runners reverse their direction on the track during workouts, but occasionally that maneuver will help.

Popliteus Tendinitis

Mayfield[24] describes this syndrome - characterized by pain on the lateral aspect of the knee just above the joint line and anterior to the lateral collateral ligament - caused by popliteus tendon tenosynovitis. The pain is aggravated by weight bearing, is felt particularly when the knee is flexed from 15° to 30°, and is increased with downhill running. Because of the intra-articular position of the popliteus tendon, this pain penetrates more deeply than does the pain in some other syndromes.

Tenderness is felt just anterior to the lateral collateral ligament, just above the joint line. We test for popliteus pain by flexing the affected knee to 90° and putting the lateral malleolus of the affected leg on the opposite knee. This position produces stress on the popliteus tendon, and palpation produces pain. Occasionally, one sees small radiodensities in the area of the popliteus tendon, but this is uncommon.

The general management of this condition includes proper foot positioning by whatever means needed, and decreasing activity. Oral anti-inflammatory agents and ice application after running are usually enough to handle the condition. If the pain persists, the condition may be confused with a peripheral tear of the lateral meniscus, and arthroscopy is indicated. If arthroscopy reveals no meniscal tear and inflammation around the popliteus tendon, a local injection of steroid into that area helps. The runner then has to rest for at least two weeks. Conservative measures usually suffice.

Medial Collateral Bursitis

Brantigan and Voshell[25] described the "no name, no fame bursa," located between the superficial and deep portions of the medial collateral ligament at the medial joint line (Figure 6-18). Occasionally, runners have pain in this area that may be difficult to distinguish from the pain of peripheral meniscal tear or even of inflammation of the pes anserinus bursa. With inflammation of Voshell's bursa, the runner may have pain even when sitting, particularly if he is in cramped quarters and is forced to keep his knees at 80° to 100° of flexion. There should be no effusion, and tenderness is localized to the area along the superficial portion of the medial collateral ligament just below the joint line.

Occasionally, injecting a small amount of local anesthetic in the interval between the two portions of the medial collateral ligament, being careful not to put it into the joint, will cause the pain to disappear, and thus confirm the diagnosis.

The hallmarks of treatment are rest and oral anti-inflammatory agents, plus ice applications after running. If the pain does not disappear after a suitable period, a local injection of steroid into the area may rapidly relieve symptoms, but the runner should not run for 14 days, to allow for the full effect of the steroid and repair of the damaged tissues.

Stress Fracture of the Proximal Tibia

Although stress fractures are common in runners, such fractures are not common at the knee level, although they have been described in both the medial aspect of the proximal tibia[26] and the medial tibial plateau.[27] With a stress fracture in this location, the runner complains of localized pain increased by running and relieved by rest. Ordinary walking is not painful. The diagnosis may be difficult because of the other anatomic entities within the area, such as the pes anserinus bursa with the proximal tibial stress fracture and intra-articular pathology with the tibial plateau stress fracture, which may confuse the issue.

Findings on a early radiograph may be negative, but radiographs repeated 4-6 weeks after the onset of pain should show some condensation of the trabecular bone or periosteal new bone formation, confirming a stress fracture. If the history and physical examination are suggestive of a stress fracture but radiographs remain negative, diagnosis can be confirmed by a bone scan; this should show the very localized "hot spot" from the increased radionuclide uptake, and confirm the diagnosis.

The only treatment for stress fractures is rest. It is our practice to tell the runners to stay off the road completely until localized tenderness has resolved and repeat radiographs have shown maturation of the repair process. If they resume running before the localized tenderness disappears, the pain recurs and symptoms are prolonged over a longer interval.

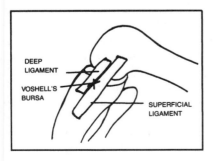

Figure 16-8. The Voshell's bursa (x) between deep and superficial medial collateral ligament.

Hamstring Injuries

Injuries to the hamstring muscles and tendons are common in a variety of running sports. The most common injury is a strain, which occurs in the muscle belly substance or at the muscle-tendon junction. Total rupture of a hamstring muscle or tendon is unusual but is occasionally seen in sprinters or hurdlers. More commonly seen is a partial tear of the muscles. After an acute episode, there is localized swelling with deep hemorrhage, plus pain with palpation or any attempted stretching of the hamstrings. Full extension of the knee or a long stride causes pain within the hamstrings.

The acute treatment should be directed at complete rest plus applying ice packs to the affected area. After the acute pain has resolved, we start the patients on a regimen of hamstring stretching exercises, keeping their exercises within the limits of pain tolerance. An anti-inflammatory agent should be helpful in relieving some pain and spasm, and we have found that the combination of ice application and gentle stretching is the most efficacious method. As the pain and spasm recede, runners begin to stretch more fully and finally progress to a full series of stretching exercises. Early in their rehabilitation they start light progressive resistance strengthening exercises of the hamstrings, and gradually progress with the strengthening program.

The major problem with runners having hamstring pulls is that they return to action too quickly, making them subject to recurrent injuries. We keep them out of training until the hamstring tenderness has completely resolved and they are able to stretch the hamstrings as well or better than they could before injury. They also must have full strength of their hamstrings. The runner and his coach may have to recognize that missing part or all of a season is necessary to prevent the runner from sustaining permanent damage. Once the injury has healed, the runner must be assiduous in stretching his hamstring muscles to prevent a recurrent tear. It is important for both the quadriceps and the hamstring muscles to be strengthened, so that there is no imbalance of the muscle-tendon units about the knee.

REFERENCE

1. Apple DF: Knee pain in runners. South Med J 72:1377- 1379, 1979.
2. Brubacker CE, Jones SL: Injuries to runners. Am J Sports Med 2:189-198, 1974.
3. Baugher WH, Balady GJ, Warren RF, Marshall JL: Injuries of the musculoskeletal system in runners. Contemp Orthop 1:45-54, 1979.
4. Buchbinder MR, Napora NJ, Biggs EW: The relationship of abnormal pronation to chondromalacia of the patella in distance runners. J Am Podiatry Assoc 69:159-162, 1979.
5. Ellison AE: Skiing injuries. Clin Symposia 29:18- 37, 1977.
6. Hughston JC: Subluxation of the patella. J Bone Joint Surg 50A:1003-1026, 1968.
7. Labelle H, Laurin CA: Radiological investigation of normal and abnormal patellae. J Bone Joint Surg 57B:530, 1975.

8. Merchant AC, Mercer RL, Jacobson RH, Cool CR: Roentgenographic analysis of patellofemoral congruence. J Bone Joint Surg 56A:1391-1396, 1974.

9. DeHaven KE, Collins HR: Diagnosis of internal derangements of the knee; the role of arthroscopy. J Bone Joint Surg 57A:802-810, 1975.

10. Gray RG, Gottlieb NL: Intra-articular corticosteroids: An updated assessment. Clin Orthop 177:235-263, 1983.

11. Broukhim B, Fox JM, Blazina ME, DelPizzo W, Hirsh, L: The synovial shelf syndrome. Clin Orthop 142:135-138, 1979.

12. Iino S: Normal arthroscopic findings in the knee joint in adult cadavers. J Japan Orthop Assoc 14:467, 1939.

13. Mizumachi S, Kawashima W, Okamura T: So-called synovial shelf in the knee joint. J Japan Orthop Assoc 22:1, 1948.

14. James SL, Bates BT, Ostering LR: Injuries to runners. Amer J Sports Med 6:40-50, 1978.

15. Kennedy JC: The Injured Adolescent Knee. Baltimore, Williams & Wilkins, 1979.

16. Larson RL, Cabaud HE, Slocum DB, James SL, Keenan T, Hutchinson T: The patellar compression syndrome: surgical treatment by lateral retinacular release. Clin Orthop 134:158- 167, 1978.

17. Slocum DB, James SL, Larson RL: Surgical treatment of the dislocating patella in athletes. Presented at the Annual Meeting of the American Orthopedic Association, Hot Springs, VA, 1973.

18. Maquet P: Mechanics and osteoarthritis of the patellofemoral joint. Clin Orthop 144:70-73, 1979.

19. Curwin S, Stanish WD: Tendinitis: Its etiology and treatment. Chapter 5: Jumper's Knee, p 99-113. Lexington, MA, Collamore, 1984.

20. Kaufer H: Mechanical function of the patella. J Bone Joint Surg 53A:1551-1560, 1971.

21. Blazina ME, Kerlan RK, Jobe FW, Carter VS, Carlson GJ: Jumper's knee. Orthop Clin No Am 4:665-678, 1973.

22. Renne JW: The iliotibial band friction syndrome. J Bone Joint Surg 57A:1110-1111, 1975.

23. Noble CA: Iliotibial band friction syndrome in runners. Am J Sports Med 8:232-234, 1980.

24. Mayfield GW: Popliteus tendon tenosynovitis. Am J Sports Med 5:31-36, 1977.

25. Brantigan OC, Voshell AF: The mechanics of the ligaments and menisci of the knee joint. J Bone Joint Surg 23:44- 66, 1941.

26. Colt EWD, Spyropoulos E: Running and stress fractures. Br Med J 2(6192): 706, 1979.

27. Schmidt Brudvig TJ, Gudges TD, Obermeyer L: Stress fractures in 295 trainees: A one-year study of the incidence as related to age, sex, and race. Military Med 148:666-667, 1983.

CHAPTER 7

Tendinitis and Plantar Fasciitis in Runners

William J. Clancy, Jr., M.D.

Introduction

The term tendinitis appears to be confusing and perplexing. It is frequently used incorrectly to describe inflammatory reaction involving either the tendon and/or the tendon sheath. *Dorland's Medical Dictionary* defines tendinitis as an inflammation of the tendon, and tenosynovitis and tenovaginitis as an inflammation of the tendon sheath.[1] *Blakiston's New Gould Medical Dictionary* defines tendinitis as an inflammation of the tendon usually at the point of its attachment to bone, tenovaginitis as an inflammation of the tendon and its sheath, and tenosynovitis as inflammation of the sheath of a tendon.[2]

For the various injuries to the tendon and its surrounding tissue to be adequately diagnosed and treated, a consistent and accurate classification system based on documented pathologic findings is imperative. The literature is presently deficient on documentation of the various pathological entities. To date, Puddu's classification of tendon injuries appears the most complete.[3] Our operative and clinical findings, however, as well as those found in a review of the literature, suggest that a more detailed classification than that presented by Puddu, et al, should be developed.[3-12]

The classification system presented in this chapter is intended to be simplistic, functional, and to correspond to the pathologic findings noted by the author and those reported in the literature (Table 7-1).

Tenosynovitis and tenovaginitis refer to an inflammation involving the paratenon or tendon sheath without any involvement of the tendon itself. The primary causes are either from tissue friction or from an external mechanical irritation. We have seen several cases of pes tenosynovitis secondary to repetitive motion over an osteochondroma on the proximal tibia, Achilles tenovaginitis from an exostosis on the posterior tibia, and flexor hallucis tenosynovitis from an osteochondroma on the talus. All were relieved by excision of the bony prominence. External causes of tenosynovitis of the dorsum of the foot are not uncommon in runners and basketball players who tie their shoelaces too tightly, thus trapping the extensor sheaths. Achilles tenovaginitis is not infrequently seen when an inexperienced person mechanically crimps the Achilles tendon sheath while taping an ankle.

Friction between the tendon and tendon sheath and/or the tendon sheath and the surrounding tissue may lead to an inflammatory reaction within the tendon sheath and surrounding tissue. Snook[12] noted this entity at surgery in the Achilles tendon in several runners. If this inflammatory reaction becomes chronic, the secondary vascular changes in the paratenon could possibly lead to tendon degeneration, because the tendon receives its blood supply almost exclusively on a segmental basis through the mesotenon or vascular septa of the paratenon.[13-16]

Tendinitis in this classification refers to a primary injury or symptomatic degeneration within the tendon, or a combination of both with a secondary symptomatic inflammatory reaction occurring within the paratenon (R. Ljungqvist, personal communication). There are two potential causes. As is well documented, repeated loading of the musculotendinous unit leads to fatigue of the muscle, shortening, and decreased flexibility, which may result in increased loading of the tendon during the state of eccentric loading. For example, the gastro-soleus muscles in distance runners must undergo eccentric contraction to allow for heel strike. If this muscle group is tight from fatigue, then theoretically the Achilles tendon is subjected to increased loading. It is of interest that patients with acute and chronic Achilles tendinitis are more often symptomatic not on heel-off, but at heel strike, and the symptoms are diminished if they run with elastic tape extending from their heel to their calf.

Table 7-1
Classification of Tendon Injury

I. Tenosynovitis and tenovaginitis—an inflammation of only the paratenon, either lined by synovium or not.

II. Tendinitis—an injury or symptomatic degeneration of the tendon with a resultant inflammatory reaction of the surrounding paratenon.
  1. acute—symptoms present less than two weeks.
  2. subacute—symptoms present longer than two weeks but less than six weeks.
  3. chronic—symptoms present six weeks or longer.
    a. interstitial microscopic failure
    b. central necrosis
    c. frank partial rupture
    d. acute complete rupture

III. Tendinosis—asymptomatic tendon degeneration due to either aging, accumulated microtrauma, or both.
  1. interstitial   3. acute rupture
  2. partial rupture

The second cause is that of repetitive active loading of the musculotendinous unit, leading to collagen failure. This fatigue, or stress failure of the tendon, could be considered analogous to stress fractures of bones as seen in runners. Peacock,[14] and Peacock and Van Wenkle[17] showed that tenocytes are essentially end stage cells and that they are capable of only a limited repair potential. That fact may explain why many cases of chronic Achilles tendinitis treated adequately may still take up to six months of rest to become asymptomatic. Environmental factors as well as variations of normal anatomy leading to increased loading of the musculotendinous unit may predispose to the development of tendinitis.

Tendinitis can be classified as acute, subacute, and chronic. Acute tendinitis includes those in which the patient is symptomatic for less than two weeks; subacute cases include those in which the patient has had symptoms less than six weeks; and those in which the patient has had symptoms longer than six weeks would be termed chronic. The terminology is based both on the expected inflammatory response of tissue in general and on the expected clinical prognosis based on the length of symptoms.

The subclassification of chronic tendinitis is based on the changes found at surgery in 27 athletes with chronic tendinitis involving the Achilles tendon (21), the posterior tibial tendon (3), the anterior tibial tendon (1), and the peroneal tendons (2). The subclassifications are: 1. interstitial microscopic failures, 2. central necrosis, 3. partial rupture. Of those patients with interstitial failure, about one-third had a definite nodular deformity palpable on examination. The pathologic findings covered the gamut of collagen degeneration, including mucoid degeneration, splaying of fibers with acellularity, fibrocartilage metaplasia, calcification, and bone metaplasia (Figures 7-1 to 7-3).

Hypocellularity, acellularity and absence of inflammatory response were quite common in most cases. An inflammatory response was noted to be present

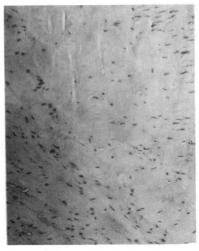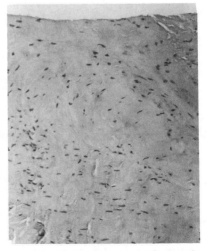

Figure 7-1 and 7-2. Photomicrograph of biopsies from two cases of chronic Achilles tendinitis, demonstrating areas of collagen degeneration containing splaying of fibers and loss of cellularity.

essentially in only those with a gross partial rupture. In two patients, central necrosis[6] was found in which the outer tendon appeared completely normal. In one patient a large partial rupture was found, and in the other there was complete disruption without any tissue filling the defect (Figures 7-4 and 7-5). The partial ruptures were obvious when the tendon sheath was incised (Figure 7-6).

Tendinosis, a term first described by Puddu, et al,[3] refers to degenerative lesions of tendon tissue without any alteration of the paratenon, and without clinical symptoms. This finding has been noted by many authors.[4,5,8] The changes may consist of either mucoid, fatty, hyaline, and/or fibrinoid degeneration, cartilage metaplasia, calcification, and bone metaplasia. These changes were initially noted when biopsies were taken of acute ruptures of the Achilles tendon in previously asymptomatic patients.[4,8] It is uncertain whether these changes were purely due to aging, accelerated aging, accumulated microtrauma, or a combination of these factors. With time and repetitive loading, these patients may develop clinical symptoms, and the condition would then be termed tendinitis. As previously noted, a number of patients with Achilles tendinosis may develop acute spontaneous subcutaneous ruptures of the Achilles tendon.

Treatment

In general, those patients with acute tenosynovitis and tenovaginitis respond readily within ten days to rest, local heat application or contrast baths, and oral

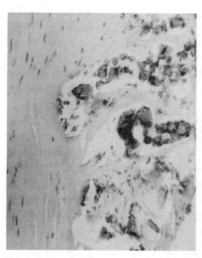

Figure 7-3. Photomicrograph of a biopsy of a case of chronic Achilles tendinitis showing calcific replacement of an area of collagen degeneration.

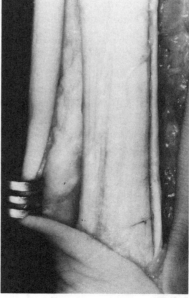

Figure 7-4. Apparently normal-appearing Achilles tendon in a patient with chronic Achilles tendinitis.

anti-inflammatory medication. One must look for internal or external mechanical causative factors. In those cases that have not resolved within a reasonable amount of time, the judicious use of a local steroid injection about the sheath, but not directly into the tendon, may be considered. One must be sure that the entity is definitely tenosynovitis and not a true tendinitis, because the risk of potential rupture from masking the symptoms of the underlying tendon problem or the direct effect of cortisone on diminishing the tensile strength of the tendon may lead to rupture.

Those with acute tendinitis usually will be totally asymptomatic within two weeks with a program of rest, localized heat application or contrast baths, and stretching. The role of oral anti-inflammatory agents has not been well documented in this entity. When the involved area is no longer tender to palpation, the athlete may resume his training program on a graduated basis. To prevent recurrence, one must try to evaluate any predisposing factors such as errors in the training program, any adverse environmental factors, and any significant variations of anatomy.

Subacute tendinitis, in which symptoms are present for up to six weeks, usually takes about six weeks to resolve on the above program. Patients recovering from subacute tendinitis should not return to training until the area is no longer tender to palpation.

Patients with chronic tendinitis, whose symptoms are present for six weeks or longer, will usually need at least six weeks and frequently much longer for their symptoms to abate so that they can resume training without recurrence. Those with obvious tendon deformity should still be treated conservatively for at least three to six months before surgery is recommended. Surgery is generally not

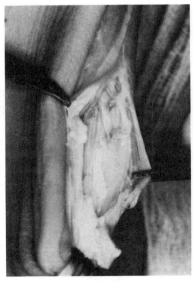

Figure 7-5. A longitudinal incision of an Achilles tendon in a patient with chronic Achilles tendinitis.

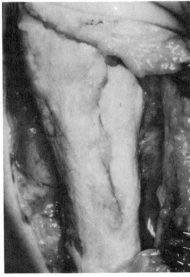

Figure 7-6. An obvious partial rupture of an Achilles tendon within which there is significant replacement.

recommended in those with chronic symptoms and without tendon deformity unless they are still symptomatic after six months of a good conservative program.

Surgery consists of incising the tendon sheath and examining the tendon by palpation. In the normal-appearing tendon, several longitudinal incisions are made into the tendon in the area of previously noted tenderness. If there are no gross pathologic changes, a biopsy is taken and the subcutaneous tissue and skin are closed over drains. The longitudinal incisions are used for a two-fold purpose: first, to see if there is any area of central necrosis or rupture; and second, to stimulate a healing reaction. If a significant area of degeneration is found, it is excised. If the defect is not too large, the tendon is closed. If the defect is significant, the plantaris tendon is resected as proximally as possible, and then interwoven through the defect (Figure 7-7). If an exceptionally large area of calcification is present or an area of multiple ruptures is found, as occasionally seen in the Achilles tendon, then the entire area of the tendon is resected, even if this procedure necessitates resecting a segment of tendon. A Bosworth turndown flap then is done (Figure 7-8).

Those who have had only an incision placed in the tendon, or had a small defect resected and closed, are placed in a short leg cast for two weeks. If the Achilles tendon was the site of surgery, the cast is maintained for three to four weeks to allow for healing of the poorly vascularized skin and subcutaneous tissue. Early controlled motion is the desired goal where possible.

Archilles tendinitis is by far the most common tendinitis seen. The athlete usually notes the onset of pain with crepitance just above the heel counter usually

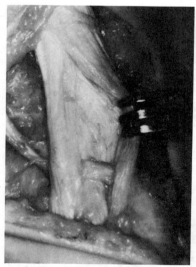

Figure 7-7. After the area of degeneration was resected, the plantaris was interwoven through the tear.

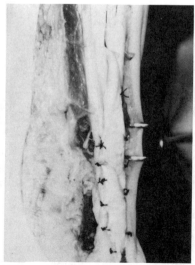

Figure 7-8. A Bosworth turndown procedure is used as replacement for a segmental resection of an area of complete degeneration in case of chronic Achilles tendinitis.

several hours after a run. The pain is usually most noticeable on climbing stairs and perhaps on normal walking for the first two to three days, then the symptoms are present only on running, usually just at heel strike. On examination, some crepitance may be present to active motion. Only one small painful area will be present to palpation, and it will be only the size of the breadth of the examining finger tips. It is usually about two or three centimeters above the superior lip of the calcaneus. Examination of the opposite normal Achilles will demonstrate a distinct difference in pain.

A thorough history should be taken to determine whether there has been any change in the surface or in training patterns that may be predisposed to the injury. The most common errors are a significant increase in mileage over a short time, a significant increase in an interval program, an increase in hill running, or a recent layoff from running with a too rapid return to the previous level of running. During the physical examination, one should look for predisposing factors that are highly associated with Achilles tendinitis, such as heel valgus, pronation, femoral anteversion, or a tight gastro-soleus muscle group.

Retrocalcaneal bursitis is frequently misdiagnosed as Achilles tendinitis or insertional tendinitis, a rare entity. Although the athlete may complain of pain at the insertion of the Achilles tendon into the calcaneus, carefully pressure on both sides of the calcaneus should reduplicate his symptoms. Local injection of steroid and xylocaine into this area between the upper one-third of the calcaneus and the Achilles tendon should temporarily alleviate all symptoms. It is important to note that the Achilles tendon inserts far inferiorly on the calcaneus. In general, a significant number of our patients with retrocalcaneal bursitis have a cavus foot deformity with or without an exostosis of the superior lip of the calcaneus. Repeated episodes of retrocalcaneal bursitis dictate an osteotomy of the superior lip, which has been performed in eight runners with excellent results. Posterior tibial tendinitis, like peroneal tendinitis, is fortunately only infrequently encountered in the runner. Those with posterior tibial will present with pain located at the posterior inferior edge of the medial malleolus. Occasionally, they may have some tenderness more proximally. This is often misdiagnosed as shin splints, but one should note that no muscle is attached to the posterior tibial tendon at this point.

Posterior tibial tendinitis is usually seen early in the beginning of a training program and is highly associated with running on asphalt or concrete surfaces. Foot pronation is the most common anatomic variation seen with this entity. Treatment is essentially the same as that for Achilles tendinitis. If symptoms have been present for four weeks, roentgenograms should be obtained to make sure it is not a stress fracture of the distal tibia or medial malleolus. If significant foot pronation is present, flexible foot orthotics with a medial heel wedge can be beneficial.

Peroneal tendinitis is even more uncommon than Achilles or posterior tibial tendinitis and is usually seen early in a training program. The area of maximum tenderness is generally just distal to the lateral malleolus but not as far as the base of the fifth metatarsal. If the symptoms are present just behind the lateral malleolus, one must be sure it is not a stress fracture of the distal fibula, which is one of the most common locations for stress fractures in a runner. The periosteal inflammatory reaction of a distal fibula stress fracture may cause an inflammatory reaction of the peroneal sheath. Roentgenograms at four weeks will document a stress fracture, if present. Treatment is essentially the same as that for Achilles and posterior tibial tendinitis.

In my opinion, the above tendinitises in most cases represent a primary injury to the tendon with a secondary inflammatory reaction of the paratenon, causing the symptoms of pain and crepitance. The use of steroids is rarely if ever indicated in these conditions, because it can mask the symptoms, directly decrease the tendon's tensile strength, and inhibit the tendon's healing response.

Extensor tenosynovitis, which presents as a swollen forefoot with crepitance on extension and flexion of the toes, represents a tenosynovitis of the extensor tendons usually secondary to tying the shoelaces too tightly. With localized heat or contrast baths, and oral anti-inflammatory agents, the symptoms should subside significantly within several days. A soft spongy pad, along with an application of vasoline to the forefoot, should enable the runner to resume running in a few days, even if some discomfort is still present.

It must be remembered that a stress fracture of one of the metatarsals can cause the same symptoms and edema of the dorsum of the foot. Careful palpation of each metatarsal shaft should render the correct diagnosis almost immediately, long before an x-ray would be positive — generally three to four weeks after onset of symptoms.

Plantar Fasciitis

Plantar fasciitis is a term used to describe a painful condition located about the posterior medial surface of the foot just distal to the attachment of the plantar fascia to the calcaneus. This extremely disabling entity is seen far more commonly in distance runners than sprinters or middle-distance runners.

Initially, the symptoms are of gradual onset, and of extremely low intensity. The athlete is usually able to carry on with his training program for several weeks to several months without alteration in intensity or distance. With time, though, the pain becomes more noticeable and the athlete is forced to change his gait pattern by keeping the foot in a rather supinated or inverted posture from foot strike through to toe off. That position appears to minimize the symptoms. The athlete may be able to continue his level of training for several more weeks or months before the pain becomes so severe that he can no longer train. The pain is generally most severe after running, and early in the morning after rising. It is not uncommon for the athlete to feel or complain of a nodularity in the proximal medial plantar fascia.

Physical examination will usually reveal that the maximal area of tenderness is located over the medial edge of the plantar fascia just distal to the insertion of the calcaneus. In some, the maximal area of tenderness may be present just at the plantar fascia insertion into the calcaneus. These patients almost always have pain to palpation of the posterior inferior origin of the abductor hallucis muscle, possibly, as has been theorized, as a result of the overuse of the abductor hallucis muscle in its role to aid in producing forefoot supination to decrease the loading on the plantar fascia.

I believe that plantar fasciitis is an inflammatory reaction that is the result of a fatigue failure in the plantar fascia, somewhat analogous to the pathological concept of chronic tendinitis. This belief is based on the results of tissue biopsies in over 30 cases of chronic plantar fasciitis in runners who were surgically treated.[18] All specimens demonstrated the typical findings of collagen degeneration, as previously described.

This injury must be differentiated from the more common nerve entrapment syndromes. The nerve entrapment syndromes to be considered are entrapment of the medial and lateral plantar nerves (tarsal tunnel syndrome), entrapment of the calcaneal nerve and entrapment of the nerve to the abductor digiti quinti. Those with a nerve entrapment syndrome frequently complain of a burning pain with paresthesias on the medial side of the heel. Unfortunately, electrodiagnosis studies are not as diagnostic as reported. They are frequently negative except in those with long-standing nerve entrapment. These patients can be distinguished from those with plantar fasciitis in that they do not have pain to direct palpation of the plantar fascia.

Treatment

Once the diagnosis is made, the athlete is removed from running, but is allowed to bike or swim to maintain his cardiovascular conditioning. He is fitted with an orthotic device with a one-eighth inch medial heel wedge to decrease the loading of the plantar fascia. The patient is seen at six-week intervals. When there is no longer any pain to palpation of the plantar fascia, and no noticeable symptoms in the morning, a graduated running prescription is given. The orthosis is kept in the running shoe for the next several months.

In general, if the patient is seen within several weeks after the onset of symptoms, it usually takes a minimum of six weeks of rest before his foot is no longer tender to palpation and running can be resumed. Many cases may take as long as three months to resolve. In those who have had symptoms for several months, and who have continued to train, it will take at least three months, and often six months, for the symptoms to resolve.

Those who are still symptomatic after four to six months of appropriate treatment should be considered for surgical release of their plantar fascia. The surgery can be done as an outpatient procedure under Bier block. It consists of a one-inch longitudinal incision made along the medial aspect of the plantar fascia insertion (Figure 7-9). The abductor hallucis fascia (Figure 7-10) and the plantar fascia are completely released with a meniscotome (Figure 7-11). A bulky dressing with or without a posterior mold is applied and worn for ten days. The patient is then started on a gentle static stretching program and allowed to start swimming. At three weeks he is allowed to start biking. At four weeks, five minutes of continuous jump roping is begun and is increased to ten minutes at the fifth week. At six weeks, he is allowed to start a graduated running program every third day. At eight weeks he can resume a daily running program.

This surgical procedure has been done on ten runners with chronic resistant plantar fasciitis with excellent results. All returned to running within eight weeks, and have had no recurrences.

Tendinitis and plantar fasciitis are significant disabling problems that unfortunately require a significant rest from the patient's desired activity. To achieve a good result, the physician must understand the underlying pathology and investigate any predisposing factors. Because significant time is required for these entities to resolve, the physician and the athlete must have good communication so that the athlete will adhere to the recommended programs.

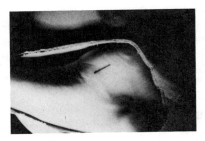

Figure 7-9. The medial plantar incision for release of the plantar fascia.

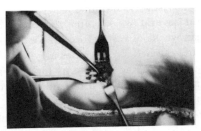

Figure 7-10. Isolation of the fascia overlying the abductor hallucis and the extension of the plantar fascia.

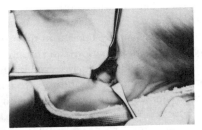

Figure 7-11. Utilization of a meniscotome for release of the plantar fascia.

REFERENCES

1. Dorland's Illustrated Medical Dictionary, Twenty- fifth Edition. Philadelphia, WB Saunders Co, 1974.
2. Blackiston's New Gould Medical Dictionary, Fourth Edition. New York, McGraw-Hill Co, 1979.
3. Puddu G, Ippolito E, Postacchini F: A classification of Achilles tendon disease. Am J Sports Med 4:145- 150, 1976.
4. Arner O, Londholm A, Orell S: Histological changes in subcutaneous rupture Achilles tendon. Acta Chir Scand 116:484- 490, 1958.
5. Arner O, Lindholm A: Subcutaneous rupture of the Achilles tendon. Acta Chir Scand (Suppl) 239, 1959.
6. Burry HC, Pool CJ: Central degeneration of the Achilles tendon. Rheumatol Rehabil 12:177-181, 1973.
7. Clancy WG, Neidhart D, Brand RL: Achilles tendinitis in runners: A report of five cases. Am J Sports Med 4:46-57, 1976.
8. Davidsson L, Solo M: Pathogenesis of subcutaneous tendon rupture. Acta Chir Scand 135:209-212, 1969.
9. Denstad TF, Roassa A: Surgical treatment of partial Achilles tendon rupture. Am J Sports Med 7:15-17, 1979.
10. Fox JM, Blazina ME, Jobe FW, et al: Degeneration and rupture of the Achilles tendon. Clin Orthop 107:221-224, 1975.
11. Ljungqvist R: Subcutaneous partial rupture of the Achilles tendon. Acta Orthop Scand (Suppl) 113:1-86, 1968.
12. Snook GA: Achilles tendon tenosynovitis in long- distance runners. Med Sci Sports 4:155-157, 1972.
13. Lagergren C, Lindholm A: Vascular distribution in the Achilles tendon. Acta Chir Scand 116:491-495, 1958.
14. Peacock EE: A study of the circulation in normal tendons and healing grafts. Ann Surg 149:145, 1959.
15. Schatzker MD, Branemark PI: Intravital observation on the microvascular anatomy and microcirculation of the tendon. Acta Orthop Scand (Suppl) 126, 1969.
16. Smith JW: Blood supply of tendons. Am J Surg 109:272- 276, 1965.
17. Peacock EE, Van Wenkle W: Surgery and biology of wound repair. Philadelphia, WB Saunders Co, 1970.
18. Snider MP, Claney W G and McBeath AA: Plantar fascia released for chronic plantar faxcutis in runners. Am J Sports Med 11:215-219, 1983.

CHAPTER 8

Exertional Compartment Syndromes

Scott J. Mubarak, M.D.

Introduction

A compartment syndrome is due to increased tissue fluid pressure in a closed fascial space compromising the circulation to the nerves and muscles within the involved compartment. The initial insult causes hemorrhage, edema, or both to accumulate in the closed fascial compartments of the extremities. The noncompliance of the compartment's fascial boundaries causes an increase in intracompartmental fluid pressure that, in turn, produces ischemia. Without immediate decompression of the compartment, the indwelling muscles and nerves may be permanently damaged, resulting in a Volkmann's contracture (Figure 8-1). The syndrome is most commonly caused by fracture, severe contusion, drug overdose with limb compression, or postischemic swelling. Rarely, intense use of muscle, as during strenuous exercise, may initiate compartment syndromes.

The exercise-initiated compartment syndromes are divided, by clinical findings and reversibility, into two forms. An acute syndrome exists when intramuscular pressure is elevated to such a level and is of such a duration that immediate decompression is necessary to prevent intracompartmental necrosis. The clinical findings and course are the same as compartment syndromes initiated by a fracture or contusion, except the event occurs after strenuous activities without external trauma. The second form, a chronic compartment syndrome, exists when exercise raises intracompartmental pressure sufficiently to produce small-vessel compromise and therefore ischemia, pain, and, on rare occasions, neurologic deficit. These symptoms dissappear when the activity is stopped, and reappear during the next period of exercise. If, however, the exercise is continued despite pain (ie, with continued ischemia), a chronic compartment syndrome may proceed to an acute form that requires decompression. An example of the latter is when a military recruit exercises under duress beyond his own limits of pain tolerance.

History

Anterior compartment syndrome initiated by exertion was probably first described by Dr. Edward Wilson, the medical officer on Captain R. R. Scott's ill-fated race to the South Pole[1] (Figure 8-2). Scott, Wilson, and three others failed in their attempt to reach the South Pole before the Norwegian, Roald Amundson. On the return trip from the pole, Dr. Wilson had severe pain and swelling in the area of the anterior compartment, which he accurately described in his diary. The following, dated January 30, 1912, is an excerpt from his diary:

"My left leg exceedingly painful all day so I gave Birdie my ski and hobbled along side the sledge on foot. The whole of the tibialis anticus is swollen and tight, and full of tenosynovitis, and the skin red and oedematous over the shin."

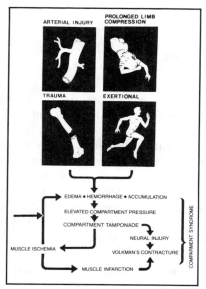

Figure 8-1. Pathophysiology of a compartment syndrome. Multiple cases may initiate a compartment syndrome: untreated, a Volkmann's contracture will result. Immediate surgical intervention is necessary to break this cycle. Strenous exercise may initiate an acute compartment syndrome. (From Mubarak SJ, Hargens AR: Symposium on Trauma to the Leg and its Sequelae. St. Louis, CV Mosby, 1981).

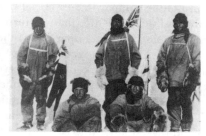

Figure 8-2. Dr. Edward Wilson (fourth from left) and Capt. R.R. Scott (third from left) pose by the Norwegian flag at the South Pole in early January, 1912. These explorers perished on the return trip from the South Pole. Dr. Edward Wilson was hobbled by the effects of an anterior compartment syndrome. With permission from Peter Brent: Captain Scott, Sat Review Press, New York, 1974.

Over the ensuing days his leg gradually became less painful as his general medical condition deteriorated. Dr. Wilson perished along with Scott and the others in the expedition on their return trip from the South Pole.

Thirty years passed before exertional anterior compartment syndrome of the leg became recognized as an entity. In a lecture in 1943, Vogt[2] described a case of ischemic muscle necrosis after marching (Table 8-1). In 1944, Horn[3] added two more cases, one involving the anterior and lateral compartments, and an isolated one of the anterior compartment. That same year, Sirbu, et al.[4] described a case of the anterior compartment syndrome resulting from a long march. He performed a fasciotomy and termed the disorder "march synovitis." Over the next 15 years, many isolated cases of acute anterior compartment syndromes of the leg resulting from exertion were reported.[5-10] Only two cases of the acute syndrome with lateral compartment involvement[11] and one case involving the superficial posterior compartment have been reported.[12]

Mavor,[13] in 1956, was probably the first to report a chronic form of the anterior exertional compartment syndrome. His affected patient had recurring pain in his anterior compartment associated with numbness and a muscle hernia. Fasciotomy relieved him of his problem. The existence of a chronic syndrome was questioned by Griffith[14] and later by Grunwald and Silberman.[15] Nevertheless, subsequent reports by various authors and the pressure studies of French and Price[16] confirmed the existence of this entity. In his monograph on this subject, Reneman reported on more than 61 chronic cases, also with pressure documentation.[17]

A chronic form involving other compartments of the leg has been described, although tissue pressure documentation is lacking. Reneman reported on seven cases of the chronic syndrome involving both the lateral and anterior compartments.[17] Kirby reported on a patient with bilateral chronic superficial posterior compartment syndromes; his patient's symptoms were relieved by fasciotomies.[18] Three additional cases of chronic syndromes in the superficial posterior compartment were reported by Snook.[19] Eleven cases of exertional syndromes involving the deep posterior tibial compartment were reported by Puranen.[20]

Table 8-1

Historical Description of Exertional Compartment
Syndromes of the Leg

Compartment	Acute Form	Chronic Form
Anterior	Wilson, 1912 Vogt, 1943 Horn, 1944 Siru, et al, 1944	Mavor, 1956
Lateral	Blandy & Fuller, 1957	Reneman, 1968
Superficial Posterior	Mubarak, et al, 1978	Kirby, 1970
Deep Posterior	—	—

Isolated chronic cases involving the second interosseous compartment of the hand[21] and the volar compartment of the foream[22] have also been documented.

Pathogenesis

The exact pathogenesis of the exertional tibial compartment syndrome is unknown. Elevated compartment pressure is the immediate cause of muscle and nerve ischemia in acute compartment syndromes. Furthermore, studies in our laboratory and by others[16, 23-28] have shown that patients with chronic syndromes have elevated pressures in the involved compartments at rest, and higher pressures during and after exertion sufficient to precipitate symptoms. The factors responsible for the elevation of compartment pressure in certain persons after exercise remains speculative. The pressure rises in the compartment due to: 1) the limitation of the compartment size (rigid container); and 2) an increase in the volume of the contents of the compartment (Table 8-2).

The rigid container in the usual case is the anterior compartment of the leg. This area is enclosed in a noncompliant osteofascial envelope made up of the anterior compartment fascia, the interosseous ligament, the tibia, and the fibula (Figure 8-3). Because room for expansion is minimal, fluid accumulation in this space will cause a rise in pressure.

TABLE 8-2
Probable Factors in the Pathogenesis of the
Exertional Compartment Syndrome

A. Limited Compartment Size
  1) Thickened Fascia

B. Increased Volume of Compartment Contents
  1) Acutely—Muscle swelling due to increased capillary permeability and intracellular edema
  2) Acutely—Restricted venous of lymphatic outflow
  3) Acutely—Hemorrahge due to torn muscle fibers
  4) Chronically—Muscle hypertrophy

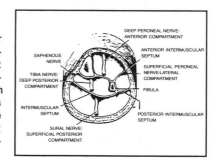

Figure 8-3. The leg consists of four compartments. Each contains a peripheral nerve. The anterior compartment is most frequently involved with exertional compartment syndromes. With permission from Mubarak SJ, Owens CA: Double incision fasciotomy of the leg for decompression in compartment syndromes. J Bone Joint Surg 59A:184-187, 1977.

During exercise, two interesting phenomena occur. First, during a strong isometric or isotonic contraction, intramuscular pressure rises sufficiently to render the muscle ischemic while the contraction is maintained. This fact has been noted by a number of authors using a variety of indirect methods of estimating tissue pressure,[29-35] but was confirmed by direct measurement of the muscle during contraction in our laboratory, using the wick catheter.[36-38] The pressure rises acutely during a muscle contraction, probably both by a mechanical means and because of a cessation of blood flow out of the muscle.

Second, with prolonged exercise, muscle increases acutely in bulk by as much as 20%.[39] Linge[40] demonstrated acute hypertrophy in untrained rats after five hours of exercise. These findings are probably due to increased capillary permeability resulting in fluid accumulation in both the intracellular and extracellular spaces. Other possibilities have been suggested to account for the volume increase in the compartment of subjects under exercise conditions. Anomalies of venous or lymphatic return may exist in patients with the chronic syndrome.[17] Unaccustomed exercise may lead to hemorrhage from torn muscle fibers as an additive source of fluid accumulation.[5,41] Finally, in the chronic state, muscle hypertrophy occurs with repeated exercise or conditioning. Whatever the cause, the pressure rises and therefore fluid must accumulate in the compartment interstitial spaces to cause either chronic and/or acute compartment syndromes after exertion.

Exertional Tibial Compartment Syndrome: Acute Form

Background and Clinical Presentation

Excessive use of muscles as a cause of an acute compartment syndrome is extremely uncommon. Less than 100 cases are documented in the literature, and during the past 13 years of our study of over 150 patients with acute syndromes, only three cases were initiated by exercise.

Most cases of the acute syndrome developed in patients performing tasks (forced marches or prolonged runs) to which they were unaccustomed. In some cases the patient had symptoms of a chronic compartment syndrome for months before the acute episode (17% in Reneman's experience).[23] The initial symptom of this acute compartment syndrome is severe pain over the involved compartment. The pain is initiated during the exercise, or develops within 12 hours after the exercise. As the pain increases, numbness and weakness are noted, and medical attention is sought.

The clinical findings in acute compartment syndromes initiated by exertion are identical to those of an acute syndrome of any cause (Figure 8-4). There will be increased pressure and pain over the involved compartment or compartments. Stretching the involved muscles of that compartment will exacerbate this pain. Muscle weakness (paresis) and a neurologic deficit will be present. A careful sensory examination using two-point discrimination can be helpful in documenting which compartments are involved. Capillary fill and pedal pulses (dorsalis pedis and posterior tibial) are routinely intact, though palpation may be difficult because of ankle and foot edema. A Doppler evaluation can be useful in this situation. This finding is true because even, though intracompartmental pressure may be high enough to cause ischemia to muscle and nerve, it is only rarely high enough to occlude a major artery.

The clinical findings for each of the isolated compartments of the leg are listed (Table 8-3). Note that a lateral compartment syndrome will usually involve both superficial and deep peroneal nerves that originate in this compartment.

Laboratory Investigations

Tissue pressure measurement: This is the best objective test for determining the need for fasciotomy. The wick catheter and slit techniques, which we have used over the past 13 years, provide an accurate and reproducible means of determining tissure pressure under equilibrium conditions.[36,42] Other techniques are available and have been found to be valuable in the diagnosis of acute compartment syndromes.[43-45]

If the intracompartmental pressures are greater than 30 mm Hg (normal 0-8 mm Hg) in association with the appropriate clinical findings, surgical decompression should be done immediately.[46-47]

Table 8.3
Typical Findings of Acute Compartment Syndromes of the Leg

	Anterior	Lateral	Superficial Posterior	Deep Posterior
Sensory Deficit	Deep Peroneal Nerve	Superficial and Deep Peroneal Nerves	Sural Nerve	Tibial Nerve
Muscle Weakness	Tibialis Anterior Toe Extensors	Peroneus Longus and Brevis	Gastrocnemius and Soleus	Tibialis Posterior Toe Flexors
Pain with Stretch	Foot and Toe Flexion	Foot Inversion	Foot Dorsiflexion	Toe Extension
Pedal Pulses	Intact	Intact	Intact	Intact

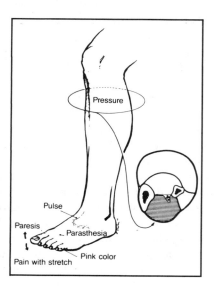

Figure 8-4. Early findings of an acute compartment syndrome illustrated in the anterior compartment. Modified from Mubarak SJ, et al: Laboratory diagnosis of orthopaedic diseases: Section I—Muscle pressure Measurement With The Wick Catheter. Practice of Surgery, Hagerstown, MD, Harper & Row, Inc, Chapter 20N, 1978.

Electromyography and nerve conduction: Matsen used electromyography and nerve conduction occasionally to serially monitor a decline in nerve function,[48] which is suggestive, but not diagnostic, of a compartment syndrome. We have not found this testing to be of much value in the acute syndrome. The problem by definition is increased pressure in the compartment, and the treatment is decompression. Thus, measurement of the pressure is the most direct means of diagnosing this pathologic state and evaluating the adequacy of surgical decompression. When a neurologic deficit is present postoperatively, electromyography may be helpful in establishing whether the patient is improving.[49,50]

Arteriography and doppler: These tests are only used to more fully evaluate the arterial supply to the limb. If a possible arterial injury coexistent with the compartment syndrome is suspected, these tests should be used. With only a compartment syndrome, the arteriographic finding may show small-vessel (arteriolar) cut-off created by the pressure elevation.

Differential Diagnosis

The acute compartment syndrome must be differentiated from a direct nerve contusion (neurapraxia) and an arterial injury. Because either of these two may coexist with a compartment syndrome, tissue pressure measurement and arteriography are extremely important diagnostically. Problems such as a large subcutaneous hematoma or an abscess present with swelling and often moderate pain; however, without neurologic deficit, these problems are usually easily differentiated from a compartment syndrome.

Treatment for Acute Compartment Syndrome

The treatment is the same as for any acute compartment syndrome: immediate surgical decompression. We use the double-incision technique, using one or both incisions, as necessary, to decompress the involved compartments. The details of this technique are described elsewhere.[24,51] The incisions are left open and the limb is splinted. At five to seven days, delayed primary closure or skin grafting is performed.

Exertional Tibial Compartment

Syndrome: Chronic Form
Background and Clinical Presentation

The chronic form of exertional tibial compartment syndrome is much more common than the acute form. Reneman[23] reported the largest series (61 cases) with nearly all involving only the anterior compartment. Symptoms were bilateral in 95% of his patients and in about 61% of our patients.[52] Most of Reneman's patients were from the military, whereas our patients ranged from casual joggers to enthusiastic marathoners. Most of our patients were male.

In most cases, the patient notes recurrent pain over the anterior or lateral compartment area, which is initiated by exercise and has been present for several months. The exercise may vary from a prolonged walk or march to a marathon run. For a given patient the onset of the pain is reproducible for a specific speed and distance. Usually the patient must discontinue his run and rest for a few minutes. Some persons, however, can continue the run at a reduced speed, whereas others who discontinue their exercise immediately may be bothered by symptoms for hours.

The pain is described as a feeling of either pressure, aching, cramping, or a stabbing sensation over the anterior compartment. Occasionally, associated symptoms include numbness on the dorsum of the foot, weakness, or an actual foot drop.

The findings on physical exmination before exercise are few. Findings from neurocirculatory examinations are normal. Usually the muscles are well developed in all compartments. It is best to ask the patient to perform his or her usual run or exercise that initiates the problem. A postexercise sensation of increased fullness over the anterior compartment may be noted, but the neurocirculatory status will usually remain normal. Occasionally, hypesthesia on the dorsum of the foot will be documented. Changes in the pedal pulses after exercise require further workup of the vascular system.

Muscle hernias, noted in 60% of Reneman's cases,[23] may be clinically more obvious after exercise. We have encountered these fascial defects in 39% of our patients.[52] Most are located in the lower one third of the leg, overlying the anterior intramuscular septum between the anterior and lateral compartments (Figure 8-5). In this location the fascial defect may represent an enlargement of the orifice through which a branch of the superficial peroneal nerve (medial dorsal cutaneous nerve) exits the lateral compartment. We have encountered this situation on multiple occasions. The muscle herniation may cause superficial peroneal nerve irritation and even neuroma formation (Figure 8-6).[17,53]

Laboratory Investigations

Tissue pressure measurement: The needle technique was first used by French and Price in 1962 to study chronic syndromes.[16] Reneman, using the same tech-

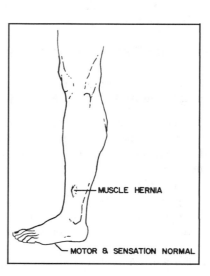

Figure 8-5. Muscle hernias are commonly associated with chronic exertional compartment syndromes and neurologic examination is usually normal.

nique, investigated a large number of patients. He found that the intramuscular pressures at rest, immediately after exercise, and at six minutes after exercise, exceeded normal control subjects of comparable age.[17] He could not measure the pressures continuously during exercise, with this technique.

Using the slit catheter technique, we observed similar changes in pressure between the two groups, with the additional advantage of continuous monitoring during the exercise. The slit catheter is inserted into the involved compartment under sterile conditions and local anesthesia. It is taped into position, and pressure measurements are determined during complete rest in the supine position. The subject's foot is then attached to an isokinetic exerciser (Orthotron, Lumex Corporation) using the foot attachment apparatus (Figure 8-7). A standard setting is used for all patients. The subject is instructed to dorsiflex and plantarflex the foot once every two seconds, until the activity must be stopped because of pain or fatigue. The pressures are continuously recorded by the slit catheter connected to a pressure transducer and strip recorder. We have found this method of exercise the most standard, although on occasion we have used a treadmill or had the patient run his usual distance to initiate the pain. Reinsertion of the slit in these circumstance must be rapid because the intramuscular pressures fall quickly.

In normal subjects, resting supine, the mean pressure of the anterior compartment is 4 ± 4 mm Hg. During exercise, pressure rises to more than 50

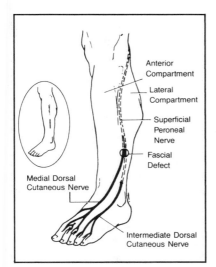

Figure 8-6. Relationship of superficial peroneal nerve branches to the fascial defect commonly seen with chronic exertional compartment syndromes. With permission from Garfin S, et al: Exertional anterolateral compartment syndrome. J Bone Joint Surg 59A:404-405, 1977.

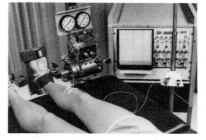

Figure 8-7. The wick catheter has been inserted into the right anterior compartment of a patient with a suspected chronic compartment syndrome. The foot is attached to an isokinetic exerciser. Intracompartmental pressures are continuously recorded by the wick catheter connected to a pressure transducer and strip recorder.

mm Hg. Moreover, intramuscular pressure rises and falls with each muscular contracture and relaxation. When the patient stops the exercise because of fatigue or pain, intramuscular pressure begins to fall. In normal subjects the pressure will decline below 30 mm Hg immediately, and at five minutes pressure will be back to the pre-exercise rest levels (Figure 8-7).

Intramuscular pressure measured at rest is usually greater than 15 mm Hg in patients with the chronic syndrome. During exercise these pressures rise to greater than 75 mm Hg. At times the pressure during exercise may exceed 100 mm Hg. At completion of the exercise, intramuscular pressure will remain greater than 20 mm Hg for five minutes or longer and usually symptoms of pain and possibly paresthesia are present (Figure 8-8). We have used these findings as our laboratory confirmation of the chronic compartment syndrome. In these patients we recommend fasciotomy, which should normalize both resting and postexercise intramuscular pressure.

Differential Diagnosis

Intermittent claudication due to partial femoral artery obstruction: By history, this condition is identical to exertional tibial compartment syndrome, except that the patients tend to be a little older than the chronic syndrome patients. The diagnostic clue in this entity is that the pedal pulses present at rest disappear with exercise. An arteriogram will confirm this diagnosis.[54]

Stress fractures of the tibia or fibula: This diagnosis can be made clinically by noting local tenderness over the bone at the fracture site. Although the radiographs will initially be negative, changes will usually be found ten to fourteen days after the onset of pain. A bone scan will usually be positive at the onset and may be beneficial in the diagnosis.

Tenosynovitis: Tenosynovitis of the dorsiflexors of the foot is characterized by crepitus, erythema, and pain on movement of the tendons localized to the dorsum of the foot and ankle (see Chapter 7).

Infection: Cellulitis, pretibial fever,[55] and tropical diseases[56] may initially suggest a compartment syndrome. In most cases the patients will be febrile with the loss

Figure 8-8. Illustrative anterior compartment pressures recorded with the wick catheter during exercise of a normal subject and a patient afflicted with a chronic anterior compartment syndrome. The resting pressure of the chronic syndrome is elevated over that of the normal control. During exercise the pressure rises to greater than 75 mm Hg for more than five minutes in the patient with the chronic syndrome.

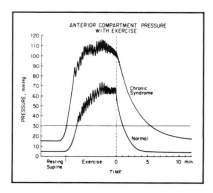

of function secondary to pain. Infections are rarely confused with the chronic syndrome.

Shin splints: These are usually defined as the pain associated with activity at the beginning of training, after a relatively inactive period.[57] The pain and tenderness are usually located over the anterior compartment and clear in a couple of weeks as the athlete becomes conditioned. Reneman believes that shin splints may represent a mild form of the chronic compartments syndrome.[17]

Medial tibial syndrome: This has been classified by various authors as a stress fracture,[58] deep posterior compartment syndrome,[20] or a shin splint.[57,59,60] Because the cause is unknown, the terminology selected by Puranen is probably most appropriate for this affliction.

The syndrome is usually seen in runners, but has been noted in athletes participating in tennis, volleyball, basketball, and long jumping. The pain is recurrent and associated with repetitive strenuous exercise. It is located along the medial border of the distal tibia. It increases after running a given distance and decreases with rest. Pain is often present, even without exercise, when the posteromedial edge of the distal tibia is palpated.

The physical findings are highly specific. There is a localized area of tenderness over the posteromedial edge of the distal one-third of the tibia (Figure 8-9). This area is often exquisitely tender. The posterior compartment muscles are sometimes atrophied. No motor, sensory, or circulatory disturbances are found. On examination of the patient after exertion, the painful area will be more symptomatic. Injection of xylocaine into this area will relieve the pain and allow the patient to exercise without discomfort.

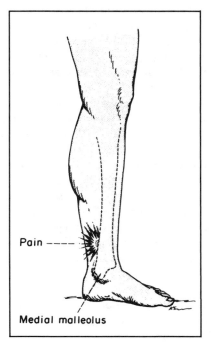

Figure 8-9. Clinical findings of the medial tibial syndrome. There is a localized area of tenderness over the posteromedial edge of the distal one third of the tibia (arrow).

Initially, radiographs are always normal. If the duration of the pain exceeds three to four weeks, hypertrophy of the cortex and possibly some periosteal new bone formation may be noted. Devas[58] presented a series of patients with evidence of a stress fracture of the tibial cortex in this area. Bone scanning may show a mild uptake or have entirely normal results.[20, 61, 62, 63] Even when positive, however, the bone scan uptake is not as increased as with a stress fracture.

Tissue pressure has been measured using the needle technique by D'Ambrosia, et al.[64] In their series, rest pressures in 14 athletes were all within normal limits. Eriksson and Wallensten also have noted "normal" pressure studies in patients with the medial tibial syndrome.[65] Similarly, in a series of 14 patients whom we have studied with this symptom complex, the rest and postexercise pressures have remained well within normal limits. Our mean rest pressure was 88 mm Hg, and immediately postexercise, the mean pressure was 9 mm Hg. During exercise, the pressure rose to an average of 55 mm Hg.[24]

Devas was one of the first to report on patients with the medial tibial syndrome. He believed that this entity represented an incomplete fracture involving one cortex of the tibia.[58] Fourteen of his patients had radiographic changes in the lower one-third of the tibia medially. In nine he was able to demonstrate an actual fracture line, and in five others, only periosteal reaction. Jackson and Bailey[60] supported the opinion of Devas that the medial tibial syndrome represented an atypical stress fracture. Although only one of their athletes had a fracture line, follow-up films on many others showed periosteal new bone formation and the cortical hypertrophy typical of this entity. Clement[65] believed that the syndrome represented a periostitis, and that with continued stress or overloading a typical stress fracture could result.

Puranen,[20] without pressure measurement documentation, theorized that the medial tibial syndrome represented a deep posterior compartment syndrome. His rationale was primarily based on the mild uptake shown on strontium bone scans and negative radiographic findings in these patients. Puranen noted that the radiographs of typical stress fractures would be more obvious than with this syndrome. Furthermore, he had excellent results in all 11 patients in whom he had done deep posterior compartment fasciotomies. Nevertheless, since then, the intramuscular pressure studies of D'Ambrosia, et al,[63, 64] Wallensten, and from our laboratory, refute the possibility that the medial tibial syndrome is a deep posterior compartment syndrome.

Biopsy material from two of our patients who underwent fasciotomies showed, on microscopic examination, inflammation and a vasculitis in the area of tenderness (Figure 8-10).[61] This finding, the mildly positive bone scan results, and the radiographic appearance lend support for periostitis as the cause. As Devas[58] noted, however, inflammation is a common finding in the region around a stress fracture. In summary, the available information on the medial tibial syndrome indicates that it most likely represents a stress reaction to the fascia, periostium, and bone at this location of the leg, and is not a compartment syndrome.

The treatment of this entity is in wide dispute. It is obviously highly resistant to the usual measures. Andrish, et al,[59] in a prospective study of shin splints, tried a variety of therapeutic measures. Most of their patients had the findings of the medial tibial syndrome. Aspirin, phenobutazone, heel cord stretching, heel pads, and cast immobilization did not improve their overall results. Rest remained the treatment of choice for this particular entity. Jackson and Bailey[60] reported no success with taping or arch supports, and found that aspirin and local injection of steroids also were not beneficial. They found that a well-cushioned shoe was subjectively the most beneficial. Clement,[65] in a report of 20 patients, recommended a two-phase approach. First, he prescribed rest, including crutches and anti-inflammatory medication, then a graduated exercise program using isometric and isotonic exercise. The most divergent approach was that of Puranen.[20] He did posterior compartment fasciotomies in the 11 patients he reviewed and reported satisfactory results in all patients.[20]

We have taken an approach of treating these patients conservatively. The common denominator with all treatment modalities is rest and then resumption of sporting activities in a graduated fashion. With time, most will improve. Taping, arch supports, and altering shoe wear may help. Occasionally, in the more recalcitrant cases, deep posterior compartment fasciotomies are performed. Generally, patients report excellent improvement after this procedure.

Treatment of Chronic Compartment Syndrome

Once the diagnosis of a chronic exertional compartment syndrome of the leg has been extablished by history, examination, and pressure measurements, fasciotomy is usally required. In many instances, however, when the diagnosis and treatment is outlined to the patients, they will prefer to limit running or alter their exercise program. With the chronic form, fasciotomy is not urgently needed as it is with an acute compartment syndrome. Reneman[23] noted ten patients who declined his recommended surgical decompression, and all were symptomatic at 10 to 12 months follow-up. Most patients in our experience who desire to maintain a given level of jogging or running will require fasciotomy.

Mavor[13] was the first to successfully treat a chronic compartment syndrome with fasciotomy. Reneman,[17] who has the largest experience, uses a blind technique for decompression of the anterior compartment. He notes this technique is not useful in the lateral compartment because of the location of the superifical peroneal nerve. Reneman used a diathermic wire to burn through the fascia to minimize the skin incision. We prefer a more direct approach and can accomplish a satisfactory fasciotomy of both the anterior and lateral compartments through a two-inch skin incision.

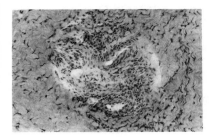

Figure 8-10. Photomicrograph (200X) of fascia overlying deep posterior compartment of a patient with the medial tibial syndrome. This illustrates the inflammation and vasculitis noted in this entity.

The necessary instruments for this procedure include right-ankle retractors (Army-Navy), a 12-inch Metzenbaum scissors, and/or a fasciotome. We have developed a commercially available fasciotome (made by Down Surgical Company, Toronto, Ontario, Canada) that was modified from the instruments suggested by others.[67-69] The fasciotome is designed to incise the fascia without the need for a long skin incision.

For either anterior or lateral compartment involvement, both compartments are decompressed. The skin incision is the mid-portion of the leg halfway between the fibula and the anterior portion of the tibial crest. The usual length is two inches (Figure 8-11).

After making the skin incision, the edges are undermined proximally and distally to allow for wide exposure of the fascia. After such exposure, almost the full extent of the compartment fascia should be visible. This step is extremely important when a small incision is used. A transverse incision is then made through the fascia, through which the anterior intermuscular septum that separates the anterior compartment from the lateral can be seen (Figure 8-12). This septum must be identified to enable location of the superficial peroneal nerve, which lies in the lateral compartment next to the septum. Then, by means of the long Metzenbaum scissors or the fasciotome, the anterior compartment is opened (Figure 8-13). Visualization is aided by retraction with the right angle retractors. The scissors are pushed, under direct vision, with the tips opened slightly in the direction of the great toe distally, and proximally towards the patella. If the tip of the scissors is suspected to have strayed from the fascia, the instrument is left in place and a small incision is made over the scissors' tip. If the

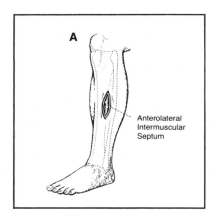

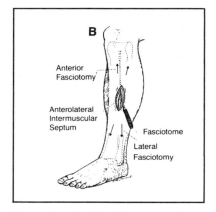

Figure 8-11A. Anterolateral fasciotomies in the absence of a fascial hernia. (A) Incision approximately 5cm long is placed between the tibial crest and the fibular shaft, over the anterolateral intermuscular septum. In the absence of a fascial hernia, the incision is in the midportion of the leg.

Figure 8-11B. (B) After the indentification of the intermuscular septum, fasciotomies of the anterior and lateral compartments are performed. (From Fronk J; Mubarak SJ; Hargens AR; Lee YK; Gershuni DH; Garfin SR; Akeson WH; Management of chronic exertional anterior compartment syndrome of the lower extremity.

fasciotomy is incomplete, further release can be performed through an accessory incision.

The lateral compartment fasciotomy is made in line with the fibular shaft (Figure 8-13). The scissors or fasciotome is directed proximally towards the fibular head and distally towards the lateral malleolus. In this way, the fascial incision is posterior to the superficial peroneal nerve. The incision is closed with an intradermal running stitch. A light dressing is applied.

Muscle hernias are frequent in the lower one-third of the leg in the area overlying the anterior intermuscular septum, which is the site of emergence through the fascia of one or both sensory branches of the superficial peroneal nerve. If such a muscle hernia is present, the skin incision should be located over the muscle hernia so that one can explore the fascial defect and identify the superficial peroneal nerve (Figure 8-14A-D). Through this approach one can easily decompress both the anterior and lateral compartments. Closure of this defect is never indicated because of the risk of precipitating an acute compartment syndrome.[49,70,71]

The patient is usually discharged the following day. Light exercises are begun within ten days and are gradually increased according to the patient's abilities. Follow-up measurements on patients who have had surgical decompression show a more normal tissue pressure during exercise. In Reneman's experience, the pressure at rest and after exercise does not completely return to normal limits. In the few patients whom we have had an opportunity to study postfasciotomy, the

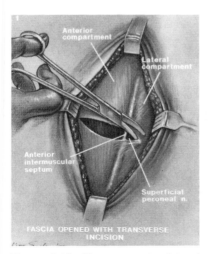

Figure 8-12. Close-up anterolateral incision: Step 1. With permission from Mubarak SJ, Hargens AR: Diagnosis and Management of Compartment Syndromes. AAOS: Symposium on Trauma to the Leg and Its Sequelae. St. Louis, CV Mosby, 1981.

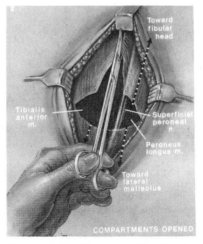

Figure 8-13. Close-up of anterolateral incision: Step 2. With permission from Mubarak SJ, Hargens AR: Diagnosis and Management of Compartment Syndromes. AAOS: Symposium on Trauma to the Leg and Its Sequela. St. Louis, CV Mosby, 1981.

tissue pressure measurements were essentially the same as those of normal runners (Table 8-4).

TABLE 8-4

Anterior Compartment Pressures in Patient with
Bilateral Chronic Exertional Compartment Syndromes:
Effect of Fasciotomy

	Resting Pressure	Postexercise*
	Right/Left	Right/Left
Preoperative	15/16 mm Hg	28/28 mm/Hg
Postfasciotomy (one year)	8/10 mm Hg	16/16 mm Hg
*5 minutes		

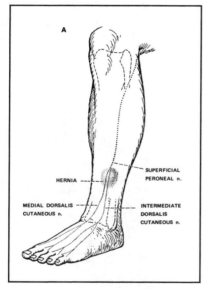

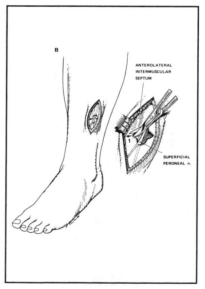

Figure 8-14A. Anterolateral fasciotomies in the presence of the fascial hernia. (A) The incision is placed directly over the fascial defect, with attention to the superficial peroneal nerve and its branches.

B. (B) The defect enlarged across the intermuscular septum (1) to gain entry into both compartments.

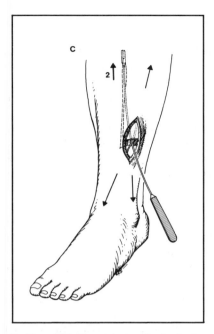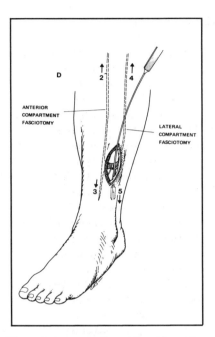

C. (C and D) Complete longitudinal release of the anterior compartment is achieved by passing the fasciotome in the direction of the patella proximally (2) and distally in the direction of the great toe(3). In the lateral compartment, the fasciotomy is carred out posterior to the fibular head (4) and lateral malleolus (5) (From Fronek J; Mubarak SJ; Hargens AR; Lee YF; Gershuni DH; Garfin SR; Akeson WH: Management of chronic exertional anterior compartment syndrome of the lower extremity. Clinical Orthopaedics and Related Research. 220:211, 1987).

REFERENCES

1. Freedman, B. J.: Dr. Edward Wilson of the Antarctic: A biographical sketch, followed by an inquiry into the nature of his last illness. Proc Roy Soc Med 47:7-13, 1953.
2. Vogt, P. R.: Ischemic muscular necrosis following marching. Read before Oregon State Med Soc, September 4, 1943.
3. Horn, C. E.: Acute ischemia of the anterior tibial muscle and the long extensor muscles of the toes. J Bone Joint Surg 27A:615-622. 1945.
4. Sirbu, A. B., Murphy, M. J., White A. S.: Soft tissue complications of fracture of the leg. Calif West Med 60:53- 56, 1944.
5. Carter, A. B., Richards, R. L., Zachary, R. B.: The anterior tibial syndrome. Lancet 2:928-934, 1949.
6. Hughes, J. R.: Ischemic necrosis of the anterior tibial muscle due to fatigue. J Bone Joint Surg 30-B:581-594, 1948.
7. Kornstad, L.: Tibialis-anterior syndrome. Nord Med 53:694, 1955.
8. Kunkel, M. G., Lynn, R. B.: The anterior tibial compartment syndrome. Can J Surg 1:212-217, 1958.
9. Severin, E: Unwandlung des musculus tibialis anterior in Narbengewebe nach uberanstrengung. Acta Chir Scand 89:426, 1944.
10. Tilloston, JF, Conventry MB: Spontaneous ischemic necrosis of the anterior tibial muscle; report of a case. Proc Mayo Clin 25:223, 1950.
11. Blandy JP, Fuller R: March gangrene. J Bone Joint Surg 39-B:670-693, 1957.
12. Mubarak SJ, Owen CA, Garfin SR, et al: Acute exertional superficial posterior compartment syndrome. Am J Sports Med 6:287-290, 1978. Mavor GE: The anterior tibial syndrome. J Bone Joint Surg 38B:513-517, 1856.
13. Griffiths DL: The anterior tibial syndrome: A chronic form? J Bone Joint Surg 38B-438-439, 1956.
14. Grunwald A, Silberman Z: Anterior tibial syndrome. JAMA 171:132-2210, 1959.
15. French EB, Price WH: Anterior tibial pain. Br Med J 2:1290-1296, 1962.
16. Reneman RS: The Anterior and the Lateral Compartment Syndrome of the Leg. The Hague, Mouton, 1968.
17. Kirby NG: Exercise ischemia in the fascial compartment of the soleus. J Bone Joint Surg 52B:738-740, 1970.
18. Snook GA: Intermittent claudication in athletes. J Sports Med 3:71-75, 1975.
19. Puranen J: The medial tibial syndrome. Exercise ischemia in the medial fascial compartment of the leg. J Bone Joint Surg 56B:712-715, 1974.
20. Reid RL, Travis RT: Acute necrosis of the second interosseous compartment of the hand. J Bone Joint Surg 55A:1095- 1097, 1973.
21. Tompkins DG: Exercise myopathy of the extensor carpi ulnaris muscle. Report of a case. J Bone Joint Surg 59A:407-408, 1977.
22. Reneman RS: The anterior and the lateral compartmental syndrome of the leg due to intensive use of muscles. Clin Orthop 113:69-80, 1975.
23. Mubarak SJ and Hargens, AR: Compartment syndromes and Volkmann's Contracture. Philadelphia, WB Saunders, 1981.

24. Logan, JG, Rorabeck, CH and Castel GSP: The measurement of dynamic compartment pressure during exercise. Am J Sports Med 11:220, 1983.

25. Matsen FA, III: Compartmental Syndromes. New York, Grune and Stratton, 1981, pp 133-142.

26. McDermott AGP, Marble AE, Yabsley RH, and Phillips, B: Monitoring dynamic anterior compartment pressures during exercise. Am J Sports Med 10:83, 1982.

27. Quarfordt, P, Christenson, JT, Eklof, B, Ohlin, P, and Saltin, B: Intramuscular pressure, muscle blood flow, and skeletal muscle metabolism in chronic anterior tibial compartment syndrome. Clin Orthop 179:284, 1983.

28. Anrep GV, Blalock A, Samaan A: The effect of muscular contraction upon blood flow in skeletal muscle. Proc Roy Soc London (Biol)114:223-245, 1934.

29. Ashton H: The effect of increased tissue pressure on blood flow. Clin Orthop 113:15-26, 1975.

30. Barcroft H, Millen JLE: The blood flow through muscle during sustained contraction. J Physiol 97:17-31, 1939.

31. Grant RT: Observations on the blood circulation in voluntary muscle in man. Clin Sci 3:157-173, 1938.

32. Hill AV: The pressure developed in muscle during contraction. J Physiol 107:518-526, 1948.

33. Kjellmer I: An indirect method for estimating tissue pressure with special reference to tissue pressure in muscle during exercise. Acta Physiol Scand 62:31-40, 1964.

34. Wells HS, Youmans JB, Miller DG, Jr.: Tissue pressure (intracutaneous, subcutaneous, and intramuscular) as related to venous pressure, capillary filtration, and other factors. J Clin Invest 17:489-499, 1938.

35. Mubarak SJ, Hargens AR, Owen CA, et al: The wick catheter technique for measurement of intramuscular pressure: A new reseach and clinical tool. J Bone Joint Surg 58A:1016-1020, 1976.

36. Owen CA, Schmidt, DA, Hargens AR, et al: Intramuscular fluid pressure during isometric contraction. Am J Sports Med, submitted.

37. Muhavak SJ, Schmidt DA, Owen CA, Hargens, AR, et al: An assessment of isometric quadricepts exercises. Unpublished data.

38. Wright S: Applied Physiology, Tenth Edition. London, Oxford Univ Press, 1961.

39. Linge B Van: Experimentele Spierhypertrofie Bij de Rat. Van Garkum, Assen, 1959.

40. Pearson C, Adams RD, Denny-Brown D: Traumatic necrosis of pretibial muscles. New Eng J Med 231:213-217, 1948.

41. Rorabeck CH, Castle P, Hardy D, and Logan J: Compartmental pressure measurements: An experimental investigation using the slit catheter. J Trauma 21:446, 1981.

42. Brooker AR, Pezenshki C: Tissue pressure to evaluate compartmental syndrome. J Trauma 19:689-691. 1979.

43. Matsen FA, Mayo KA, Sheridan GW, et al: Monitoring of intramuscular pressure. Surg 79:702-709, 1976.

44. Whitesides TE, Haney TC, Morimoto K, et al: Tissue pressure measurements as a determinant for the need of fasciotomy. Clin Orthop 113:43-51,

1975.

45. Hargens AR, Romine JS, Sipe JC, et al: Peripheral nerve conduction block by high muscle compartment pressure. J Bone Joint Surg 61A:192-200, 1979.

46. Hargens AR, Ronnie JS, Sipe JC, et al: Peripheral nerve conduction block by high muscle compartment pressure. J Bone Joint Surg 61A:192-200, 1979.

47. Mubarak SJ, Owen CA, Hargens AR, et al: Acute compartment syndromes: Diagnosis and treatment with the aid of the wick catheter. J Bone Joint Surg 60A:1091-1095, 1978.

48. Leach RE, Hammon G, Stryker WS: Anterior tibial compartment syndrome: Acute and chronic. J Bone Joint Surg 49A:451-462, 1967.

49. Leach RE, John DA, Stryke WS: Anterior tibial compartment syndrome. Arch Surg 88:187-192, 1964.

50. Mubarak SJ, Owen CA: Double incision fasciotomy of the leg for decompression in compartment syndromes. J Bone Joint Surg 59A:184-187, 1977.

51. Fronek J, Mubarak SJ, Hargens AR, Lee YF, Gershuni DH, Garfin SR, and Akeson WH: Management of Chronic Exertional Anterior Compartment Syndrome of the Lower Extremity. Clin Orthop 220:217-227, 1987.

52. Garfin SR, Mubarak SJ, Owen CA: Expertional anterolateral compartment syndrome. J Bone Joint Surg 59A:404- 405, 1977.

53. Kennelly BM, Blumberg L: Bilateral anterior tibial claudication. JAMA 203:487-491, 1968.

54. Daniels BW, Grennan HA: Pretibial fever. JAMA 122:361- 365, 1943.

55. Browne SG: The anterior tibial compartment syndrome. Differential diagnosis in a Nigerian leprosarium. Br J Surg 49:429, 1962.

56. Slocum DB: The shin splint syndrome: Medical aspects and differential diagnosis. Am J Surg 114:875-881, 1967.

57. Devas MB: Stress fractures of the tibia in athletes or "shin soreness." J Bone Joint Surg 40B:227-239, 1958.

58. Andrish JT, Bergfeld JA, Walheim J: A prospective study on the management of shin splints. J Bone Joint Surg 56A:1697-1700, 1974.

59. Jackson DW, Bailey D: Shin splints in the young athlete: A nonspecific diagnosis. Physician Sports Med 4:35-51, 1975.

60. Mubarak SJ, Gould RN, Lee YF, Schmidt DA and Hargens AR: The medial tibial stress syndrome. A cause of shin splints. Am J Sports Med 10:201, 1982.

61. Puranen, J and Alavaikko, A: Intra compartmental pressure increase on exertion in patients with chronic compartment syndrome in the leg. J Bone Joint Surg 63A:1304, 1981.

62. Wallensten, R: Results of fasciotomy in patients with medial tibial syndrome or chronic anterior-compartment syndrome. J Bone Surg 65A:1252, 1983.

63. D'Ambrosia RD, Zelis RF, Chuinard RG, et al: Interstitial pressure measurements in the anterior and posterior compartments in athletes with shin splints. Am J Sports Med 5:127- 131, 1977.

64. Clement DB: Tibial stress syndrome in athletes. J Sports Med 2:81-85, 1974.

65. Rorabeck CH, Bourne TB and Fowler PJ: The surgical treatment of exertional compartment syndrome in athletes. J Bone Surg 65A:1245, 1983.
66. Bate JT: A subcutaneous fasciotome. Clin Orthop 83:235- 236, 1972.
67. Mozes M, Ramon Y, Jahr J: The anterior tibial syndrome, J Bone Joint Surg 44A:730, 1962.
68. Rosato FE, Barker CF, Roberts B, et al: Subcutaneous fasciotomy, description of a new technique and instrument. Surg 59:282, 1966.
69. Paton DF: The pathogenesis of anterior tibial syndrome. J Bone Joint Surg 50B:383-385, 1968.
70. Wolfort FG, Mogelvang LC, Filtzer HS: Anterior tibial compartment syndrome following muscle hernia repair. Arch Surg 106:97-99.

CHAPTER 9

Injuries to the Foot

G. James Sammarco, M.D.

Introduction

The foot is the first body part to touch down and the last to leave the ground when running. The forces it transmits are often in excess of two times the body weight. The special construction of the five forefoot rays, mid-foot, and hind foot, and their bony, ligamentous, and muscular complement provides necessary stability for heel strike, stance, and toe off. The scope of this chapter includes conditions of the foot, the treatment and rehabilitation.[1]

The difference in function between the foot and the hand in running is that the foot is weight bearing, providing stability and locomotion to the body, whereas the hand is used for balance and coordination.[2-4] The bony structures of the foot two hallux phalanges, 12 phalanges of the lesser toes, five metatarsals, three cuneiforms, cuboid, talus and calcaneus, function as a unit, in sequence, and individually, to provide this. When conditions of this structure prevent mobility, painful conditions arise which alter performance.[5]

The function of the first metatarsal allows it to bear weight, as well as be flexible. The larger size of its proximal joint attests to this function. The head of the first metatarsal is rounded and articulates on its plantar aspect with two sesamoids. The hallux phalanges are also weight bearing bones. The length of the first metatarsal, and its position relating to the lesser metatarsals, is significant, since a foot with a shortened first metatarsal, the so called Morton's foot, allows increased loads to occur beneath the lesser metatarsal heads. Likewise, a significant metatarsus primus varus also permits increased loads to be borne beneath the head of the second metatarsal, a common cause of metatarsalgia, by giving a functionally shortened first metatarsal with respect to the lesser metatarsals.

The second metatarsal is anchored securely in Lisfranc's joint at the middle cuneiform. This most rigid part of the forefoot allows the most stress to be carried through the second ray. When considerable loads are carried on the ball of the foot for long periods of time, this bone may hypertrophy. This should not be mistaken on X-ray for a stress fracture.

The third, fourth, and fifth metatarsals are increased in their mobility respectively. The fifth is especially important because the high stresses carried here, predispose the bone to the risk of acute and fatigue fractures. This is due to its position, its tendinous attachments, and because it carries relatively increased loads with respect to the adjacent metatarsal.

The phalanges of the lesser toes are small, generally non-weight bearing, and carry smaller loads. The proximal phalanx is at risk of fracture or dislocation from direct trauma since runners wear light shoes with an unprotected toe. The metatarsophalangeal joint is supported by strong collateral ligaments, a heavy plantar plate, and a thin dorsal capsule, as are the interphalangeal joints. Such structures permit the transfer of stresses through soft tissue, and prevent hyperextension during toe-off. Muscle function is important, since a delicate interplay between intrinsic and extrinsic muscles is necessary to provide maximum stability and control. The pull of long and short flexors and other intrinsic muscles stabilize these joints, allowing the foot to conform to the ground during the complex maneuvering required to maintain stability. Conforming to an uneven surface is complicated by the use of a shoe. A soft rubber soled shoe shapes itself more than a rigid soled shoe, allowing the forefoot more control. A more rigid soled shoe protects the foot from surface irregularities at the expense of intrinsic muscle control, substituting, instead, the extrinsic foot muscles, the peroneus longus and brevis, tibialis posterior, the triceps surae, extensor hallucis longus, extensor digitorum longus, and tibialis anterior.

Injuries to soft tissues in runners may be acute or chronic in nature, and are often due to overuse. Nerve entrapment, as well as neuromata, including interdigital neuroma (Morton's neuroma), are common. Vascular problems are uncommon.

The plantar intrinsic foot muscles are divided into four layers. These layers control the toes. The extrinsic muscle flexor, digitorum longus, receives origins and insertions from the lumbricales and quadratus plantae respectively, along with a tendinous slip from the flexor hallucis longus, making it the most complex single muscle in the leg and foot.

The other extrinsic muscles are also complicated. All have a muscle mass lying in the calf. Their tendons pass beneath various retinacula, through the tarsal and other canals across the multiple joints of the ankle and foot. Tendinitis, attenuating tears, and rupture of these tendons is chronic and can cause significant disability as well as time away from sport.

Problems such as corns and callouses are often indicators of bigger problems, including osteophytes, bunions, and subluxing toes. Paronychia, ingrown toenails, and fungus infections are also responsible for time away from running and will be considered herein.

Fractures of the Fifth Metatarsal

Neck Fracture

Acute fractures of the neck of the fifth metatarsal are common.(Figure 9-1) The mechanism occurs through inversion of the foot. Although pain is acute, it is not uncommon for a runner, in the heat of competition, to ignore the injury, only to find swelling, tenderness, and the inability to walk after a race. X- rays show a transverse or spiral type fracture with or without comminution.

This is treated with a compression dressing and protected weight bearing, with crutches. Such fractures, have been known to take several months to heal. If reduction is necessary, closed manipulation is recommended. However, if displacement is significant, open reduction, with crossed pins or intramedullary fixation, is recommended. Postoperative treatment includes a short leg weight-bearing cast. After four weeks, following cast removal, a foot and ankle flexibility program is begun.(Table 9- 1) (Figure 9-2) A healed displaced fracture with malunion causing pain when the foot is placed into a shoe may require osteoplasty.

Shaft Fracture

Fractures of the shaft are associated with direct trauma, as well as the inversion injuries.(Figure 9-3) Long spiral fractures of the shaft are usually extensions from fractures in the neck region. These fractures are usually treated for four weeks with cast or compression dressing and limited weight bearing with crutches. If surgery is required, internal fixation with compression screws or intramedullary rod with circumferential braided 2-0 Dacron suture is recommended. Postoperative immobilization in a cast for six weeks is then necessary, followed by a rehabilitation program

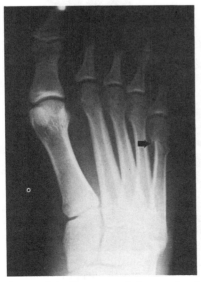

Figure 9-1. Fracture of the neck of the fifth metatarsal. This may easily be treated by immobilization.

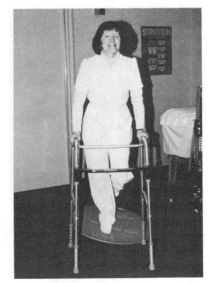

Figure 9-2. Photograph demonstrating the use of the foot and ankle exerciser board used in rehabilitation.

Base Fracture

In recent years controversy has arisen as to the etiology of fifth metatarsal base fractures. Acute fractures of the metatarsal base are often the end result of a developing stress fracture in that area. Mild pain along the lateral foot is often ignored by the runner, who feels that this is due to strain or tendinitis, since these tend to occur more commonly in running sports than do acute fractures. Taking such a fracture lightly, with only a short period of immobilization, can have disastrous prolonged consequences.[6,7]

When the fracture is completed by a single episode of trauma, it is treated as an acute injury. This is unfortunate. X-rays show a transverse fracture through the base of the fifth metatarsal.(Figure 9-4) The fracture is complete and non-displaced but appears chronic in nature, with sclerosis and rounded edges and the cortex is often thickened. Immobilization in the short leg weight bearing cast is the treatment of choice. Healing may require from three to five months. This is followed by a supervised rehabilitation program. Return to running prior to complete healing can lead to refracture. If this occurs, open reduction is indicated. Techniques for bone grafting of this fracture, with or without a compression screw fixation, have been described. Following healing and rehabilitation, the return to running should be gradual, slowly increasing distance, wearing new shoes, and running on softer surfaces, such as cinders or turf.

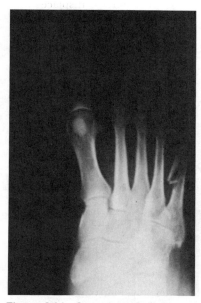

Figure 9-3A. Comminuted displaced fracture of the fifth metatarsal neck and shaft with shortening. Delayed healing and a predictable malunion with shortening are indications for an open reduction.

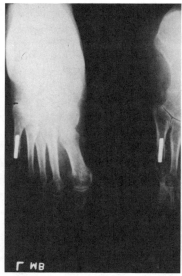

B. Intramedullary fixation of a fracture restores length and function.

Styloid Fracture

Fracture of the fifth metatarsal styloid is the result of the inversion of the foot against a contracting peroneus brevis muscle. Avulsion of the styloid process occurs with or without part of the articular surface.(Figure 9-5) X-rays show the characteristic avulsion of the styloid apophysis. Infifth metatarsal apophysis, diagnosis may be difficult.

Although immobilization in a compression dressing, with limited weight bearing and a wooden clog, is recommended for a period of four weeks, occasionally the athlete may opt for a short leg cast, to decrease the pain with the convenience of not having to use crutches. Although uncommon, delayed union and non-union do occur. Repair of the non-union with local bone graft and a compression lag screw are indicated in such circumstances, but immobilization following this should be in a cast until healing is complete. This may require two months. Running is then gradually resumed after a rehabilitation program, which includes whirlpool, a foot and ankle flexibility program, and the exerciser board.

Acute Fractures of the Middle Metatarsals

Fractures of the middle metatarsals can occur in the neck, shaft or base. Acute fractures of the neck are due to direct trauma. Although dorsal and lateral displacement are common, open reduction is indicated only if displacement is significant enough so that the weight bearing characteristics of the forefoot are significantly altered.

Multiple fractures also occur, and open reduction with internal fixation may be necessary. Axial pin fixation through the toe or intramedullary fixation is the treatment of choice. Immobilization subsequent to open reduction includes a light compression dressing and a wooden clog, with limited weight bearing. Running is restricted until clinical and radiographic healing are in evidence, usually two to three months. Such fractures should not be confused with stress fractures of the second and third metatarsals.

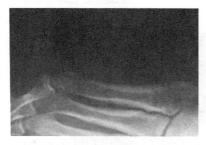

Figure 9-4. Fracture of the base of the fifth metatarsal. Although considered an acute condition, it is often the result of completing a stress fracture.

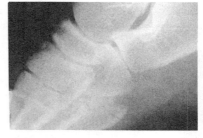

Figure 9-5. Fracture of the fifth metatarsal styloid with articular surface involvement.

Fracture of the Toes

Fractures of the phalanges occur most commonly by striking an object, such as a curb or tree. These are not common since the runner usually wears a shoe. Crush injuries occasionally occur and may be troublesome since the crush involves soft tissues, bone, and neurocirculatory structures.[8] Treatment of phalangeal fractures includes elevation for the first 48 hours and buddy taping to the adjacent toe. A stiff soled shoe is then recommended for three weeks. Running is permitted when x-ray evidence of fracture healing is evident.

The most common fracture occurs in the proximal phalanx.(Figure 9- 7) If displaced, closed manipulation is performed using 1% Lidocaine. A small gauze pad is placed between the toes to maintain alignment before buddy taping. Crush injuries to the phalanges involve more than just bone injury. Loads may have been quite high, and all tissues injured. Subungual hematoma can occur, with loss of the toenail, as well as fracture blisters. x-ray often reveals no fracture, but only evidence of soft tissue swelling. A compression dressing is advised, with elevation of the toes. As edema subsides, buddy taping is then permitted. Active range of motion is encouraged after 72 hours and running may be resumed within two weeks, or as symptoms warrant.

Fractures of the first metatarsal and phalanges are uncommon due to the mobility of the joint, its size, and strength. In children, fractures often occur through the epiphyseal plate at the proximal end of the bone. Treatment here requires the application of a short leg cast for three weeks, followed by restricted weight bearing for an additional two weeks. An avulsion fracture of the distal phalanx of the hallux occurs at the insertion of the flexor hallucis longus. The

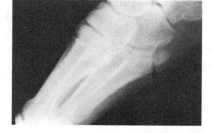

Figure 9-6. An x-ray of an inversion fracture of the fifth metatarsal styloid, with avulsion of the metatarsal apophysis. Diagnosis may be difficult.

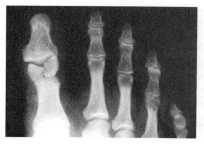
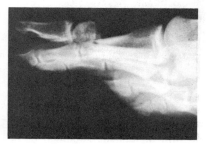

Figure 9-7A and B. An x-ray of a displaced intraarticular fracture of the hallux proximal phalanx. Closed reduction failed and open reduction was required. One may expect postoperative stiffness in such cases.

mechanism involved is that of sudden muscle contraction during the push off phase of gait against a passively extending interphalangeal joint. The fracture usually involves a portion of the articular surface. If displacement of the tendon with its bone fragment is significant, open reduction is indicated. However, for non-displaced fractures a wooden clog and limited weight bearing is permitted for a period of three weeks. Comminuted fractures through the hallux interphalangeal joint are usually caused from a direct injury, and open reduction is often necessary.

Fracture of the Mid Foot

Lisfranc and Chopart Fractures

Occasionally, a severe flexion injury to the foot occurs, disrupting the tarsometatarsal joints. Such fracture dislocation at Lisfranc's joint is due to sudden plantarflexion of the metatarsals, forcing a disruption at the proximal joint.[9] The mechanism was originally described as a stirrup injury, due to a fall from a horse.

A disruption may occur through any or all of the five tarsometatarsal joints. Diagnosis may be difficult, with the only symptom being pain. Standard x-rays may be negative. An Axial CAT scan across Lisfranc's joint will reveal chip fractures and disruption of the joint itself.(Figure 9-8) The metatarsals tend to ride dorsally.

Disruption through Chopart's joint usually occurs due to injuries creating forces of greater magnitude, such as a sudden, unrestrained fall. This occurs through a plantarflexion/inversion mechanism. Here also, x-rays may show no fracture. A bone scan and Axial CT scan are helpful in making the diagnosis, if the symptoms of a sprain do not subside within 3 weeks. Treatment of such fracture subluxations are complicated and vary from simple taping and anti-inflammatory medication to open reduction with partial or complete arthrodesis of the joints. Each case is individual and must be treated as such.

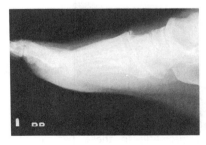

Figure 9-8A. Lateral X-ray of a foot with Lisfranc fracture. Slight dorsal displacement of the metatarsals is noted.

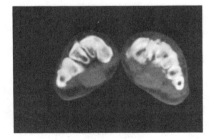

B. Scan showing disruption of the left tarsometatarsal joint, with fracture fragments present dorsally and plantarly. Prognosis is guarded, since open reduction is required for anatomic reduction and post-traumatic arthritis can be expected.

Stress Fracture

Stress fracture is covered in Chapter 4 in this book. However, any discussion of injuries to the runners foot would be incomplete without mention of it. A stress fracture occurs through time related use, rather than through significantly increased loads on a particular bone. Symptoms occur over several weeks. Often x-rays fail to show a fracture, and the runner is treated for "tendinitis." Early symptoms are diffuse pain becoming localized in two to three weeks. The stress fracture usually develops in that part of the bone carrying the highest load per unit area, although stress fractures in all bones and joints have been reported, including the phalanges, metatarsals, navicular, cuboid, talus[10] and calcaneus. (Figure 9-9)

The second and third metatarsals carry the highest forefoot loads due to their more rigid proximal joints. Therefore, this is the most common area for stress fracture. The base of the fifth metatarsal is also common since a secondary pathway for load distribution occurs in that area. Symptoms usually occur as the runner is increasing his distance or his endurance. A bone scan performed after at least two weeks of symptoms often demonstrates a "hot spot," ie, increased uptake in the region of the fracture.(Figure 9-10) However, it is not uncommon for a bone scan to remain negative for several months before showing localized uptake.

Articular surface involvement can also occur with stress fracture. Treatment includes limited weight bearing with the use of crutches and often a short leg cast.

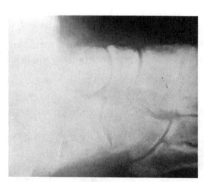

Figure 9-9. Oblique x-ray of the foot, showing stress fracture of the cuboid revealed after three months of symptoms. Bone scan became positive six weeks after symptoms began. Running was permitted three months after diagnosis was made.

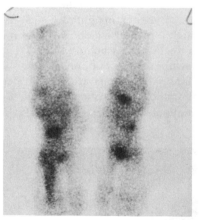

Figure 9-10. Bone scan showing increased uptake at the left second tarsometatarsal joint and at the right navicular. The runner was symptomatic in these two areas, but not in the left ankle. X-ray ultimately revealed some reaction of the proximal left second metatarsal. Restriction of running with swimming as a substitute for three months was required for healing to occur.

Treating a stress fracture of the phalanx should be the same as an acute fracture, buddy taping for three weeks with restriction of running during that time. Inadequate treatment prolongs symptoms and prevents running for an unnecessarily extended period of time. On occasion, open repair, with bone grafting and internal fixation, is necessary. This is particulary true in fractures of the base of the fifth metatarsal and navicular. It is not uncommon for a runner to be plagued with recurrent symptoms if he begins running too early. Without proper reconditioning and a gradual increasing of endurance, speed, and distance, a recurrence may be expected.

Afflictions of Joints

Turf Toe

Acute and chronic stresses occur across all the joints of the foot. These stresses can be on the dorsal or plantar regions, causing metatarsalgia, or through medial/lateral stresses with injury to the collateral ligaments. Turf-toe is a condition whereby forced abduction and extension of the hallux results in injury to the medial collateral ligaments of the hallux metatarsophalangeal joint.(Figure 9-11) Although common in contact sports such as football and soccer, runners develop this condition because of the soft-toed shoes they wear. Worn shoes and rough terrain are contributing causes. Tenderness and redness is present beneath the medial hallux at the metatarsophalangeal joint of the hallux. X-rays may be negative or show an avulsion fracture or periosteal reaction on the medial side of the first metatarsal head. Treatment includes buddy taping to the second toe, wearing a stiffer soled shoe for a period of two weeks, and restricting running until symptoms subside. A foot orthosis with rigid extension beneath the hallux is also recommended. Repeated stress causes continued ligament injury and leads to calcification of the ligaments. Although this calcification is usually asymptomatic, it can contribute to hallux rigidus.

Hyperflexion Injury

Hyperflexion of the hallux: tripping occurs when the toe is caught and pulled downward on a curb or other fixed object, causing acute hyperflexion at the interphalangeal or metatarsophalangeal joint. The tight dorsal capsule is partially avulsed. Joint motion is painful. X-rays may show a chip fracture where the medial collateral ligament has been avulsed from the metatarsal. A compression

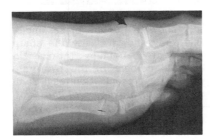

Figure 9-11. Oblique x-ray of a foot showing turf-toe soft-tissue swelling, with a small chip fracture (Arrow). (Not clearly demonstrable in photo.)

dressing is applied for three to five days, after which buddy taping and a gentle active range of motion is started in a stiff soled shoe. Return to running can begin as early as two weeks after injury. Anti-inflammatory medication, whirlpool, and a flexibility program using the foot and ankle exerciser board, ie, Baps Board®, are helpful in returning the runner to preinjury status.

Sesamoiditis

In running, high loads beneath the first metatarsal head often cause sesamoiditis. The etiology of this condition is complex involving several factors including length of metatarsals stress within the ball of the foot, the running pattern, the hardness of the running surface, the condition and thickness of the sole of the shoe, the constitutional resilience of the skin and soft tissues in the foot, and the timing of running.[11-15] Pain develops beneath the sesamoid. When examining the foot with the hallux in neutral position, tenderness is located beneath the affected sesamoid. If the hallux is dorsiflexed at the metatarsaphalangeal joint, the area of tenderness moves distally with the sesamoid. This confirms the diagnosis. X-rays may be negative for the first several months, but a bone scan can show increased uptake over the affected sesamoid within three weeks. X-ray views of the foot should include the sesamoid view, ie, a tangential view of the sesamoid, with the hallux dorsiflexed.(Figure 9-12) An oblique view of the sesamoids is also helpful. On the oblique view the X-ray tube is angled 45° toward the distal foot showing the two individual sesamoids in profile rather than superimposed. X-ray findings include enlargement and fragmentation of the involved sesamoid, not to be confused with bipartite sesamoid.(Figure 9-13) A compression fracture may be seen on the tangential sesamoid view or axial scan.

Treatment of sesamoiditis includes a horseshoe-shaped pad about the first metatarsal head. This is taped to the skin prior to putting on a sock. In addition,

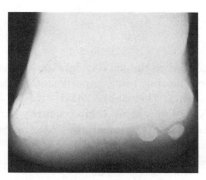

Figure 9-12. Sesamoid view x-ray of the foot showing fibular sesamoid enlargement and suggestion of disruption of its central structure. Exquisite tenderness was noted beneath the bone. Running was restricted for one month. A "U" shaped plantar pad was prescribed and swimming was substituted as an alternative exercise.

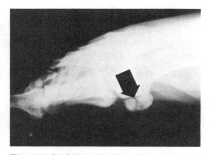

Figure 9-13. x-ray lateral view of foot showing fracture of sesamoid. The x-ray shows clearly the sharp edges of a fracture. (Arrow) No rounded corners of the two fragments are present. (Courtesy: Sammarco, G.J., *Disorders of the Foot.* Chapter 59. Jahss, M., ed. W. B. Saunders Company, Philadelphia, 1982. p.1656)

anti-inflammatory medication and instruction in a flexibility program for the foot is prescribed. A minimum of three weeks is required for symptoms to subside. During this time, running is decreased and an alternative non-weight bearing exercise pursued, such as swimming. Occasionally, symptoms are persistent and progressive over a period of several months and may require a partial or complete surgical excision of the sesamoid. If this is necessary, the runner should be advised of the possibility that, as a result of complications, including postoperative pain, termination of running as a sport may occur, since the natural energy absorbing mechanism of the foot will be altered.

Hallux Rigidus

Hallux rigidus occurs at the first metatarsal phalangeal joint. Naturally limited range of motion, as well as chronic inflammation and abnormal stresses, may contribute to degeneration of the joint. Flattening occurs with scarring, which further restricts motion.(Figure 9-14) Joint motion is greatly decreased and pain occurs during toe off. On physical examination, palpable medial osteophytes give the appearance of a bunion, along with limited painful motion. Pain increases after exercise. A serum uric acid test should be obtained to rule out gout, since this condition can present without evidence of arthritic changes or synovitis. Also, an acute gout attack may be precipitated following exercise leading to misdiagnosis since the joint appears red and tender following a run. X-rays show osteophytes dorsally, medially, and laterally, with decreased joint space, and sclerosis of the subchondral bone.

The simplest conservative treatment is a metatarsal pad. This benefits the patient in the early stages. Oral anti-inflammatories, an exercise program of prerunning flexibility, and elevation of the foot following running are treatment adjuncts, when indicated. The use of a semi-rigid orthosis with an extension beneath the hallux is also recommended. Surgical treatment includes cheilectomy, in which all osteophytes are removed from the proximal and distal sides of the joint, through a medial incision. It is important to remove at least 20% of the dorsal aspect of the joint, to ensure complete dorsiflexion is restored at the time of surgery. It may also be necessary to debride the sesamoids and release the plantar capsule from the metatarsal. If cheilectomy is unsatisfactory or fails,

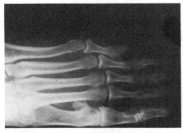

Figure 9-14A. Anterior posterior x-ray of a foot with hallus rigidus.

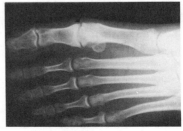

B. Oblique x-ray of a foot with hallus rigidus. Decreased joint space and sclerosis with flattened articular surface lead to stiffness and pain.

compression arthrodesis of the metatarsophalangeal joint is indicated. This will decrease the pain at the joint but may transfer loads distally and laterally in the forefoot, and the patient should be advised accordingly.

Keller bunionectomy brings the risks of proximal migration of the sesamoids and postoperative metatarsalgia. Prosthetic arthroplasty is not recommended in the runner.

Metatarsus Primus Varus, Hallux Valgus and Bunion

The pathomechanics of bunion are complex and incompletely understood. Our present knowledge indicates a complex etiology involving several components including intermetatarsal relationships, bone and joint shape, tendon alignment, hereditary factors, footwear, stress patterns, and many others. A union often occurs independently, as a large osteophyte on the medial aspect of the first metatarsal head at the attachment of the collateral ligaments. Since this can be mistaken as a strain injury or turf toe, a history of repeated symptoms without trauma after running, helps make the diagnosis.

Conservative measures are the treatment of choice for most bunions and hallux valgus. A bunion pad may be placed on the bunion. This is a large, firm, sponge rubber pad, with an oval-shaped large "donut hole" into which fits the tender bunion. This distributes the load evenly about the tender osteophyte. Associated metatarsus primus varus and hallux valgus require the use of lamb's wool placed between the first and second toes.(Figure 9-15) If surgery is required, and metatarsus primus varus and hallux valgus are not significant, a simple sliver bunionectomy will suffice. The runner should always be counseled as to the risks and consequences of surgery, and this must be weighed against the symptoms. All osteophytes should be removed. A prominent metatarsal head, medially, with hallux valgus, may require a distal metatarsal osteotomy, ie, Chevron type.[16-18] If significant metatarsis primus varus is present, along with hallux valgus and bunion, and a major forefoot reconstruction is considered, the runner must be informed of the higher risk of postoperative pain and stiffness in the hallux, since postoperative complications may lead to cessation of running.[19]

Joint Problems in the Lesser Toes

Hypermobility: Problems of the joints in the lesser toes include hypermobility of the metatarsophalangeal joint. Symptoms include metatarsalgia in the second or third toe metatarsophalangeal joint. No redness or swelling is noted. It may be

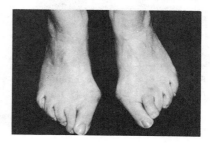

Figure 9-15. Metartarsus primus varus, hallux valgus and bunion. Surgery is considered only if prolonged symptoms are unrelieved by conservative measures, and running has ceased because of this.

associated with flexible hammer toe deformity. Physical examination reveals laxity of the metatarsophalangeal joint in the dorso/plantar plane at the affected joint. Tenderness may be present beneath the metatarsal head. X-rays show no evidence of arthritis.

A metatarsal pad with relief beneath the metatarsal head is the treatment of choice. This may be incorporated into a full insole orthosis. Severe, disabling symptoms over several months may warrant surgical excision of the proximal 20% of the proximal phalanx. To insure proper position of the toe after an excision of the proximal portion of the phalanx, a .045 smooth Kirschner wire is inserted axially through the toe into the metatarsal. This pin should pass through the long flexor of the toe at the metatarsophalangeal joint, which is pulled up during its insertion. The pin is removed after four weeks. The purpose of piercing the long flexor tendon with the pin is to insure scarring of soft tissues surrouding the proxial phalanx at the joint. This prevents dorsal migration of the toe following surgery. The use of a foot orthosis after surgery is recommended for several months.

Acute Synovitis of the Metatarsal Phalangeal Joint: Acute synovits of the metatarso-phalangal joint occurs most commonly in the second toe and is treated with buddy taping to the adjacent toe, anti-inflammatory medications, and rest after exercise. If conservative therapy fails, synovectomy is performed through a dorsal incision, retracting the extensor tendons and excising the synovium dorsally, medially, and laterally. The compression dressing is applied postoperatively for a period of ten days. Running is not permitted until complete healing has occurred, approximately one month.

Avascular Necrosis: Avascular necrosis most commonly occurs in the second or third metatarsal heads. Its etiology is still unknown, but recent case reports have indicated that it may be related to trauma in the adult. Symptoms are insidious, occurring over months. As with most metatarsalgia, the pain increases with exercise. Avascular necrosis manifests on X-ray by a lucent line just beneath the subchondral bone.(Figure 9-16) As time progresses, the metatarsal head collapses and osteophytes form medially and laterally. The joint stiffens and becomes painful in dorsiflexion and plantarflexion.

Treatment of early symptoms includes a metatarsal pad with relief beneath the metatarsal head, incorporated in a full insole orthosis, along with anti-inflammatory medication and a physical therapy flexibility program. If symptoms do not subside, surgical excision of the proximal 20% of the proximal phalanx through a dorsal incision and cheilectomy of the metatarsal head is recommended. A smooth .045 Kirschner wire is inserted axially through the toe through the long flexor tendon into the metatarsal. The tendon is pulled up into the wound with a nerve hook and pierced by the Kirschner wire to insure that plantar tissues are held firmly against the phalanx and joint. This prevents postoperative dorsal migration of the toe. The pin remains in for four weeks, after which a rehabilitation program is begun and running resumed. In the author's experience, prosthetic arthroplasty, simple cheilectomy, and total excision of the metatarsal head have not been successful surgical treatments in high performance athletes.

Tendinitis

Tendinitis occurs in any of the tendons, after a laying off period, or following increased training for a race.

At the ankle, the inflammation most commonly occurs in the tibialis posterior, peroneal or Achilles tendon. Pain occurs at the beginning of the run, but while running, it decreases. Eventually the pain restricts the runner from running the full distance desired. Swelling occurs along the tendon, medially or laterally at the ankle, or about the Achilles tendon, 3 cm above its insertion into the calcaneus. Tears of these tendons can occur with degeneration of the central fibers. The tibialis posterior tendon can be avulsed from its insertion at the navicular tuberosity.[20] In addition, tenderness, swelling, and red discoloration of the overlying skin may also indicate symptoms of accessory tarsal navicular.

Acute tendinitis of the flexor hallucis longus occurs in the posterior medial compartment of the ankle. As the tendon becomes inflamed, it binds as it passes through the tarsal tunnel, causing pain in the arch and at the posterior ankle. Stenosing tenosynovitis can occur in the tendon canal just proximal to the sesamoids. Symptoms of a functional hallux rigidus may be present due to restricted motion of the tendon. Treatment includes anti-inflammatory medication, a flexibility program, and changing running shoes, as necessary. Steroid injections are not recommended, in as much as direct injection of cortisone into a tendon can lead to rupture. The tendons tear with longitudinal rents and are chronic, occurring near the malleoli and just posterior to them. A bone scan is helpful in differentiating these conditions from stress fracture. Rarely does an acute complete rupture of a tendon occur.

If surgical repair is necessary, a longitudinal incision is made directly over the tibialis posterior or peroneal tendon, taking care to avoid the cutaneous nerves of the region. The incision for achilles tendinitis is made parallel to the medial

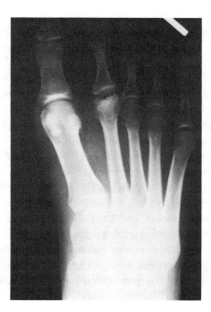

Figure 9-16. X-ray of the foot showing avascular necrosis of the second metatarsal head.

border of the tendon. The tendon sheath is opened and the tendon explored through a fiber splitting incision, and degenerated tissue rejected. A tenosynovectomy is performed if necessary. The tendon is repaired with an internal running suture of 5-0 braided Dacron. The knots are buried in each end. Occasionally multiple longitudinal rents may be present. These may be repaired in the same manner. A cast is applied postoperatively for a period of six weeks, followed by a rehabilitation program. Chronic pain of six months, with gradual collapse of the medial longitudinal arch, may indicate complete rupture of the tibialis posterior. Here, a reconstruction of the tendon with tendon transfer is recommended.

The flexor hallucis longus may be avulsed from its insertion. When this occurs, the tendon may retract into the forefoot. Repair of this uncommon injury requires reattachment of the tendon distally through drill holes in the distal phalanx. Such an injury may also occur with fracture.

Cysts of the Joints

Cysts can result from repeated trauma. They present at the metatarsal phalangeal joints. The mass forms in the web space, causing widening of the adjacent toes. Physical examination reveals a rubbery, moveable mass. Simple excision of such a cyst is recommended. A flexibility program is started as soon as healing occurs. The runner is then permitted to return to activity.

Interdigital Neuroma

Neuroma is a common cause of metatarsalgia of the common digital nerve located between the third and fourth metatarsal heads, and, less commonly, between the second and third metatarsal heads. Paresthesias is felt distally in the medial and lateral aspects of the respective toes, and burning may be felt beneath the metatarsal heads. The interval between the third and fourth metatarsals and distal web space has a unique anatomic relationship between nerves, vascular supply, and load bearing soft tissues, which may influence symptoms. Diagnosis may be made by compressing the metatarsal heads in the examiner's hand, medially and laterally. This may reproduce the characteristic paresthesias in the toes and pain. Dorsal and plantar pressure between the metatarsal heads likewise produces symptoms. Pain may often be elicited while pressing in the web space distal to the metatarsal heads.

Conservative treatment for interdigital neuroma consists of using a ¼-inch-thick metatarsal pad cemented into the running shoe with rubberized glue just behind the metatarsal heads to alleviate pressure. The padding beneath the affected metatarsal heads is relieved giving a "U" shaped appearance to the firm felt pad. Oral anti-inflammatory medication and a flexibility program are also prescribed. If these measures fail to relieve the symptoms, surgical excision is recommended.(Figure 9-17) Surgery is performed through a 3 cm dorsal incision, with meticulous care taken not to injure the cutaneous nerves. The transverse metatarsal ligament is divided for clear visualization and to relieve pressure on any nerve fiber beneath it. Both ends of the neuroma are clearly visualized before resection. The neuroma is resected from proximal to distal, dividing each digital nerve distal to the bifurcation. The author uses loop magnification to insure clean dissection of tissues. The specimen should be examined at surgery to ensure the entire neuroma has been removed. A 3-0 absorbable suture is used to approximate deep tissues, and the skin is closed with 4-0 subcuticular absorbable suture. A flexibility program is started after ten days and running is permitted as symptoms permit.

Proper Digital Neuroma: The proper digital nerve passes as a branch of the medial plantar nerve distally and medially into the forefoot and adjacent medially to the tibial sesamoid. Here, it is at risk of compression and a neuroma can form. Symptoms include pain, paresthesias, and a burning sensation along the medial aspect of the hallux and beneath the head of the first metatarsal. Symptoms can mimic tibial sesamoiditis but a positive Tinel's sign over the nerve at or proximal to the sesamoid confirms the diagnosis. Likewise, dorsiflexing the hallux draws the tibial sesamoid forward. If the pressure under the ball of the foot in the same area repeats the symptoms, this also helps confirm the diagnosis. Treatment includes a metatarsal pad, with a bunion flare, placed behind and medial to the first metatarsal head and sesamoid to relieve pressure.

If disabling symptoms persist for several months, excision of the neuroma is recommended. The incision is made medial and dorsal to the first metatarsal plantar pad and extends back into the midfoot.(Figure 9-18) Care is taken to avoid the weight bearing metatarsal pad. The digital nerve is identified at the plantar medial aspect of the proximal phalanx and followed proximally to the neuroma. Weight bearing is restricted for two weeks, followed by a rehabilitation

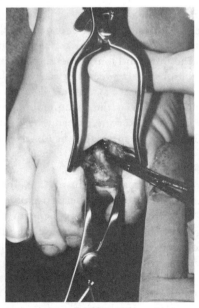

Figure 9-17A. Operative photograph showing interdigital neuroma. The neuroma is immobilized through a 3 cm dorsal incision.

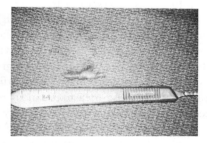

B. Operative specimen. One cm of the common digital nerve is excised with the neuroma to insure all of the tumor is removed.

program including the foot and ankle exerciser board. A metatarsal pad is worn following healing, and running is permitted after six weeks, as symptoms subside.

Injury to Dorsal Cutaneous Nerves: The cutaneous branches of the superficial and deep peroneal nerves are located on the dorsum of the foot, over the intertarsal and the tarsometatarsal joints of the medial two rays. A snugly tied running shoe compresses one or both nerves against osteophytes and ligaments from below causing pain and paresthesia. The superficial peroneal nerve lies dorsal to the deep peroneal nerve. Symptoms of compression of the superficial nerve may be in any one of its branches, medial or lateral to the first web space. However, symptoms in the first web space itself of pain, numbness, or paresthesias implicate the cutaneus branch of the deep peroneal nerve. Padding over the area where a positive Tinel's sign occurs may alleviate the symptoms. This may be made of felt or firm rubber foam, and can be placed against the tongue of the shoe or taped to the foot. A donut hole is made large enough to relieve the area of tenderness. Anti-inflammatory medication is prescribed.

If symptoms do not abate in several months, surgical exploration of the nerves is indicated. A linear incision is made over the dorsal aspect. Great care is taken to identify the vascular structures. These nerves are small and the distal branches may be difficult to define. The superficial nerve is identified proximal to the tarsometatarsal joint and followed distally through each of its branches. The deep peroneal nerve lies beneath a fascial layer and is closely associated with the dorsalis pedis artery. Once located, this is followed distally. If a neuroma is found it is resected along with any osteophytes beneath it. Injection of the nerve branches with saline is performed using a 30 gauge needle inserted beneath the perineurium. A subcuticular closure is reinforced with steri-strips. Running is restricted until healing is complete and symptoms have abated. A rehabilitation and flexibility program are prescribed as soon as healing has occurred. The area is padded when running is resumed.

The Sural Neuritis: The sural nerve passes posterior to the lateral malleolus, coursing forward and above the styloid of the fifth metatarsal. Occasionally pressure on the lateral aspect of the foot causes neuritis in this area. A positive Tinel's sign will localize the area of tenderness. A donut shaped pad, thick enough

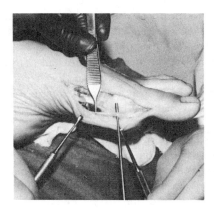

Figure 9-18. Operative photograph of neuroma of the proper digital nerve located beneath probe, at medial border of the tibial sesamoid. Excision completely relieved the symptoms.

to relieve pressure around the area, is recommended, along with anti-inflammatory medication and a flexibility program. Surgical excision is recommended if symptoms do not abate within several months.

Vascular Injury

The foot is a highly vascular structure. The arterial supply passes through the plantar aspect of the foot to the deep arterial arch, flowing distally into arterial arcades, then into common digital arteries and ultimately into small digital arteries. Communicating arteries join the plantar arteries to the smaller dorsal system. Repeated trauma can cause an aneurysm. It may manifest as a tumor between the metatarsal heads in a communicating artery. Pain and a space-occupying mass cause difficulty in fitting shoes. Surgical excision is recommended. Running is permitted when healing is complete at three weeks, as the patient tolerates, without evidence of recurrence.

When there are intermittent episodes of generalized pain throughout the foot, other conditions, including vasculitis and Raynaud's disease, should be considered. An arthritis profile should be obtained to rule out generalized conditions such as rheumatoid arthritis or systemic lupus erthematosus. The runner should not be advised to cease running, but rather to run for exercise as symptoms permit. Appropriate shoes with a softer sole and orthoses should be prescribed to allow activity as tolerated.

Calcaneodynia: The Syndrome

Calcaneodynia is a common syndrome. Although discussed elsewhere, I would like to present some observations which are presented concerning the condition. There are several aspects to calcaneodynia.[21-26] A stress fracture can occur at the inferior tuberosity of the calcaneus at the attachment of the plantar facia and flexor digitorum brevis. Symptoms of plantar heel pain begin insidiously over a period of several weeks and continue to grow in intensity until running is decreased despite heel pads or heel cups.

Treatment for this condition includes a foot orthosis with a cut out under the tender area in the center of the heel in the region of tenderness. The height of the heel pad in this region should be at least 1 cm thick and the cutout 3 cm in diameter and deep enough that the center area does not touch the skin. Anti-inflammatory medication, a slow stretching warm-up, and a decrease in running distance are prescribed. A bone scan is recommended, if symptoms are persistent, to determine if a stress fracture has occurred. If this is positive, a CT scan of the heel may be necessary to determine the nature and extent of the lesion.(Figure 9-19) The CT scan may be negative in spite of isotope localization at the inferior calcaneal tuberosity found in the bone scan indicating a periostitis rather than stress fracture. The use of a foot orthosis is recommended until symptoms subside. This may take six to eight months.

A second form of calcaneodynia occurs as plantar fasciitis. Here, through repeated mini-trauma and tensile forces on the plantar fascia, small microruptures occur, with subsequent scarring of the fascia over several months. The pain increases as the microrupture attempts to heal develop a thick fibrous scar in the substance of the proximal plantar fascia just distal to or medialto its attachment on the calcaneus.[27-29] On physical examination tenderness is noted in the plantar fascia in the middle of the medial region of the heel, just distal to the proximal attachment of the fascia. Symptoms can be increased when the toes are extended to tense the fascia while pressure is applied over the tender area.(Figure 9-20) Symptoms can persist for years and may be resistant to all conservative treatment.

The primary treatment of choice consists of a foot orthosis with a large cutout in the area of tenderness of the plantar fascia. Anti-inflammatory medication and a flexibility program are also recommended. A soft heel cup may also be tried. If symptoms persist more than six to eight months, an injection of corticosteroid is made into the area of discreet tenderness within the fascia itself. A recalcitrant plantar fasciitis with symptoms present one year, causing cessation of running as a sport faciitis are indications for surgical intervention through a medial and plantar incision. Avoiding the heel pad, meticulus dissection is made to the plantar fascia, which is then dissected both on its superficial and deep layers. The fibrous "olive" of grey-edged scar within the substance of the fascia is excised and the fascia is released, under direct vision, from medial to lateral.[38] The entire scarred area is then removed and examined. If a bone spur is present, this is also carefully removed.(Figure 9-21) The subcutaneus tissue is reapproximated with 3-0 absorbable suture and the wound is closed with 4-0 sub-cuticular absorbable suture, with steri-strips and a compression dressing. Following healing of the skin, a foot and ankle flexibility program is begun. A foot orthosis, with relief beneath the heel, is worn postoperatively. As symptoms of pain decrease, running is again permitted. This may require several months.

The third form of calcaneodynia includes the entrapment of branches of the medial calcaneal nerve or nerve to the abductor digiti quinti muscle. When such entrapment occurs, a positive Tinel's sign can be elicited over branches of the nerve as they pass along the medial aspect of the heel beneath the abductor hallucis muscle.(Figure 9-22)[31-33] This produces pain and paresthesias into the heel and occasionally along the anterior medial aspect of the heel pad. Treatment of choice is a foot orthosis with a cutout over the anterior medial heel region in the specific region where tenderness occurs. An elevated longitudinal arch is

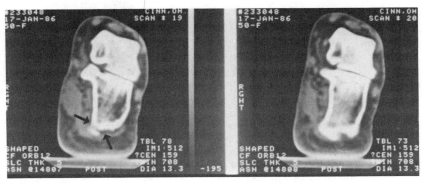

Figure 9-19. CT scan showing stress fracture of the calcaneus. No heel spur was present on x-ray.

recommended to bring the heel into subination, thereby decreasing the amount of pronation applied to the heel during the stance phase of gait. Anti-inflammatory medication and a flexibility program are recommended, including heel cord stretching, as well as a flexibility and a power building program for the intrinsic muscles of the foot.

If these measures fail after a trial of several months, a corticosteroid preparation mixed with 1% Lidocaine through a 25 gauge needle is injected into the area of triggering. This represents both a therapeutic and diagnostic test. Symptoms may be completely relieved with a single injection, but a repeat injection may be required one month later.

If the second injection fails, and symptoms have been present for more than one year along with a cessation in running, surgical exploration of the medial calcaneal nerve and nerve to the abductor digit quiniti should be performed. These nerves pass beneath the origin of the abductor hallucis muscle. Both of these nerves are small and familiarity with the anatomy of this area is necessary under loop magnification. The nerves are followed proximally above the arborization and distally as well, particularly in the area where symptoms occur. Often a tight band of ligaments and fascia surrounds the nerve. This is released and the nerve is meticulously freed from the surrounding tissues. The skin is closed with a 4-0 sub-cuticular absorbable suture and steri-strips are applied. Although the skin may heal within two to three weeks, full healing and ability to return to a full flexibility program may require 8 to 12 weeks. Running is then permitted with appropriate semi-rigid foot orthosis, including a high medial longitudinal arch, as symptoms permit.

Skin and Nails

The skin on the sole of the foot is six to eight millimeters thick. The skin on the dorsal foot is quite thin and flexible, and can be less than 1 millimeter thick.

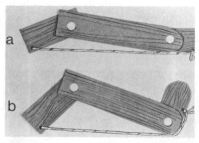

Figure 9-20. Diagrams showing function of plantar fascia.
A. The plantar fascia (rope) is attached at the calcaneus and toes (end links of wood).
B. As toes are extended, the fascia tightens, raising the arch of the foot and compressing joints to create a single stable unit from several tarsal and metatarsal bones.

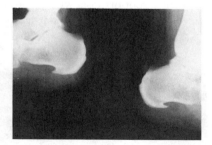

Figure 9-21. Lateral x-ray of patient with heel spurs. This lies deep to the attachment of the plantar fascia, but may trap the nerve branch of the medial calcaneal nerve beneath it.

Skin responds to stress and thickens, forming a callous where increased loads are applied. This is evident in the high arched foot, as with mild cavus deformity. This foot tends to be stiffer, with callouses developing on the heel and the ball, more readily than a foot with a flexible pes planus. Because of this, metatarsalgia and calcaneodynia tend to be more common. Beneath the skin is a layer of subcutaneous tissue containing compartmentalized fat. This structure absorbs energy during heel strike and push off. With age and increased use, thinning of the fat pad can occur. This is a common contributor to both metatarsalgia and calcaneodynia. Because high, normal, and shear stresses often cause symptoms when running, thick socks and soft soled, shock absorbing running shoes have become popular.

Clavus

As callous forms beneath the metatarsal head, the dermis thickens and may penetrate internally, as well as externally, causing a hard knot.(Figure 9-23)[34] This clavus is quite uncomfortable and the runner may shave it with a razor blade. A horseshoe or donut shaped metatarsal pad incorporated in an orthosis is recommended. This usually relieves pain. If failure of such treatment over several months requires further treatment, excision of the clavus under a local anesthetic with an elliptical incision is recommended. The wound is opened only to the dermis layer. Care is taken to preserve the subcutaneous fat since violation of the fibrous septae leads to excessive scarring. The wound is closed with 4-0 monofilament nylon mattress sutures. The sutures are removed after three weeks. During this time running is not permitted. Recurrent clavus beneath a single metatarsal head may require metatarsal plantar condylectomy. The runner should be counseled concerning risks and complications of surgery.

Corns

Hard corns occur over the dorsum of the proximal or distal interphalangeal joint. Here, a hard cornified layer of epidermis forms. This is caused by continued

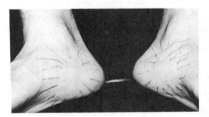

Figure 9-22. Photograph demonstrating radiating paresthesia when Tinel's sign is present over the medial calcaneal nerve, because of entrapment in the fibrous tunnel as it passes beneath the abductor hallucis and the plantar fascia.

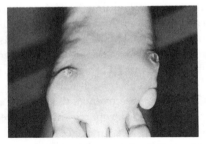

Figure 9-23. Photograph of the sole of the foot. Note the clavus beneath the first and fifth metatarsal heads. Simple padding around this helps relieve pressure, as well as shaving with a razor.

pressure on the toe by the shoe. Several layers of corn pads, relieved in the middle, easily treat this condition. Shaving the cornified layers with a razor also helps. Thin commercial corn pads may be stacked one atop the other to give better relief of pressure. Changing shoe size and width are also recommended.

Hard corns may be accompanied by a fixed or flexible hammer toe deformity. Should the symptoms of corns progress and be resistant to treatment, and a shoe cannot be modified to accommodate the toes, surgical correction of the hammer toe is recommended.

Soft corns characteristically occur between adjacent toes in this area (moisture collects), and the skin macerates from pressure between the toes causing, ulcers to form. A foam rubber pad, at least ¼-inch-thick (3 mm), shaped in a horseshoe, and relieved around the ulcer, is recommended as treatment. The joined portion of the pad (bottom of the "U") is placed distal to the corn and the adjacent toes are buddy taped. Osteophytes may occur at the proximal interphalangeal joint, giving rise to a soft corn in the overlying skin as it lies against the adjacent toe. If this is the case, the prominent osteophyte is excised through a linear incision made dorsal to the flexion crease of the toe. The osteophytes are removed with a rongeur. Subcuticular wound closure with absorbable suture is recommended. Running is permitted only after complete healing of the wound.

Occasionally, soft corns become infected and develop an abscess. The abscess may dissect into the web space. In this closed space, diastasis of the toes occurs as the abscess forms a mass. Incision and drainage with appropriate cultures is recommended. Oral antibiotics, based on culture taken pre-operatively and intraoperatively, is maintained for 10 days. The runner is permitted to return to activity following healing, usually within two weeks.

Blisters and Skin Fissures

Plantar skin which is constitutionally unable to sustain high, normal, and shear stresses of running can develop blisters. Blistering occurs between the layers of maturing dermal cells and the cornified layer permitting tissue fluid to collect. These form in areas of high stress, that is, beneath the hallux, tips of the toes, the ball of the foot, the heels, or on the sides of the first and fifth metatarsal heads. The best treatment for this condition is prevention, slowly increasing the distances, maintaining good foot hygiene, and using proper shoes. Should a blister form, the fluid filled area should be padded and the running decreased until it heals. The heavy skin overlying the blister should not be removed prematurely since this acts as protection and the fluid beneath bathes the inflamed dermis. The foot should be padded afterward and appropriate shoes purchased which fit well and have good shock absorbing characteristics.

To prevent recurrence, the affected part of the foot is taped with a single layer of paper tape (micropore)®. This decreases the friction in the ball of the foot, at the foot and sock interface, thereby decreasing high shear on the skin. An additional recommendation is the use of thin socks beneath the normally absorbent athletic socks. This also decreases the shear forces.

Fissures are uncommon and usually occur at flexion crease lines, secondary to high tensile forces on the skin. They are treated in a similar manner as blisters. Good hygiene is appropriate. These should not be confused with fissuring caused by tinea pedis.

Conditions of the Nails

Tenia Pedis and Onychomyosis

Fungal infections of the foot are common, occurring in the web spaces causing fissuring which may occur in any area where moisture collects. Here the moisture provides a growing medium. Although annoying, this is not a disabling problem and is best treated with anti-fungal cream (Loprox) applied twice daily after gentle bathing. Eczema and contact dermatitis can also occur. Proper diagnosis is essential in these conditions and a dermatological consultation is helpful. Treatment with hydrocortisone ointment is prescribed only after correct diagnosis is made.

Fungus of the nails causes them to thicken, delaminate, and loosen. This can cause repeated ingrown toenails and the thickening can cause pain from pressures on the upper part of the shoe. Such an infection is difficult to cure. Loprox cream® applied twice a day, along with griseofulvin, taken for a period of one year, is recommended. Socks must be clean, old shoes discarded, and bathrooms disinfected. Removal of the loose, painful nail and obtaining new shoes, as well as discarding old socks, is helpful in controlling the condition. The fungus is extremely difficult to eliminate and its spores can lie dormant for years. Recurrence of the infection is common. If permanent removal of the toenail is required, a local anesthesia about the base of the toe is recommended. The nail is elevated with scissors and a small incision is made on either side of the nail. Care is taken to remove the entire nail back to the germinal region of the nail. When this is completed, using electro-cautery, the germinal region is destroyed. An adaptic® dressing is applied with a light compression dressing. Following permanent removal of the nail, nine months is required for all tenderness of the nail bed to subside, but running may be resumed when the wound is healed. Padding is recommended over the nailbed to relieve pain until normal toughening of the skin has developed and tenderness has ceased.

Ingrown Toenail

Ingrown toenail is a common cause of infection and is often due to improper trimming of the nail or nail breakage. It occurs at the medial or lateral hallux nail border. If the nail edges are cut back behind the medial and lateral skin margins, lateral borders continue to grow beneath the skin distally. This allows infection to occur and affects performance. Treatment involves incision of the nail including its germinal portion.(Figure 9-24) This is done under local anesthesia with an adaptic® dressing applied afterward. Running is permitted after the wound heals in two weeks. Removal of the entire nail is not necessary. Removing the entire nail requires a prolonged period of protection, up to one year, until regrowth. Right, this is curretted and packed with gauze to ensure drainage.

Permanent partial removal of the nail by ablating the germinal portion using silver nitrate stick or electrocautery is indicated with repeated episodes of infection.

Paronychia

Paronychia is a soft tissue infection around the nail margin, often involving the base of the nail as well as its medial and lateral borders. Incision and drainage is performed with a No. 15 Bard-Parker blade above and parallel to the nail, under local anesthetia.(Figure 9-25) At the time of drainage, appropriate cultures are taken and the patient is placed on antibiotics. An adaptic® and light compression is applied. The dressing is changed in 48 hours and the foot is soaked in a saline solution twice a day for 15 minutes. Running is permitted following healing.

Black Toe

Repeated trauma to the great toenail can cause chronic subungual hematoma. This is usually asymptomatic and requires no treatment. Chronic hematoma beneath the nail gives a blackened color to the nail, known as black toe. The nail may elevate and cause mild pain. Padding around the nail is helpful. Removal of the toenail is not recommended since it requires at least nine months to regrow, during which time the nail bed is tender. Following an acute crush injury, however, if considerable blood collects beneath the nail, swelling,

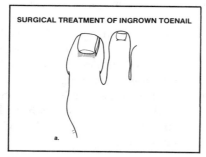

Figure 9-24A. Ingrown toenail. Twenty percent of the nail is removed including the germinal area beneath the cuticle. (By permission: Sammarco, G.J.: *Surgery of the Skin,* M. Harahap, ed. Warren Green, St. Louis, 1985)

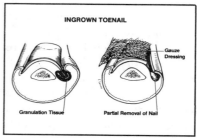

B. A cross section of the toe through the toenail. Left, granulation tissue is present beneath the nail.

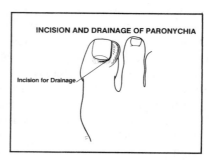

Figure 9-25. The incision is made just above the nail curving over the germinal region. (By permission: Sammarco, G.J.: *Surgery of the Skin,* M. Harahap, ed. Warren Green, St. Louis, 1985)

tenderness, and pain occur. It is easily drained using a drill or a paperclip with the end heated red hot in an alcohol flame.(Figure 9-26) This is passed through the nail permitting the collection of the blood to be evacuated.

Prevention and Treatment of Running Injuries

FOOT AND ANKLE FLEXIBILITY PROGRAM

Maintaining proper flexibility is an important part of any athletic program. Habits learned as a youngster tend to become ingrained in the adult. Even when running has been interrupted for a number of years, the preparation for it is not completely forgotten. This aspect of pre-run conditioning is therefore important, even in the youthful athlete because of its ramifications to an adult runner and especially following injury.

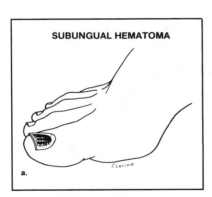

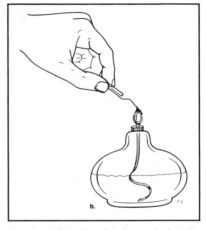

Figure 9-26A. Diagram of the foot with subungual hematoma.

B. A paperclip is heated in an alcohol lamp until it glows red hot.

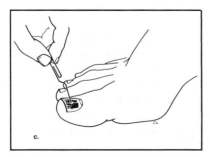

C. The hot end then passes easily through the nail, allowing blood to escape and relieving pressure on the toe. (By permission: Sammarco, G.J.: *Surgery of the Skin,* M. Harahap, ed. Warren Green, St. Louis, 1985)

Rehabilitation of the runner's foot and ankle following injury is based on the principles of early mobilization, returning range of motion and function to preinjury status and ultimately decreasing pain. Disabling injuries to the ankle are often the cumulative result of several minor episodes followed by one major episode. Problems of the foot, however, include categories of acute and chronic injuries as well as static deformity and overuse.

The flexibility program presented here is designed for rehabilitation following injury or surgery. A therapist often assists the runner in instruction. The program is also self explanatory and designed for easy comprehension. There are both weight bearing and non-weight bearing exercises. The runner will progress from the full program to a more abbreviated one as improvement in function progresses.

Table 9-1
Flexibility Program for the Foot and Ankle
Non Weight Bearing

Do each exercise 10 times a day. Increase repetitions of each exercise by 5 each day up to a total of 30 repetitions. Do program 3 times daily.

Exercise slowly and to the maximum stretch.

1. Sit on floor with legs straight in front. Place a towel around the ball of the foot. Grasp both ends of the towel with hands and pull foot toward knee. Stretch to the count of 5. Release.

   Same as above except pull more with right hand to bring foot to the right, then pull with left hand to bring foot to the left.

   Repeat with the knee bent about 30°.

2. Sit on the floor with your legs straight out. Flex the foot upward toward your face and curl the toes under at the same time. Now point the foot downward and bring the toes up at the same time. The sequence is: Foot up, toes down; foot down, toes up.

   Sit on the floor with legs straight out in front, putting the foot flat against the wall. With heel and the ball of the foot flat against the wall, pull toes toward your face. Hold to count of 5, relax.

   Do same exercise with the knee bent 30°.

3. Sit in chair with knee bent and foot flat on floor under knee. Keep heel and ball of foot on floor, raise toes. Keeping toes up, slide foot back a few inches, relax toes. Raise toes again and slide foot back a few more inches. Keep raising the toes and sliding foot back until you can no longer keep the heel on the floor while raising the toes. Bring this foot back out to starting position.

   Repeat from starting position, raise heel - keeping toes flat on the floor, then press down again. Lean upper body forward for increased stretch.

   Same position as above, slide foot forward as far as you can, keeping both the toes and heels in contact with the floor. At this point, keep the heel in place and knee straight. Flex foot up toward the knee, then point the foot and press toes onto the floor. Keep stretching and pointing the foot.

   Repeat from starting position, except keep the toes curled as you stretch and point the foot.

4. Sitting with the knees parallel, foot flat on the floor; pull the inside edge of the foot toward you (supinate), keeping the outside edge on the floor. Hold to the count of 5. Flatten the foot, then bring the outside edge of the foot toward you (pronate), keeping the inside edge on the floor, including the big toe. Hold to the count of 5. Do not let the knee move during this exercise. Sitting with feet flat on floor. Claw the toes and inch foot forward as toes claw, then release. Separate the toes between clawing. Inch out as far as possible, then slide back and start again.

5. Sitting with feet flat on the floor, raise the big toe, then the second, progressing to the little toe. Reverse and go from the little toe to the big toe. Sitting with feet flat, slightly lift heel, putting weight on the lateral borders of the feet. Roll from the little toe to the big toe, then back to the heel without letting the heel touch the floor. You are making a complete circle around the ball of the foot. Repeat and reverse.

Progressive Weight Bearing

1. Using two chairs for suport, stand with one foot 12 inches in front of the other, feet flat on floor. Rock forward onto the front foot so that the weight is on this foot, leaving the back foot in contact with the floor, toes on the floor, heel lifted. Rock all the way back so that the front foot is on the heel and toes are pulled back. Change position of feet and repeat.
   Between two chairs, stand on the good leg; swing affected leg all the way back, knee flexed, foot pointed, then swing leg forward to an extended leg, foot and toes pulled toward you (dorsiflexed). Keep repeating.

2. With your back to the wall, feet directly under shoulders, weight evenly distributed. Slowly bend knees and do not raise heels. Go to the point of maximum stretch and hold 5 counts, then rise up and repeat.
   Standing as above, at the bottom of the knee bend roll onto the balls of the feet to the maximum arch, roll down, then straighten legs. Repeat.

3. Standing on a step with feet parallel, heels hanging off the edge so that the calves are maximally stretched. Pull all the way up onto the toes, slowly, then lower all the way down to maximum stretch. Repeat up to 10 times. Repeat with feet turned out, then turned in. Progress to using 5- to 10-pound ankle weights.

4. Standing with all the weight on one leg, keep the knee straight and raise to a fully arched foot, slowly, then lower down. Repeat up to 20 times.
   Standing with all the weight on one leg, bend knee and keep heel down, then straighten knee and pull up to a full arch. Slowly lower the heel, keeping knee straight. Repeat.

5. Standing, rock back on heels, claw toes - walk on heels and then walk with toes clawed around pencils.
   Walk on heels with 1- to 3-pound ankle weights wrapped around forefoot.

6. Standing, raise and lower the inner sides of feet with the toes clawed.
   Stand with feet parallel, on the balls of the feet. Weight on the outer borders of the feet, knees about four inches apart. Roll the weight from fifth metatarsal to big toe in a circular motion. The heels stay off the floor. Do this exercise with the feet turned in, then with the feet turned out.

REFERENCES

1. Jacobs, S.J., Berson, B.L.: Injuries to runners: A study of entrants to a 10,000 meter race. Am J Sports Med 14(2):pp. 151-155, 1986.
2. Cavannagh, P.P.: The biomechanics of lower extremity action in distance running. Foot Ankle 7:197-216, Feb. 1987.
3. Mann, R., Hagy, J.: Biomechanics of walking, running and sprinting. Am J Sports Med 8:345-350, 1980.
4. Mann, R.A.: Rupture of the posterior tibial tendon. AAOS Instructional Course Lectures Vol. XXXIII, pp. 302-309, 1984.
5. Lutter, L.: Cavus foot in runner. Foot Ankle 1:225-228, 1981.
6. Acker, J.H., Drez, D. Jr.: Nonoperative treatment of stress fractures of the proximal shaft of the fifth metatarsal (Jones' fracture) Foot Ankle. 7:152-156, Dec. 1986.
7. Lehman, R.C., Torg, J.S., Pavlov, H., Delee, J.C.: Fractures of the base of the fifth metatarsal distal to the tuberosity: A review. Foot Ankle 7:245-253, Feb., 1987.
8. Jahss, M.H.: Traumatic dislocations of the first metatarsophalangeal joint. Foot Ankle 1:15, 1980.
9. Anderson, L.D.: Injuries of the forefoot. Clin Orthop 122:18-27, 1977.
10. Hontas, M., Haddad R., Schlesinger, L.: Conditions of the talus in the runner. Am J Sports Med 14(6): 486-489, Nov.- Dec., 1986.
11. Jahss, M.H.: The sesamoids of the hallux. Clin Orthop 157:88-97, 1981.
12. Lehman, R., Gregg, J., Torg, E.: Iselin's disease. Am J Sports Med. 14(6):494-496, Nov.-Dec., 1986.
13. Lillich, J., Baxter D.: Common forefoot problems in runners. Foot Ankle 7:145-151, Dec., 1986.
14. Parra, G.: Stress fractures of the sesamoids of the foot. Clin Orthop 18:281, 1960.
15. Richardson, E.G.: Injuries to the hallucal sesamoids in the athlete. Foot Ankle 7:229-245, Feb., 1987.
16. Corless, S.R.: A modification of the Mitchell procedure. J Bone Joint Surg 58B:138, 1956.
17. Johnson, K., Cofield R., Morrey, B.: Chevron osteotomy for hallux valgus. Clin Orthop 142:44-47, 1979.
18. Lillich, J., Baxter, D.: Bunionectomies and related surgery in the elite female middle-distance and marathon runner. Am J Sports Med 14(6):491-493, Nov.-Dec., 1986.
19. Mann, R.A., Coughlin, M.J.: Hallux valgus and complications of hallux valgus in surgery of the foot. (Mann, R.A. ed.) 5th ed., CV Mosby, St. Louis, MO. pp. 65-131, 1986.
20. Mann, R., Moran, G., Dougherty, S.: Comparative electromyography of the lower extremity in jogging. Am J Sports Med 14(6):501-510, Nov.-Dec., 1986.
21. Blechschmidt, E: The Structure of calcaneal padding. Foot Ankle 2:260-283, 1982.
22. Bordelon, R.L.: Subcalcaneal pain. Clin Orthop 177:49- 53, 1983.
23. Leach, R.E., Seavey, M.S., Salter, D.K.: Results of surgery in athletes with

plantar fasciitis. Foot Ankle 7:156-162, Dec., 1986.

24. Snook, G.A., Chrisman, O.E.: The management of calcaneal pain. Clin Orthop 82:163, 1972.

25. Tanz, S.: Heel pain. Clin Orthop 28:169-178, 1963.

26. Waller Jr., J.F.: Hindfoot and midfoot problems of the runner. Symposium on the Foot and Leg in Running Sports. St. Louis, CV Mosby Co., 1982, pp. 64-72.

27. Furey, J.G.: Plantar fasciitis: The painful heel syndrome. J Bone Joint Surg 44A:180-182, 1962.

28. Gillett, H.G.: Interdigital Clavus. Clin Orthop 142:103-109, 1979.

29. McBride, A.: Plantar fasciitis. AAOS Instructional Course Lectures Vol. XXXIII. pp. 278-282, 1984.

30. Parks, J.C.: Injuries to the hindfoot. Clin Orthop 122:28-36, 1977.

31. Leach, R.E., DiIorio, E., Harney, R.A.: Pathologic hindfoot conditions in the athlete. Clin Orthop 177:116-121, 1983.

32. Kech, C.: The tarsal tunnel syndrome. J Bone Joint Surg 44A:180-182, 1962.

33. Lutter, L.: Surgical decisions in athletes' subcalcaneal pain. Am J Sports Med 14:6, 481-485, Nov.-Dec., 1986.

34. Murphy, P.C., Baxter, D.E.: Nerve entrapment of the foot and ankles in runners. Clin Sports Med 4:753-762, 1985. 122:28-36, 1977.

35. Leach, R.E., DiIorio, E., Harney, R.A.: Pathologic hindfoot conditions in the athlete. Clin Orthop 177:116-121, 1983.

36. Kech, C.: The tarsal tunnel syndrome. J Bone Joint Surg 44A:180-182, 1962.

37. Lutter, L.: Surgical decisions in athletes' subcalcaneal pain. Am J Sports Med 14:6, 481-485, Nov.-Dec., 1986.

38. Murphy, P.C., Baxter

CHAPTER 10

Heat Injury in Runners: Treatment and Prevention

Peter G. Hanson, MS, M.D.

Introduction

Heat injury has become a major medical problem in warm-weather road races. An estimated 25 million persons currently participate in fun runs and competitive road races in the United States each year. Many local events attract 500 to 1,000 runners, whereas major road races draw 5,000 to 20,000 participants.[1]

The incidence of clinically significant injury is estimated at 0.1% to 2.0% of race participants when ambient temperatures are 24° to 27°C (75°-80°F).[1-4] Even this seemingly small fraction could represent 50 to 200 heat casualties, and quickly overwhelm the medical facilities of a medium-sized city.[5] In addition, a much greater percentage of subclinical heat morbidity probably goes unreported. Therefore, medical personnel who provide care for participants in road races must develop plans to prevent and treat potential heat-injury cases.

This chapter summarizes the clinical physiology and initial management of heat injury in runners, and suggests some possible strategies for preventing heat injury in road races.

Temperature Regulation in Runners

Body Temperature

During steady-state exercise, body temperature in runners normally increases to a range of 38° to 40°C (100°-104°F) (Figure 10-1). The elevation in body temperature is actively regulated to maintain a state of controlled hyperthermia, which is also compatible with optimum biochemical activity, blood flow, and oxygen transport for muscle contraction.

The runner is, however, also vulnerable to heat injury as a consequence of the complex interplay between increased heat production, dehydration, and circulatory and metabolic failure that may occur with substantial exercise. The critical thermal maximum core temperature for humans appears to be 42°C (107.6°F).[6] Sustained temperatures above this level result in thermal injury and clinical heat stroke. Surprisingly, some well-conditioned runners may attain rectal temperatures of 41.0° to 41.5°C (105.8°-106.7°F) with no evidence of heat stroke.[3-7]

Rectal temperature in runners is strongly influenced by the higher temperatures of venous blood returning from active leg muscles (40.5°-41.5°C; 104.9°-106.7°F) and the visceral-hepatic temperatures (41.0°-41.5°C).[8] These facts may explain the remarkable elevation in rectal temperatures measured in some runners. Esophageal temperature is probably a closer measure of core and brain temperature.[9] For clinical purposes, however, we must assume most runners will maintain body temperature within 1.5° to 2.0°C (2.7°-3.6°F) of the critical level for heatstroke.

Heat Balance

Body-heat content (H) is determined by the balance between metabolic heat production (M), additional heat gain from solar radiation (R), heat gain or loss from convection and conduction (C), and heat loss from evaporation (E) of sweat and lung water. These factors are usually expressed as a heat-balance equation:

$$H = M + R + C - E$$

For the warm-weather runner this equation is dominated by heat gains from metabolism and solar radiation, and heat loss from evaporative cooling (Figure 10-2).

Metabolic heat production is proportional to relative percent of maximal oxygen consumption (VO_2 max). An average runner usually maintains a metabolic rate equal to 75%-80% VO_2 max during races greater than 10 km.[10] Oxygen consumption and corresponding heat production may be roughly estimated from running velocity and an assumed caloric equivalent for oxygen consumption summarized below:

$$VO_2 \text{ (ml/kg. min)} = 178 \text{ (m/min} - 150) + 33$$

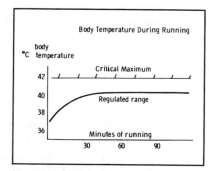

Figure 10-1. Body temperature during running.

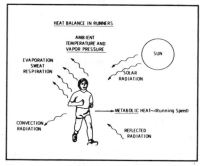

Figure 10-2. Heat balance in runners.

$$Kcal/hr = VO_2 \text{ (ml/kg. min) kg} * 5 * cal/l * 60 \text{ min.}$$

Estimated metabolic heat production for a 75-kg runner with an average velocity of 200 meters/min would be approximately 1,000 Kcal/hr.

Radiant heat gain (R) is determined by the intensity of solar insolation (I), the surface area of exposure (A), and a radiant uptake constant (a):

$$R = a * A * I$$

Radiant insolation may exceed 1,000 watts/M2 on a clear summer day. An average runner with 0.5 to 1.0 M2 of exposed (shadow) surface could gain 150 to 200 Kcal of additional heat per hour.[11]

The combined heat gains from exercise metabolism and environmental radiation would produce a progressive rise in body temperature of 2.4°C every 10 minutes in the absence of efficient body-cooling mechanisms.

Heat Loss

Temperature regulation during steady-state running depends almost entirely on increased skin blood flow and the evaporation of sweat (95%) and pulmonary water (5%). Each liter of completely evaporated water provides 580 Kcal heat loss. Sweat production and pulmonary water excretion are also proportional to the relative work intensity. Water loss may range from 1.5 to 2.5 liters per hour, depending on body size. The net effect of cooling, however, may vary greatly depending on environmental factors of ambient temperature, vapor pressure, and wind velocity. Even under ideal conditions, 20%-30% of sweat is probably lost to physical runoff.

Fluid Loss

Fluid losses of 1.5 to 2.5 liters per hour impose an additional burden to temperature regulation. Voluntary fluid intake by runners seldom replaces more than 25%-30% of these losses.[12,13] As a result, total body water depletion may approach 8%-10% for marathons.

Sweat is a hypo-osmolar filtrate (50-150 mosm/L), so that water loss greatly exceeds electrolyte loss. At high sweat rates, the concentrations of sodium and chloride do increase, whereas potassium concentration remains constant. Corresponding electrolyte losses in prolonged sweating may equal 5%-10% of extracellular sodium and 1%-2% of total body potassium.[12]

Volume depletion and electrolyte losses clearly potentiate the probability of heat injury in runners. Body temperature during exercise is significantly higher when dehydration exceeds 3% body weight.[10,14] In addition, reduced blood volume further decreases cardiovascular efficiency and cooling capacity.

Heat Acclimation

Temperature regulation and responses to exercise are dramatically improved with heat acclimation (Figure 10-3). In the acclimatized runner, sweating and increased skin blood flow are initiated at lower core temperatures, so that maximum rectal and skin temperatures are cooler for the same metabolic rate.[15]

Heart rate and cardiac output demands are also reduced in the heat-acclimatized runner. The improved cardiovascular responses are probably related to a reduction in peripheral venous volume and a corresponding increase in central blood volume secondary to cooler skin temperatures.

The apparent tolerance to higher body temperatures and efficient cooling capacity of elite athletes is reflected in the comparatively few reports of heat injury in international class runners. Highly trained runners appear to have superior cooling capacities during sustained exercise. Gisolfi found significantly lower values for rectal and skin temperatures in a group of highly trained distance runners, compared with those of well-conditioned college athletes running at the same percent VO_2 max and equal sweat rates.[16]

Novice runners, by comparison, are more likely to be unacclimated and relatively untrained for warm-weather road races. In addition, they may attempt to complete distances that exceed their training level or run at an excessive rate to finish, possibly ignoring premonitory symptoms of impending heat injury.

Heat-Injury Syndromes

Heat injury in runners should be considered as a continuum of clinical states characterized by variable combinations or hyperthermia and volume depletion. The evolution of heat injury in runners is illustrated in a simplified format (Figure 10-4).

From a state of normal temperature and fluid volume, sustained exercise produces a combination of progressive dehydration and regulated hyperthermia. Excessive early fluid depletion leads to a predominate heat exhaustion syndrome,

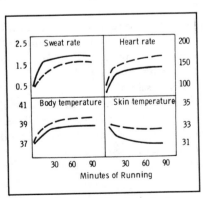

Figure 10-3. Physiological responses to steady state exercise in acclimatized (———) and unacclimatized (- - -) runners. (compiled from multiple references)

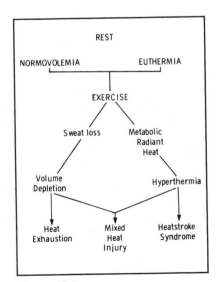

Figure 10-4.

with moderate hyperthermia. Progressive metabolic hyperthermia may produce heatstroke syndrome with mild dehydration. Most runners will show evidence of combined heat injury syndromes with significant dehydration and hyperthermia. This condition should be considered in the initial evaluation and management of apparent heat injury in runners.[17] Table 10-1 summarizes the clinical findings, initial management, and potential complications of heat injury.

Heatstroke

Heatstroke is the most serious of heat injuries that may be encountered in runners. The mechanism of exertional heatstroke probably involves the accumulated imbalance between metabolic and environmental heat gain and decreasing or impaired heat loss.[18,19] The numerous contributing factors include: progressive volume depletion, alterations in cardiac output and skin blood flow, and decreasing or impaired sweat secretion or evaporation. Exertional heatstroke may occur in the presence of active sweating.[18,20,21] Recent reports of clinical heatstroke in runners have emphasized the finding of profuse sweating.[2-5,22,23] Anhydrosis after the onset of heatstroke may be a secondary response to severe central nervous system dysfunction.

(Heatstroke in runners is usually preceded by significant disturbances in mental status, including disorientation and bizarre behavior. Any runner who exhibits this behavior pattern and loses consciousness during a road race must be suspected of having significant hyperthermia or clinical heatstroke.) It is of paramount importance to obtain vital signs and rectal temperature, to differentiate heatstroke from other possible causes of mental aberration or unconsciousness, such as hypoglycemia, cardiovascular failure, or arrhythmia. If rectal temperature exceeds 41°C, immediate thermal resuscitation should be started.

Hemodynamic status is characterized by tachycardia (heat rate 120-140 beats per minute), normal or reduced systolic pressure (140-100 mm Hg), and low or absent diastolic pressure. These findings are consistent with a high-cardiac-output, low-peripheral-resistance state.[23] Relative bradycardia and preservation of blood pressure may be seen in highly conditioned distance runners, in spite of considerable hyperthermia.

The skin is usually vasodilated and warm. As previously described, active sweating is usually found on initial examination.

Rectal temperature in heat stroke may range from 40° to 43°C; however, the temperature may be influenced by the transport time from field to hospital. An average initial temperature of 41.5°C was found in several recent reports of heat stroke in runners.[3,20,22]

Effective treatment of heat stroke includes immediate cooling, appropriate rehydration, and treatment of circulatory status. Complications and mortality in heatstroke are directly related to the delay in achieving body temperatures below 40°C. Most authorities recommend rapid cooling to 38.5°-39°C, followed by closely monitored passive cooling.[3,20,21,24] Thermal resuscitation, by means of wet ice towels applied to the neck, axilla, abdomen, and groin, may be started in the field and continued during transport to hospital.

Richards et al pointed out that spot cooling of these regions maximizes countercurrent exchange cooling to superficial great vessels, while minimizing

Table 10-1

Heat Injury Management in Runners or Athletes

	Hyperthermia-Heatstroke	Hypovolemia-Heat Exhaustion	Other "Exertional Syncope"
Clinical Findings	—Initial temp > 41°C (rectal) (May fall during transport) —Impaired consciousness—variable (Initial unconsciousness or severe disorientation) —Active sweating (may be found initially) —Cutaneous vasodilation (unless shock) —C-V: HR 120-160 BP wide pulse pressure 140-120/0 (shock may ensue)	—Initial temp 39-40°C (or less) —Mild disorientation —Active sweating —Cutaneous vasoconstriction, piloerection C-V: HR 120-140 BP 100-80/60-40 supine *Orthostatic ↓ prominent*	—Brief syncope or collapse associated with prolonged or intense exercise. May occur in cool weather (Usually "under-conditioned" person) —Temp < 39°C —C-V: HR < 120 *BP normal with mild orthostatic drop*
Initial Management	—TREAT AS TRAUMA CASE —Establish IV line —Use ECG monitor, Foley Cath —Do lab studies—STAT	—Establish IV line —Do lab studies—STAT Lytes, Glucose, U/A (expect ↑ WBC, RBC in runners)	—Determine volume status (Orthostatis ↓'s) —Check Glucose, Lytes, U/A ECG

Table 10-1 continued

CBC, Lytes, LFTS, PT, PTT
Glucose, ABG, U/A BUN/Cr.
—Initiate cooling with ice on wet towels
—Continue active cooling to 39°C (rectal)
—Give IV: ½ NS/D5W to replete ECF
  vol. *Do Not Overload*
—Give mannitol 12.5 GM IV
—Maintain urine output and C-V
  status. Use Swan-Gantz to direct
  fluid therapy if shock develops
—Avoid vasopressors

—Cool if temp = 40°C
—Give IV: 1/2 NS D5W
  Give 1 liter 30 min.
—Continue volume repletion
  based on urine output and V.S.
—Add K⁺ if depleted

—Treat as heat exhaustion

Complications

—*HOSPITALIZE FOR 48-72 HRS*
—Watch urine (hematuria, myoglobinuria)
  (Except WBC, RBC in runners
—Expect hepatocellular damage
  Max 48-72 hrs.
—Expect PT, PTT and platelets
  Max 48-72 hrs.
—DIC—may develop
—Watch for occult sepsis

—Discharge if condition is
  uncomplicated.
  Warn patient to watch for urine
  changes in subsequent 48 hrs.

*Watch for other causes of
xyncope in exercise:*
—Hypertrophic cardiomyopathy
—Mitral valve prolapse
—Dysrhythmia
—Myocarditis—myocardial infarction
—Drug abuse

cutaneous vasoconstriction which tends to reduce heat loss.[3] Immersion therapy is effective, but cardiac monitoring may be difficult, and resuscitation effects delayed or hazardous in the case of cardiac arrest or dysrhythmia.

For initial fluid therapy, a glucose-electrolyte solution, such as half-normal saline with 5% dextrose should be used. Hypoglycemia is a common finding in hyperthermic runners, and may be simultaneously corrected with glucose-containing solutions.[4,22]

Extracellular volume depletion should be corrected so that urinary output is maintained. Mannitol 25 mg may be administered intravenously, as a prophylactic measure. Excessive administration of fluids, however, should be avoided, to prevent circulatory overload and possible cerebral edema.[21,24] If severe hypotension is present, pulmonary artery wedge pressure monitoring may be required, to evaluate ventricular function and guide fluid therapy.

Basic laboratory work must include electrolytes, hepatic and muscle enzymes, uric acid, BUN and creatinine, urinalysis, coagulation studies, and CBC with platelet count. A 12-lead electrocardiogram and cardiovascular monitoring are advisable during the initial period of treatment.

Hematologic and biochemical alterations and exertional heat stroke are complex and reflect combined factors of tissue damage, dehydration, and disturbances of acid-base and renal function. Heatstroke victims should always be hospitalized and observed for 24 to 48 hours so that potential major complications may be identified and treated.

The time course and magnitude of serum enzyme concentration increase may be of prognostic value and should be closely monitored for evidence of continued hepatic or muscle damage.[6,21] Transient decrease in calcium and phosphate levels are apparently due to intracellular shifts of these ions secondary to cellular damage. Hypernatremia and hypokalemia may be found initially, probably secondary to volume depletion, although increased potassium levels may be related to muscle injury. Delayed coagulation times and thrombocytopenia are probably explained by a transient decrease in hepatic synthesis of clotting factors combined with increased peripheral platelet consumption due to tissue injury. The presence of fragmented red cells and decreased platelet and fibrinogen levels are suggestive of disseminated intravascular coagulation, which is a common complication of heatstroke. Shibolet et al emphasized that the apparent coagulopathic changes may be transient and do not require heparin therapy unless changes in laboratory values indicate continued deterioration.[21]

Acute renal failure is also a frequent complication of heatstroke. Rhabdomyolysis with myoglobinuria and hyperuricemia are probably contributing factors to renal tubular damage. This complication may be avoided by early rehydration and osmotic diuresis. The management of these complex problems in heatstroke has been detailed in several recent reviews.[3,14,20-23] Heatstroke victims should be evaluated for chronic heat intolerance after recovery. Recent reports suggest some persons remain susceptible to recurrent heat injury with exercise.[25]

Heat Exhaustion

Heat exhaustion is characterized by moderate-to-severe volume depletion, with water losses usually exceeding electrolyte losses during prolonged exercise.

Characteristic symptoms of fatigue, nausea, and headache are often severe enough to limit further participation in a road race. Significant hypovolemia may be tolerated while running, but may be followed by acute hypotension while walking or standing. Heat exhaustion victims are usually confused and irritable, but maintain consciousness while supine.

Rectal temperatures are elevated (39°-40°C), but should be below 41°C. Circulatory status is characterized by rapid heart rate (100-140 beats per minute), and prominent orthostatic hypotension. The skin is cool, with marked vasoconstriction and pallor. Active sweating should be present.

Treatment of heat exhaustion also requires fluid therapy and moderate cooling. Normal or half-normal saline with 5% dextrose may be used for initial fluid replacement. Subsequent fluid therapy may be guided by levels of serum electrolyte and glucose levels, which should be obtained on all runners who are treated in an emergency department. Adequate clinical response should be evaluated by progressive improvement of orthostatic blood pressure and urinary output.

Routine laboratory studies are consistent with acute hyperosmotic volume depletion. Hematocrit, serum sodium, creatine, and BUN levels are increased. Urine is scant and highly concentrated, with positive protein, granular casts, RBC, and WBC. Serum enzymes from muscle sources (LDH, SGOT, CPK) are moderately elevated, but such elevation may be due to exercise alone.

Most patients with heat exhaustion may be released after adequate fluid replacement. Patients should be warned to watch for unusual symptoms, especially alterations of urine appearance and output. Delayed rhabdomyolysis, with myoglobinuria and acute renal failure, is a potential complication.

Hypothermia in Runners

Road race events held in cool, wet, or windy conditions may result in post exercise hypothermia. Body core temperature rises and is maintained above normal during active running in cold weather. However, prolonged exposure, decreased heat production due to slowing pace, and increased heat loss from skin may lead to gradual hypothermia. Post exercise hypothermia is more common and usually occurs 20 to 30 minutes after running, due to the combined effects of decreased heat production and re-entry of cool blood from peripheral subcutaneous tissues.

Symptoms of mild hypothermia (rectal temperature 35° to 36°C) include intense shivering and vasoconstriction (blue lips, white fingertips). Muscle movement is stiff and skin sensation is decreased. Moderate hypothermia (33° to 35°C) causes increased shivering, depressed mental function, and further impairment of musculoskeletal movement.

Post-exercise hypothermia must be anticipated in cool, wet weather. Runners should dress appropriately, with modern outer clothing (Gortex or polypropylene) while running, and should have warm, dry clothes available at the finish line area.

Treatment of mild hypothermia includes passive warming with blankets and warm fluids, and monitoring of vital signs. More severe hypothermia may require hospital care to manage potential complications of rewarming.

Prevention of Heat Injury

Organization

The potential for heat injury may be greatly reduced by proper planning of the date, time, and route of a road race. Climatic data for the anticipated date of the road race should be carefully screened for temperature and heat-stress index. The most commonly used heat index is the "Wet Bulb-Globe Temperature" (WBGT). This index was developed for use in military training camps; it measures wet bulb temperature (WB), dry bulb temperature (DB), and metal globe temperature (GT). The WBGT index is calculated as follows:

$$\text{WBGT}^\circ\text{C} = 0.7 + 0.3\,\text{GT} + - 0.1\,\text{DB}$$

Using this index, the American College of Sports Medicine[26] established guidelines for conducting road races in warm weather conditions (Table 10-2). A maximum limit of 28°C WBGT (82°F) is recommended for races in excess of 16 km (10 mi). Despite close adherence to these guidelines, however, significant heat injuries have been reported over a wide range of distances (10 km- 42 km) and ambient temperatures (20°-28°C).

Heat Injury in Running

Another important factor in planning a road race is the route. In many instances the route is established by tradition or logistic constraints. A properly planned closed loop may be easier to monitor, and will provide a central aid station at the beginning and end of the race.

Aid stations should be positioned at 4 to 5 km (2.5 to 3 mile) intervals for all races greater than 10 km (6.2 mile). Field aid stations should provide fluids (water and hypotonic electrolyte solutions) and minor first aid (bandages, towels, and ice). Personnel assigned to field aid stations should be well versed in spotting potential heat victims.

An emergency communication system is vital for large road races. Such communication should provide contact between race officials and medical personnel at the finish, mobile emergency units in the field, and local hospital emergency rooms or fire rescue units.

Medical Coverage

Medical personnel should include physicians, nurses with intensive-care experience, and emergency medical technicians. Skilled professional personnel are best utilized in a major aid station located at the race finish. Paramedical and other knowledgeable persons may act as spotters at field aid stations.[27,28]

The major aid station at the finish should be equipped with cots, blankets, water, ice, intravenous fluids, and general medical equipment necessary for triage and initial treatment of heat injuries or other anticipated medical problems. Details of the organization and equipment needs for road race aid stations have been published.[27]

Local hospitals and emergency departments should be notified well in advance of the road race dates, so that personnel and supplies may be increased during this period of the race. Communication with medical staff in these hospitals is important for maintaining a consistent plan for management of persons with heat injury.

Advice to Runners

Printed pre-race instructions to runners should contain a section on medical self-care. Information should include recommendations for training and condi-

---

Table 10-2
The American College of Sports Medicine
Position Statement on
Prevention of Heat Injuries During Distance Running

Based on research findings and current rules governing distance running competition, it is the position of the American College of Sports Medicine that:

1. Distance races (16 km or 10 miles) should *not* be conducted when the wet bulb temperature—globe temperature* exceeds 28°C (82.4°F).
2. During periods of the year when the daylight dry bulb temperature often exceeds 27°C (80°F), distance races should be conducted before 9:00 A.M. or after 4:00 P.M.
3. It is the responsibility of the race sponsors to provide fluids that contain small amounts of sugar (less than 2.5 g glucose per 100 ml of water) and electrolytes (less than 10 mEq sodium and 5 mEq potassium per liter of solution).
4. Runners should be encouraged to frequently ingest fluids during competition and to consume 400–500 ml (13-17 oz.) of fluid 10-15 minutes before competition.
5. Rules prohibiting the administration of fluids during the first 10 kilometers (6.2 miles) of a marathon race should be amended to permit fluid ingestion at frequent intervals along the race course. In light of the high sweat rates and body temperatures during distance running in the heat, race sponsors should provide "water stations" at 3-4 kilometer (2-2.5 mile) intervals for all races of 16 kilometers (10 miles) or more.
6. Runners should be instructed in how to recognize the early warning symptoms that precede heat injury. Recognition of symptoms, cessation of running, and proper treatment can prevent heat injury. Early warning symptoms include the following: piloerection on chest and upper arms chilling, throbbing pressure in the head, unsteadiness, nausea, and dry skin.
7. Race sponsors should make prior arrangements with medical personnel for the care of cases of heat injury. Responsible and informed personnel should supervise each "feeding station." Organizational personnel should reserve the right to stop runners who exhibit clear signs of heat stroke or heat exhaustion.

It is the position of the American College of Sports Medicine that policies established by local, national, and international sponsors of distance running events should adhere to these guidelines. Failure to adhere to these guidelines may jeopardize the health of competitors through heat injury.

tioning, pre-race nutrition, and fluid intake; advice on clothing and footwear; guidelines for consumption of fluids; and recognition of heat symptoms during the race (Table 10-3). Runners should also be advised not to participate during or immediately after a febrile illness. Medication that may influence thermal regulation should also be mentioned. Immediately before the race, runners should be apprised of current ambient temperature and humidity conditions, and reminded of the symptoms of heat injury. This preparation is especially important whenever the temperature exceeds 21°C WBGT (70°F). They should be strongly encouraged to drink adequate volumes of fluid (200-300 ml) at each aid station. Alcoholic drinks should be discouraged. Finally, runners should be warned not to attempt a substantial increase in pace, to catch up or finish a race

---

Table 10-3
Warm-Weather Medical Self-Care
for Beginning Runners

Training and Preparation. You should be able to run _____*
miles at 9-11 minutes per mile pace to finish this race comfortably. Try to train _____** miles per week for at least 4 weeks before this race. Drink about 8 ounces of fluid 1 hour before the race and up to twice that amount 10-15 minutes before race time. Start warming up—stretching and jogging—about 30 minutes before race.

Race of 6 to 9 miles:	12-22 miles	26 miles
*run 3/** train 18	run 6/tr. 25	run 12/tr. 37

Temperature is a critical factor. Significant heat injury may occur at all temperatures from 65-80°F. Above 80°F, novice runners should *reduce running pace by about 1 minute per mile.* Wear only light athletic clothing (shorts, T shirt, tank top, or topless). Body temperature will normally rise to 102-103°F during race due to exercise heat production. Further increases nay occur due to radiant sun exposure, dehydration, and decreased sweat rate.

Fluid Replacement is essential to restore sweat losses. The average-size man (140-160 pounds) may lose 1.5-2.0 quarts of sweat per hour. Drink 6-8 ounces fluid at *each* aid station. Stop to drink. Even then, you may replace only 50% of sweat loss.

Problems During Run may include muscle cramps, joint pains, blisters, fatigue. Heat symptoms are most dangerous—headache, dizziness, disorientation, nausea, decrease in sweat rate, pale, cold skin. Don't try to run through these symptoms. Stop, walk or rest, ask for help.

After Running. At finish, you may become dizzy or faint on coming to a stop due to a fall in blood pressure. To prevent this, *keep moving.* But, if symptoms develop, lie down, raise legs, call for help.

Chronic Medical Problems. If you have medical problems such as asthma, diabetes, hypertension or other cardiovascular problems, check with your physician before entering a race. Wear a 'medic alert' tag and I.D.

Remember, running is fun but it can be stressful. Listen to your body. Walk when you are tired. There is always another race.

when symptoms of heat stress are present. Novice runners should be advised to voluntarily decrease their planned running pace by 1 mile/min if the ambient temperature exceeds 24°C WBGT (75°F).

Summary

Heat injury is a threat to all distance runners, regardless of experience. Sustained high metabolic rate and unavoidable dehydration are constant stresses to adequate temperature regulation. The best defense against heat injury is prevention. Heat casualties are inevitable, however, in large warm-weather races, and preparation should be adequate to handle these problems. Medical personnel who provide coverage for organized road races should familiarize themselves with the clinical syndromes of heat injury, and develop a well-coordinated plan for identification and immediate management of heat casualties.

REFERENCES

1. Williams, R.S., Schoken, D.D., More, M., et al: Medical aspects of competitive distance running. Postgraduate Medicine 70:41;1981.
2. England, A.C., Fraser, D., Hightower, A., et al: Preventing severe heat injury in runners: Suggestions from the 1979 Peachtree Roadtree Experience. Ann In Med 97:196, 1982.
3. Hart, L.E., Egier, B.P. et al: Exertional heatstroke: The runner's nemesis. CMA Journal 122:1144,1980.
4. Sutton, J.B., Coleman, M.H., Millar, A.P., et al: The medical problems of mass participation in athletic competition: The Sun City-to-Surf race. Med J Aust 2:127, 1972.
5. Nicholson, M.R., Somerville, K.W.: Heatstroke in a run for fun. Br Med J 1:525, 1978.
6. Bynum, G.D., Pandolf, K.B., Schuette, W.H., et al: Induced hyperthermia in sedated humans and the concept of critical thermal maximum. Am J Physiol 235:F227, 1978.
7. Maron, M.B., Horvath, S.W.: The marathon — A review. Med Sci Sports 10:135, 1978.
8. Rowell, L.B.: Human cardiovascular adjustments to exercise and thermal stress. Physiol Review 54:75-159, 1974.
9. Greenleaf, J.E.: Hyperthermia and exercise. Ann Rev Physiol (Environ Physiol III) 20:157, 1979.
10. Adams, W.C., Fox, R.R., Fry, A.J., et al: Thermoregulation during marathon running in cool, moderate, and hot environments, J Appl Physiol 38:1030, 1975.
11. Mitchell J.W.: Energy exchanges during exercise. In Nadel E (ed): Problems with Temperature Regulation During Exercise. New York, Academic Press, 1977, pp 11-26.
12. Costill, D.E.: Sweating, its composition and effects on body fluids. Ann Ny Acad Sci 301:160 1977.

13. Pugh, L.G.C., Corbett, J.L., Johnson, RH: Rectal temperatures, weight losses and sweat rates in marathon running. J Appl Physiol 23:345, 1967.

14. Syndham, C.H.: Heatstroke and hyperthermia in marathon runners. Ann NY Acad Sci 301:128, 1977.

15. Nadel, E: Control of sweating rate while exercising in the heat. Med Sci Sports 11:31, 1979.

16. Gisolfi, C.V., Wilson, N.C., Claxton, B.: Work-heat tolerance of distance runners. Ann NY Acad Sci 301:139, 1977.

17. Hanson, P.G.: Heat injury in runners. Phys Sports Med 1:91, 1979.

18. Gilat, T., Shibolet, S., Sohar, E.: The mechanism of heatstroke. J Trop Med 66:204-212, 1967.

19. Hubbard, R.W.: Effects of exercise in the heat on predisposition to heatstroke. Med Sci Sports 11:66, 1979.

20. Costrini, A.M., Pitt H.A., Gustafson, A.B., et. al.: Cardiovascular and metabolic manifestations of heatstroke and severe heat exhaustion. Am J Med 66:296, 1979.

21. Shibolet, W., Lancaster, M.C., Danon, Y.: Heatstroke, a review. Aviat Space Environ Med 17:280, 1976.

22. Hanson, P.G., Zimmerman, S.W.: Exertional heatstroke in novice runners. JAMA 242:154, 1979.

23. O'Donnell, T.F., Jr.: The hemodynamic and metabolic alterations associated with acute heat street injury in marathon runners. Ann NY Acad Sci 301:262, 1977.

24. Knochel, J.P.: Environmental heat illness: an eclectic review. Arch In Med 133:841, 1974.

25. Shapiro, Y., Magazanik, A., U'dassin, R., et. al.: Heat intolerance in former heatstroke patients. Ann In Med 90:813, 1979.

26. American College of Sports Medicine position statement on prevention of heat injuries during distance running. Med Sci Sports 7:VII-IX. 1975.

27. Noble, H.B., Bachman, D.: Medical aspects of distance race planning. Phys Sports Med 1:78, 1979.

28. Richards, R., Richards, D., Schofield, P.J., et. al.: Reducing the hazards in Sydney's the Sun City-to-Surf run. 1971 to 1979, Med J Aust 2:353, 1979.

CHAPTER 11

Female Runners

Lyle Micheli, M.D.

Introduction

The growing interest of women in sports competition of all kinds has attained its most dramatic expression in running and running competitions. The first Bonnie Bell Marathon championship for women only was held in Boston in 1977, with 1,329 entrants. In 1978, 4,524 women began the 10 km course, and entries were accepted until the day before the race. The 1979 Bonnie Bell championship had 5,045 entrants, and registration was closed six weeks before the race.

There are many reasons for this explosion of female runners. Women, like men, are interested in fitness as a means of improving health and preventing disease. Most current weight-reduction programs stress regular exercise in addition to caloric reduction, and even the cosmetic and beauty firms, as evidenced by the many sponsored women's races, are emphasizing the healthy and athletic look.

Whatever the reasons, more women of all ages and levels of athletic experience are taking to running, and physicians dealing with runners and running injuries are noting a dramatic increase in both the number and the variety of injuries sustained by women.[13]

Although there has been much interest in women's participation in sports in the past, two types of sports competition for women were interdicted until recently: contact sports and endurance sports, including distance running, biking, and swimming. Contact sports for women were prohibited for fear of impact injuries, and endurance sports were eliminated for fear that women, having "weaker hearts," could not sustain prolonged endurance stress.

In 1967, Kathy Switzer, the first official female entrant in the Boston Marathon, ran only after successfully evading marathon officials who attempted to physically restrain her from starting the race (which she completed). Even today, in Olympic competition, this distance bias persists. Although men compete over distances from 100 meters to the marathon distance of 43.2 kilometers, the greatest distance permitted for female competition is 3,000 meters.

One of the historic bases for this concern dates to the 1928 Olympics in Paris. Up to that time, most female competitive running was 300 meters or less. For some reason, with just three-weeks notice, an additional competition of 800 meters was added to the Olympic slate. The entrants from the various competing nations had no opportunity to train over this distance, and the results were disastrous. Only nine women completed the race, from a field of 14. People were outraged that "fair maidens" were submitted to such stress. Alarmed Olympic officials responded by permanently barring further long-distance competition for women. This interdiction has persisted even to our own times.

Female Physiology Versus Distance Running

The notion that women cannot safely sustain the cardiovascular and thermal stresses of long-distance running has been most recently addressed by a position statement of the American College of Sports Medicine (1979). In reviewing current studies of endurance training for women, it was concluded that women respond in much the same manner as men to systematic exercise training, including endurance training. Cardiorespiratory function is improved, as reflected by increased maximal oxygen uptake (VO_2 max), lowered blood pressure and pulse, and lowered percentage of body fat.[1]

In fact, Wilmore and Brown[20] studied 11 world-class female runners in 1974 and found a mean body fat of 15.2% of total body weight, which was about half that expected. In addition, the maximal oxygen uptake of this group measured 59.1 milliliters per kilogram per minute, which was much higher than that of nonrunning women, although still 16% lower than the maximal oxygen uptake of male runners of similar caliber. This difference, however, was reduced to 7.8% when expressed relative to lean body weight.

Another concern often expressed has been related to the ability of women to sustain the thermal stress of long-distance running. For many years women were thought to have less tolerance to environmental heat stress than men. That observation appeared to be particularly true when studied in association with prolonged exercise. Long-distance running carries with it the potential for significant thermal stress, even in the most favorable climatic conditions of ambient temperature and humidity. The associated water loss and hypovolemia of distance running appears to increase the susceptibility of both heat and cold injury in runners.[9]

More recent studies on thermal regulation in women have been reassuring. The observed differences in thermal stress response between men and women appear more quantitative than qualitative. Although women, on the average, require a higher skin temperature before onset of sweating, thermal equilibrium maintenance in the physically fit woman is little affected. Recent studies showed that cardiovascular fitness is an important factor in the body's ability to respond to thermal stress.[4] This relationship provides a plausible explanation for the observed differences between men and women in some of these earlier studies; in many of the studies, physically active male subjects were compared with sedentary female subjects.[19] Ironically, in one study that compared physically fit female subjects, the tested women appeared to have better heat tolerance than the control male population.[18]

When women who are trained for long-distance running are compared with matched nonathletic women, the trained women show a significantly enhanced ability to handle heat stress.[4] Thus, the properly conditioned woman apparently has an adequate ability to handle the thermal stress of long-distance running. Of course, even well-conditioned female, as well as male, runners must be wary of lack of heat acclimatization in distance running. An unusually warm and humid April Boston Marathon in 1976 took a terrible toll on northern runners who were cardiovascularly and musculoskeletally fit, but not heat acclimatized; their counterparts from warmer climates were little affected.

In summary, then, recent studies have shown that the physiologic response of highly trained women to endurance stress is similar to that of their male counterparts and far exceeds that of the untrained and physically unfit man in our society. In a further assault on historic views of male superiority and endurance fitness, Dr. Ernest Von Acken, a German physiologist, suggested that women, in addition to having a higher average percentage of fat in their body weight than do men, may have an enhanced ability to metabolize this body fat.[17] Thus, after two and a half to three hours of endurance stress, when the body supply of both muscle and liver glycogen have been depleted and lipids must be metabolized directly, the female may have a physiologic edge over the male. The main proponent of this view in our country, Dr. Joan Ullyot, herself a world-class marathoner, cites the dramatic performances of women in the ultra-marathon 50-mile competition in recent years.[17] Although this theory has yet to be proved, and although recent studies suggest that the highly trained male and female athlete are similar in their ability to metabolize lipids, such studies serve to further suggest that sex, per se, has little to do with a person's capability for high-level endurance stress. The dramatic and progressive decrease in the women's marathon record over a ten-year period reflects the untapped resources--both athletic and physiologic—in the female running population (Table 11-1).

Menstrual Problems

Studies of menstrual cycles in competitive female athletes suggested that a higher incidence of menstrual irregularity is found in these athletes than in the general population.[6] Amenorrhea and oligomenorrhea have occurred in a variety of situations characterized by loss of body weight and psychological stress.[8] Menstrual abnormalities have been recorded in ballet dancers and female athletes of all types, but endurance sports appear to have a particularly high incidence of these problems. This association may be partially explained by findings from studies being done at Harvard's Laboratory of Reproductive Science. Their studies show that lipid metabolism, and in particular, total percentage of body weight as fat, may be directly related to controlling the menstrual cycle.[8] High-endurance athletes, including women, sustain the greatest decrease in total body fat, and this factor alone may explain observations that about one third of competitive female distance runners between ages 15 and 45 experience amenorrhea or oligomenorrhea during training.[20] An additional factor may be that running long distances can result in decreased serum levels of pituitary gonadotropins in some women and may directly or indirectly contribute to menstrual irregularity.[3]

Recent studies have given further cause for concern when women who are participating in sustained heavy endurance training become amenorrheic. Drinkwater et al. found that bone density decreases significantly in these women, when compared to controls, and expressed concern that this might increase the chance of bone injury.[5] In addition, a study by Lloyd et al. suggests that women runners with menstrual abnormalities have an increased rate of musculoskeletal injury.[12] They found an injury rate of 24% in college age women athletes with irregular or absent menses, as compared to 9% for women with regular menses.

Although the long-term effects of these menstrual irregularities in young female athletes is unknown at this time, some reassurance is offered by Eriksson et al.[7] who did a recent follow-up study of competitive female swimmers in Scandinavia. These athletes were first tested in 1961 after being involved in competitive swimming for an average of 2.5 years. At follow-up, ten years later, all had discontinued high-level training and were indistinguishable physiologically from their less-athletic counterparts. Nine of the 12 had had children.

This type of information is reassuring, but we still cannot be certain that prolonged periods of endurance training accompanied by menstrual irregularities may not adversely affect subsequent gynecologic function. For the present, the safer approach would be to attempt to design training regimens and nutritional programs that avoid this development in the highly competitive female athlete.

Table 11-1

Women's Marathon Record Times (1967-1978)[16]

Year	Winning Time	Name of Winner (Country)
1967	3:15:22	Maureen Wilton (Canada)
1967	3:07:26	Anni Pede-Erdkamp (W Ger)
1970	3:02:53	Caroline Walker (US)
1971	3:01:42	Beth Bonner (US)
1971	3:00:35	Sara Berman (US)
1971	2:55:22	Beth Bonner (US)
1971	2:49:40	Cheryl Bridges (US)
1973	2:46:36	Miki Gorman (US)
1974	2:46:24	Chantal Langlace (Fr)
1974	2:43:54	Jacqueline Hansen (US)
1975	2:42:24	Liane Winters (W Ger)
1975	2:40:15	Christa Vahlensieck (W Ger)
1975	2:38:19	Jacqueline Hansen (US)
1977	2:37:57	Kim Merritt (US)
1977	2:35:15	Chantel Langlace (Fr)
1978	2:34:48	Christa Vahlensieck (W Ger)

Running Injuries

As women have become more active participants in running, some observers claim that they have a higher incidence of injuries from running than do men. Although this clinical observation has often been made by physicians caring for runners, clear support for this claim, based on sound epidemiologic information, is not available.[10, 13]

Our own experience with sports injuries in women suggest that although the rate of injury in certain women's sports programs, including running, may be relatively higher than that of similar men's programs at the initiation of such programs, this phenomenon is more likely due to undertraining and inappropriate training of a relatively greater number of under-conditioned and novice female athletes, than due to any real sexual difference in risk of injury from running.

Two examples that support this view come to mind. Four years ago, when women first began to play rugby football in the Boston area, the rate of overuse injuries from running training of these new ruggers was surprisingly high, and was actually greater than that of impact injuries sustained in this vigorous contact sport. This year, overuse injuries in these athletes are now at a minimum, reflecting, we believe, progressive improvement in the fitness level of the players, as well as a more appropriate matching of training rate and intensity.[13]

Our second example comes from the previously cited Bonnie Bell championship races held in Boston since 1977. In 1978, when we had the opportunity to provide the medical supervision for this race, seven stress fractures directly attributable to this competition were identified after the race. Last year, with more entrants, we identified only one stress fracture resulting from the race.

Running, in particular, carries with it the potential for overuse injuries from the repetitive impact between foot and ground. The female runners appeared to be sustaining more than their share of these microtrauma injuries, including stress fractures, chondromalacia patella, multiple tendinitides, bursitis about the hip and knee, plantar fasciitis, and the ubiquitous shin splints (Figure 11-1).

The occurrence of a given overuse injury in a given athlete at a specific time is usually the result of the interaction of several factors: an error in training, such as too much too fast; anatomic malalignment of the bones or joints, including the result of previous injury; imbalance of the muscle-tendon units of the extremity, either in flexibility or strength; improper equipment, such as poorly constructed running shoes; or change in running surface, such as from dirt or grass to concrete. For the past two and a half years, we have used a simple checklist, incorporating six possible causative factors, in assessing each overuse injury seen in our own Sports Medicine Clinic, and have attempted to determine which risk factors were primary or secondary in the occurrence of a given injury. (Table 11-2)

Female runners, particularly the newer ones, appear to be sustaining these injuries in high numbers. In the past, the relatively low level of athletic training and physical activity of women in our society rendered them significantly less fit. Cardiovascular fitness can be reached in a matter of months when a person is engaged in a fitness program. On the other hand, the musculoskeletal system

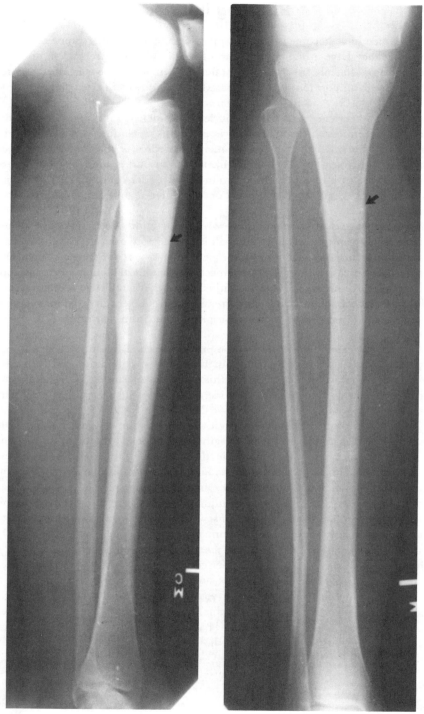

Figure 11-1. Shin splints in a young female runner who began rapid hill training over a three-week period.

and, in particular, the bones of the extremities, take much longer to remodel and strengthen themselves in response to increased physical demands.[2] Two of these overuse syndromes, in particular, are presently occurring with greater frequency in our female athletes. Although the explanation, at least in part, may be related to differences in athletic preparation and training, other factors may be working.

We did a prospective causative assessment of 53 stress fractures diagnosed in our Sports Medicine Clinic over a seven-month period (Figure 11-2). Of these fractures, 18 occurred in men and 29 in women, whereas during the same period, only 40% of our clinic population was female. We cannot know, of course, the relative population at risk during the same period, ie, the number of men and women of similar age participating in running in the Boston area, but these data suggested that women were sustaining a higher rate of stress fractures than men, in association with running.[15]

Additionally, women may have a higher risk for certain stress fractures than men. Throne and Datz found a relatively higher occurrence of pubic rami stress fractures in women than men.[16]

The other condition that is seen with a higher frequency than expected in young women athletes and runners is chondromalacia patella, or extensor mechanism stress syndrome. Once again, our ongoing prospective studies on the causative factors working in this condition often include an error in training or an associated direct blow to the extensor mechanism that initiates these symptoms. In addition, many of these athletes will have one or more of the anatomic malalignments of the lower extremity, including femoral anteversion, patella alta, genu valgum with tibia vara, or pes planus. Also associated with this condition in these women is imbalance of the muscle tendon units, especially relatively tight heelcords, perhaps reflecting the greater use by women of higher heeled shoes.

The high occurrence of chondromalacia patella in women has been suggested to be related to the greater width of the female pelvis, compared with that of the

---

Table 11-2
Risk Factors in Lower Extremity Overuse Injuries in Runners[17]

1. Training errors, including abrupt changes in intensity, duration, or frequency of training.

2. Musculotendinous imbalance—of strength, flexibility or bulk.

3. Anatomical malalignment of the lower extremities, including differences in leg lengths, abnormalities of rotation of the hips, position of the kneecap, and bow legs, knock knees, or flat feet.

4. Improper footwear: improper fit, inadequate impact absorbing material, excessive stiffness of the sole, and/or insufficient support of hindfoot.

5. Changes in running surface: concrete pavement versus asphalt, versus running track, versus dirt or grass.

6. Associated disease state of the lower extremity, including arthritis, poor circulation, old fracture, or other injury.

male.[10] We have been unable to substantiate this finding. A comparison of the distance between the femoral head and the valgus angle at the knees, taken from orthoroentgenogram studies of 25 men and 25 women from the Growth Study Clinic of our own hospital, failed to show a significant difference between male and female, particularly when further compared to body weight.

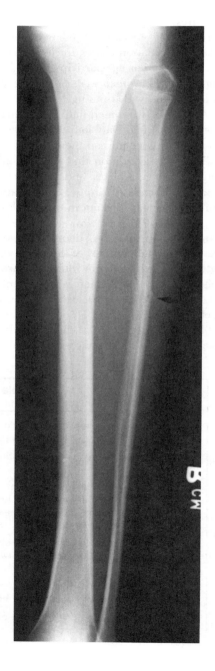

Figure 11-2. Proximal fibula stress fracture in a young female "speed" runner. Note adjacent tibial sclerosis, the probable site of a prior tibial stress fracture.

We believe that the relatively higher incidence of this complaint in the female running population is related primarily to training error and lack of long-term running conditioning. We have also been impressed with the high incidence of musculoskeletal imbalances, such as relative weakness of the quadriceps muscle, and tightness of the hamstrings and gastroc-soleus muscles in these athletes.

We have used a combined therapeutic approach in this population to manage patello-femoral stress syndromes in association with running. A specific strengthening and stretching program to compensate for musculotendinous imbalance is instituted. The program consists of static straight-leg-raising exercises done in a progressive resistive fashion with the patient in a semi-Fowler's position, supine and resting on the elbows. The exercise is done with the knee in full extension, with slow elevation of the extended leg to 45°. With this exercise, most of these patients will experience a significant decrease in pain and other complaints related to the extensor mechanism, when they are able to lift 10 to 12 pounds in three sets of 10 repetitions. We maintain this program of progressive resistive exercises until the range of 18 to 25 pounds is reached, depending on the size and age of the patient. This level of resistance is then maintained for a minimum of six months. Dynamic resistive exercise to either quadriceps or hamstrings are not begun until the static straight-leg-raising program can be done without pain and without quadriceps lag in the range of 15 to 18 pounds.

In those patients with significant anatomic malalignment, we have also used orthotic devices combining forefoot and hindfoot posting to alter the ground-foot impact. We are uncertain as yet whether these orthotic devices serve primarily to compensate for anatomic malalignment, to provide additional heel cushioning, or to alter the time course of impact absorption by the lower extremity. We use only flexible orthotics for any condition in the female distance runner. Using this combined approach of exercises with or without orthotic devices, we have been able to successfully manage more than 90% of our young women patients with patello-femoral stress syndromes.[10]

Our own clinical experience with women's running injuries suggests that careful attention to slow and progressive training, in addition to instruction in running technique, is of prime importance in preventing these injuries. Next in importance is increasing the muscular strength and endurance of the back and lower extremities by means of resistive weight training and progressively intensified running training. As important, despite the somewhat increased general flexibility of women as compared with that of men, is attention to improving the flexibility of the lower extremities in these female runners through systematic stretching exercises. Although the overall flexibility of women may in general be greater than that of men, the gastroc-soleus mechanism in particular appears to be tighter in the woman than the man, and requires special attention in the female runner.

REFERENCES

1. American College of Sports Medicine: opinion statement; the participation of the female athlete in long- distance running. Med Sci Sports 11:NO4 (Winter, 1979) suppl ix- xi.
2. Carter D, Spengler DM: Mechanical properties and composition of cortical bone. Clin Orth Rel Res 135:192-217, 1978.

3. Dale E, Gerloch DH, Martin DE, et al: Physical fitness profiles and reproductive physiology of the female distance runner. Phys Sports Med 83-95, 1979.

4. Drinkwater, BL: Physiological responses of women to exercise. Exercise Sports Sci Rev 1:125-153, 1973.

5. Drinkwater BL, Nilson K, Chestnut CH, Brenner WJ, Shoinholtz S, and Southworth RB: Bone mineral content of amenorrheic and eumenorrheic atheletes. NEJM 311:277-281, 1984.

6. Erdelyi GJ: Effects of exercise on the menstrual cycle. Phys Sports Med 4:79-81, 1976.

7. Eriksson BO, Engstrom I, Karlberg P, et al: Long- term effect of previous swim training in girls. A 10-year follow-up of the "Girl Swimmers." Acta Paediatr Scand 67:285-292, 1978.

8. Frisch RE, McArthur JW: Menstrual cycles: Fatness as a determinant of minimum weight for height necessary for their maintenance of or onset. Science 185:949-951, 1974.

9. Gilofolvi CV, et al: Work-heat tolerance of distance runners. Ann NY Acad Sci 301:139-50, 1977.

10. Haycock CE, Gillette JV: Susceptibility of women athletes in to injury. Myths vs. Reality JAMA 236:163-165, 1976.

11. Kuscsik N: The history of women's participation in the marathon. Ann NY Acad Sci 301:862-876, 1977.

12. Lloyd T, Triantafyllou SJ, Baker ER, Houts PS, Whiteside JS, Kalenak A, and Stumpf PG: Women athletes with menstrual irregularity have increased musculoskeletal injuries. Med Sci Sports Exercise. 18:374-379, 1986

13. Micheli LJ: Injuries in female athletes. Surgical Rounds 44-55, May 1979.

14. Micheli LJ, Santopietro FJ, Gerbino, PG et al: Etiologic assessment of overuse stress fractures in athletes. Nova Scotia Med Bulletin, April June 1980, pp. 43-47.

15. Micheli LJ, Stanitski CL: Lateral retinacular release for parapatellar knee pain. Am J Sports Med (in press, 1981).

16. Thorne, Datz FL: Pelvic stress fracture in female runners. Clin Nucl Med 11:828-829, 1986.

17. Ullyot J: Woman's secret weapon: Fat. Runner World 22-23, 1974.

18. Weinman KP, Slabochova EM, Bernauer T, et al: Reactions of men and women to repeated exposure to humid heat. J Appl Physiol 22:533-538, 1967.

19. Wells CL: Sexual differences in heat stress response — do they exist? Phys Sports Med 5:78-90, 1977.

20. Wilmore JH, Brown HC: Physiological profiles of women distance runners. Med Sci Sports 6:178-81, 1974.

CHAPTER 12

Neurophysiology of Stretching

William D. Stanish, M.D., FRCS(C), FACS
Cheryl L. Hubley-Kozey, MSc

Introduction

Historically, dancers and athletes have used techniques of stretching to enhance flexibility. These elite performers were intuitively aware that inadequate precompetition warm-up, including stretching, would impair body movement. Also they perceived, albeit unscientifically, that improper stretching of soft tissues could lead to early fatigue, muscle soreness, and frequently injury. The pre-performance ritual of muscle stretching of the ballerina has persisted to this day and clearly remains of unquestioned value.

The scientific arena of sports medicine, however, has approached stretching for flexibility differently. In the past, high school, collegiate, and professional athletic teams customarily spent relatively brief periods for pregame warm-up. Furthermore, many athletes were sometimes totally idle during specific games or practice, but were expected to prepare from a muscle-tendon standpoint when summoned for action. Indeed, performances were hampered and injuries were frequent when these essentially unprepared athletes were sent into competition. Epidemiologically, soft-tissue strains or pulls are still the most common injuries seen by sports medicine physicians.

The increasing prominence of sports medicine and sports science in the past 15 years has generated an attempt to provide a more scientific understanding of athletic performance and injury prevention. Fundamental to this renewed, and sometimes political, quest for enhancing athletic output, has been research into the area of muscle and tendon mechanics. These moving units were, and still are, studied under varying static and dynamic circumstances, so that we may understand more fully the traditionally appreciated value of warm-up and flexibility training. Of course, as with most research of this type, a proverbial Pandora's box has been opened. As more answers were sought regarding the science of stretching, more questions arose. Even now, only the surface is scratched in our attempt to add a scientific basis for stretching to enhance flexibility.

Contemporary research in sports science has defined and elucidated satisfactorily how best to build strength and power. Comparable definitions, however, do not exist for stretching. The collective reviews of Holland[1] and Harris[2] were valuable in pointing out the discrepancies in the research, but certain consistencies did exist. For instance, enhanced flexibility was found to be sport-specific, amplifying the fact that some athletes could be extremely flexible through the shoulders but very tight in the hip flexors and ankle regions. These excellent reviews also dispelled the concept that weightlifters became muscle-bound and sacrificed flexibility. Indeed, weightlifters and wrestlers have been reported to be remarkably flexible at certain joints,[3] while gymnasts are more flexible than age-matched normals only on selected measures.[4]

In this chapter, we will discuss the practical techniques of stretching for flexibility and also present the current knowledge on the basic physiology of muscle and tendon under stress. Many points are theoretical; however, the ingredients of this chapter are the summations of research to date on the subject of flexibility, augmented with personal clinical experience.

Muscle-Tendon Join

At Rest

The classical macrostructure of muscle has been more than adequately described in textbooks and manuscripts. Little material, however, is available on those structural elements within muscle that are responsible for its elastic properties. In 1938, A.V. Hill suggested, by theory, that muscle possesses two components responsible for its elastic recoil characteristics; an actively contracting component (CC) and a passive elastic element located in series (SEC).[5] (Hill described the mechanics of the active muscle and suggested that the tendon possesses elastic properties in series and this elastic characteristic is a result of the cross-bridges between actin and myosin). (Figure 12-1)

Further research demonstrated that there was a component of elasticity, acting in parallel (PEC) with the contracting machinery, which is said to be present in the sarcolemma and fascia.[6-9]

An excellent review article by Chapman points out the difficulty in attempting to anatomically locate these elastic structures, and concludes that they are mechanical concepts which describe the behavior of muscle.[10] They are,

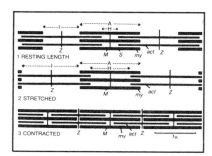

Figure 12-1. Actin-myosin crossbridges.

however, valuable in allowing us to discuss many of the important concepts relating to stretching. (Figure 12-2)

The muscle at rest can be clinically appreciated as a soft tissue with a constant desire to shorten. Athletic activities producing muscle hypertrophy will predictably produce transient, and sometimes permanent, muscle contracture, coupled with the subjective feeling of tightness. It has been our experience that if contraction is allowed to persist, the contracted soft, tissue muscle and tendon will be susceptible to injury when flexibility is demanded in the athletic challenge. Stolov and Thompson demonstrated that there is adaptive shortening of the tissue if it remains in a shortened position.[11] There is also evidence which supports the theory that the muscle tendon unit is less likely to break down if its inherent characteristics of elasticity are consistently trained through stretching exercises.

Tendons have been singularly neglected in much of the clinical and research material related to flexibility training. Tendon injuries, however, are far more frequent than intrinsic muscle injuries. Cross-sectioning of the tendon reveals progressively smaller subunits decreasing in diameter from the tendon bundle to the fibril, microfibril, and, the smallest subunit, trophocollagen. The tendon fascicle is composed of many fibers and, in the unstretched condition, it has a pleated, wavy appearance that disappears when the fascicle is stretched.

Experimentally, when a tendon is stretched, the resultant stress (ie, the load over a cross-sectional area) is not a simple linear function of the strain (ie, the increase in length over the original length × 100) applied, as can be seen in Figure 12-3. In the primary region, elongation occurs with little increase in load. This is associated with the wavy collagen fibers straightening out. As the fibers become oriented in the direction of loading, there is an increase in tissue stiffness, and the stress versus strain relationship becomes linear. Following this point, there is progressive tissue failure and damage begins to occur.

The quality of the elastic compliance of a muscle-tendon unit is proportional

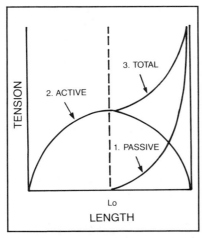

Figure 12-2. Force-length relationship.

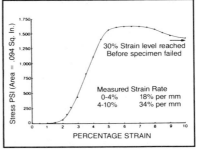

Figure 12-3. Tendon stress-strain curve.

to the ratio of muscle to tendon in the contractural unit. For example, experiments with dogs have demonstrated the higher level of elasticity in the sartorius, which is principally muscle along its entire length, with very little tendon, in contrast with the gastrocnemius, which has a long tendinous component. It is beyond the scope of this chapter to discuss in depth the complex structure and mechanical properties of tendon. The interested reader is referred to the works of Harkness[12] and Viidik.[13,14]

Clinically, as previously stated, we have noted greater numbers of tendon injuries than intrinsic muscle breakdowns, suggesting that muscle, with its superior inherent compliance, is less likely than tendon to be disrupted under comparable stress.

In Action

The literature abounds with reviews of the mechanics of concentric, isometric, and eccentric modes of exercise. Nevertheless, only a few scientists have attempted to elucidate the behavior of the elastic components of the muscle-tendon unit under varying conditions. The mechanisms and techniques of improving muscle-tendon compliance are examined here under the assumption that the neurochemical status of the contractural unit is normal. The specifics of muscle contraction will be discussed later in this chapter.

When muscle shortens during concentric movement, positive work and heat are predictable byproducts. During that type of muscle shortening, the elastic components (set in parallel, and vital to muscle compliance) shorten simultaneously. On the other hand, when the muscle-tendon is isometrically or eccentrically active at lengths greater than rest length, the PEC becomes strained like a spring and, in the latter case, the muscle is said to be performing negative work. During isometric activation there is not external work being done. In all three types of activation, the SEC, during an active lengthening (eccentric) contraction has been associated with storage of energy in this component. It is said that this stored energy could be used to enhance the force output during a concentric contraction immediately following the eccentric activation.[15,16]

Enhanced flexibility achieved through stretching allows the muscle-tendon unit greater properties of compliance. For a given load, this greater compliance allows the muscle to deform and recoil, achieving the ideals of improved work without structural breakdown.

Tension produced during a muscle contraction is transmitted via the tendon to the limb of its insertion. The tension produced is inversely related to the velocity of shortening. During isometric contraction, when the velocity of shortening is zero, the tension is greater for the same activation level than that produced concentrically. Although the entire range of velocities have not been tested, during eccentric activations the force generated is higher for the same level of activation. (Figure 12-4) The maximum concentric and isometric tensions are well below the tensile strength of tendon. Kamen reported values for eccentric tension production of 6%-11% greater than for maximum isometric contractions.[17] Harkness proposed that eccentric loads may be as much as twice maximum isometric values, if applied rapidly.[12] Therefore, neither concentric nor isometric contractions appear to be likely causes of tendon breakdown.

Similarly, passive stretch of a tendon, while the muscle is relaxed within physiological limits, cannot be considered damaging to the tendon, because the resultant strain is accommodated by the rather remarkable extensibility of relaxed muscle.

The Practical Value of Enhanced Flexibility Through Stretch

Clearly, enhanced flexibility is an important characteristic for certain athletes to achieve superior levels of athletic performance. Simultaneous with the desire for enhancing athletic performances, concern is growing over the upsurge of injuries secondary to recreational and sport challenges. The sport medicine literature is replete with reports of epidemiological injury profiles of various sports. Common to all these statistical analyses is the fact that soft-tissue injuries are most frequently encountered by sport physicians and thus are a major concern. Compounding the issue is the undeniable fact of body physiology that "form follows function" and that complete rest for an injured athlete often leads to devastating atrophy. Also, surgeons are recognizing the limitations of surgical intervention in the management of soft-tissue injuries that are commonly microscopic.

Although a causal relationship has not been established there is evidence to suggest that the risk of soft-tissue injuries to the muscle-tendon unit can be reduced with structured flexibility conditioning programs. Various types of stretching programs have been devised and will be described later; however, the common denominator of them all is enhancing flexibility.

Once a muscle or tendon has been injured, the pathophysiology of soft-tissue repair is always the same, with collagen being the final byproduct. For a high-level athlete, that circumstance is fundamentally less than ideal because of the lack of inherent elasticity within the proliferating fibrous scar.

Thus, our practice has been to use graduated stretching techniques during the post-injury rehabilitating program for muscle and tendon trauma. (Figure 12-5)

Flexibility training is certainly not the panacea in the prevention or treatment of muscle and tendon injuries. Nevertheless, coupled with astute progressive strength retraining and muscle rebalancing, we can avoid many of these common soft- tissue injuries.

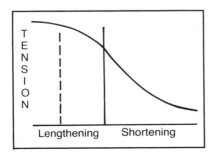

Figure 12-4. Force-velocity relationship.

Physiology of Stretching

A clear scientific explanation of the physiology of stretching continues to elude contemporary research. Many credible laboratories have worked tediously to elucidate the mechanics of stretching, in an attempt to offer practical advice and explanations regarding the most effective techniques of enhancing flexibility. Their findings somewhat clarify the physiology of stretching for flexibility.

Histologically, the muscle includes the extrafusal component which can be large or relatively small, depending on the task of that particular muscle. Simplistically, muscles are essentially divided into two fiber types which, from a laboratory standpoint, are differentiated by histochemical means. From a clinical standpoint, those muscle fibers that are slow-twitch in nature are extremely high in aerobic potential, and carry the appropriate aerobic enzymatic package. The second fiber type, which strains according to its enzyme, is identified as being critical to anaerobic function and is fast twitch in nature.

These muscles are fired and controlled by complex neural influences. They work in tandem with the intrafusal muscle spindle that controls muscle tone. This unit sets the muscle in readiness for work. The intrafusal system conducts information to the central nervous system through the afferent unit. This unit is extremely responsive to passive stretch. As a passive stretch of the extrafusal muscle system occurs, the intrafusal system is triggered and the afferent unit stimulates an alpha efferent to facilitate contraction of the extrafusal system, with a complementary inhibition to the antagonist muscle. The intrafusal system is complemented by a type 2 afferent that, paradoxically, conducts at a slower or weaker rate and coaxes the antagonist to fire, thus inhibiting the extrafusal agonist system. The intrafusal system, having been stretched, is encouraged back into readiness by the gamma efferent system. If, for any reason, the gamma

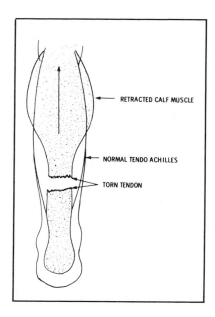

Figure 12-5. Tendon rupture.

system is obliterated, then muscle tone is rapidly reduced, and no reflex (primary monosynaptic) can occur. (Figure 12-6)

Other structures within muscle units that are responsible for muscle tone are the Golgi tendon organs (GTO). The GTO exist in series and require a major effort or contraction (usually voluntary) to be stimulated. They have an extremely high threshold and respond most effectively with a voluntary contraction of significant magnitude. As the extrafusal system contracts, the GTO fire and relax the extrafusal complex and simultaneously fire the antagonist system. If the tension is too great, then the GTO fire simultaneously to the agonist and the antagonist muscle groups, yielding dual inhibition to both these units. The entire muscle complex will reduce its electromyographic activity.

First it is generally agreed that the elongation of the muscle-tendon unit should be the primary objective of a flexibility training program. This elongation will allow the joint to move through the range of motion necessary to perform the skills of a sport with undue stress on these tissues. Second, individuals have been concerned with strengthening the muscle-tendon unit through various forms of stretching. The latter can be achieved through muscle activation, which loads the muscle-tendon unit. Eccentric contractions are advocated because the overall unit is lengthening and the tension generated is higher than that produced during a concentric, isometric,[18] or passive exercise. Since many injuries are associated with eccentric activations, the goal is to increase the strength of this unit, to withstand these very high forces.

To address the elongation of the muscle-tendon unit, we must first examine the factors which resist this elongation. The muscle can actively resist a length increase by generating tension via the contractile component.[19] This resistance can be effectively eliminated by insuring that the muscle is completely relaxed, and many stretching techniques attempt to achieve this total relaxation.

The PEC of the muscle can also resist length changes via passive tension in

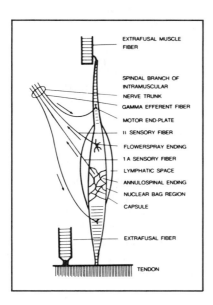

EXTRAFUSAL MUSCLE FIBER

SPINDAL BRANCH OF INTRAMUSCULAR NERVE TRUNK

GAMMA EFFERENT FIBER

MOTOR END-PLATE

II SENSORY FIBER

FLOWERSPRAY ENDING

1 A SENSORY FIBER

LYMPHATIC SPACE

ANNULOSPINAL ENDING

NUCLEAR BAG REGION

CAPSULE

EXTRAFUSAL FIBER

TENDON

Figure 12-6. Neural components.

these components upon lengthening. (Figure 12-2) This resistance can be altered by changing the tissue compliance and attempting to move the passive tension curve to the right.

The muscle-tendon unit has been described as having both plastic and elastic properties resulting in the ability to recoil (elastic) or deform permanently (plastic).[20] The type of flexibility exercises employed will depend on the identified objective for the athlete in a particular sport.

Basically, there are three stretching methods utilized — ballistic (bouncing), static, and Proprioceptive Neuromuscular Facilitation (PNF)-with many variations of each presented in the literature. Most researchers report no significant differences between the ballistic and static techniques for increasing flexibility, usually measured as joint range of motion.[21,22] The static techniques are usually advocated, as there is less likelihood of evoking a strong stretch-reflex response because the movement is performed slowly. The muscle spindle evokes a muscle excitation in response to a length increase and an increase in the rate of change in length. Therefore, the ballistic techniques would evoke a much larger reflex response because of the stretch and speed of strength. Also, the force is controlled more easily during static stretching than during the ballistic techniques, which rely primarily on momentum to generate a stretch.

The PNF techniques have been shown to be superior for increasing flexibility in some, but not all, published studies.[23-27] Recent works have cast doubt on their superior effectiveness and whether these techniques are, in fact, safe methods of stretching.[19-27] Moore and Hutton found high electromyograms (EMGs) from the muscle while it was being stretched.[26] The basic theory underlying this technique is that the contraction will result in maximum relaxation of the muscle during stretch due to reciprocal inhibition. It has been demonstrated however, that an after discharge exists[28,29] which would be reflected in the high EMG recordings from the stretched muscle as reported by Moore and Hutton. The contract-relax-antagonist-contract technique was associated with the highest level of EMG, and subjects reported pain during the stretch, as well.[26] It should be stated that pain is the body's mechanism for protection against injury and thus caution should be employed when using these techniques.

The problem with all of the above techniques is that the effects are lost shortly after the stretching ends indicating very little retention. This suggests that the type of deformation is mostly elastic, because the muscle returns to its original length after the stretching force is removed with little permanent deformation taking place.

Warren and Lehmann showed that low static forces, applied for a long duration to heated tissue, resulted in a permanent deformation of the muscle-tendon unit and, in particular, the connective tissue structures.[30-31] The increased tissue temperature is necessary to increase compliance, thus facilitating a length change with minimal risk of injury.

Many papers have addressed the effects of heat on flexibility measures, with conflicting results.[30-35] The application of the heat in some of these studies was superficial and did not necessarily heat the muscle-tendon unit. In general, those studies that attempted to increase the temperature of the muscle-tendon unit also showed an increase in flexibility, possibly relating to enhanced tissue compliance. This effect is also not retained and is lost once the tissue temperature returns to normal; therefore the stretch in association with the increase in temperature is very important.[35]

There is a great deal of practical information contained in the above summary of the literature, which can be easily transformed into advice for training the flexibility of an athlete. Before any program is implemented, however, the objectives of the program must be clearly identified. It may be single or multifaceted and, in either case, the program must reflect the needs of the athlete within the sport.

If the goal is to strengthen the muscle-tendon unit, then concentric, eccentric, or isometric exercises will load, and thus strengthen, this unit. Eccentric exercises can be used to produce greater forces for the same activation level. In order for this type of exercise to be effective, the person should not be able to lift or move the load concentrically. Care must be taken during eccentric exercise to ensure that the load is not in excess of the tissues strength capabilities.

An individual may need to increase flexibility in order to perform a skill without undue stresses on the muscle-tendon tissues. He may have to focus on a permanent deformation and movement of the passive tension curve to the right. In order to achieve this he should apply low forces for long periods of time to a heated muscle-tendon unit. Such a program may be necessary following injury, after a long layoff from participation, or if extreme flexibility is necessary to perform a skill. If active tension is resisting the length increase necessary to perform a skill, then muscle relaxation techniques should be employed. Relaxation techniques, such as static stretching or the PNF techniques that do not contract the antagonist to stretch that agonist, should be of benefit.

Preparticipation or training to maintain a certain level of flexibility should focus first on heating the muscle-tendon unit to increase its compliance. The easiest method of achieving this goal is through an active warm-up, although there are other methods of heating deep tissues. Second, static stretching for a short duration (30 sec to 1 min) or various PNF techniques could be employed to maintain the elasticity of the muscle-tendon. It must be repeated that the gains of these techiques are lost shortly after the exercises are completed. They must therefore be performed frequently to ensure maintenance of the desired degree of flexibility.

Regardless of the objective or the type of exercise used, the athlete's discomfort should be closely monitored, and the entire process must be totally pain free.

REFERENCES

1. Holland GJ: The physiology of flexibility: A review of the literature. Kinesiology Review: 49-62, 1968.
2. Harris ML: Flexibility. Physical Therapy 49(6):591- 601, 1969.
3. Leighton L: A study of the effect of progressive weight training on flexibility. Physical Mental Rebah 28:101, 1964.
4. Kirby RL, Simms FC, Symington VJ, Garber JB: Flexibility and musculoskeletal symptomatology in female gymnasts and age matched controls. Am J of Sports Med 9:160-164, 1981.
5. Hill AV: The heat shortening and the dynamic constance of muscle. Proc Royal Soc B 126:136-195, 1938.

6. Hill AV: The series elastic component of muscle. Proc Royal Soc B 137:270-280, 1950.

7. Hill AV: The mechanics of active muscle. Proc Royal Soc B 141:104-117, 1953.

8. Huxley AF, Simmons RM: Mechanical properties of the cross-bridges of frog striated muscle. J Physiol London 218:59P- 60P, 1971.

9. Hill DK: Tension to interaction between the sliding filaments of resting striated muscle. The effect of stimulation. J Physiol London 199:367-684, 1968.

10. Chapman AE: The mechanical properties of human muscle. In Turjung RL (ed): ESSR Vol. 13, McMillan Publishing Co. New York, pp. 443-501, 1985.

11. Stolov WC, Thompson SC: Soleus immobilization contracture in young and old rats. Arch Phys Med and Rehab 60:556-557, 1979.

12. Harkness RD: Mechanical properties of collagenous tissues. In Gould BS (ed): Treatise on Collagen, Vol. 2, pt A. Academic Press, pp. 247-310, 1968.

13. Viidik A: On the correlation between structures and mechanical function of soft connective tissues. Verh Anat Ges 72:75-89, 1978.

14. Viidik A: The effect of training on the tensile strength of isolated rabbit tendons. Scand Plastic Surg 1:141- 147, 1967.

15. Cavagna G, Sabiene F, Margaria R: Effect of negative work in the amount of positive work performed by an isolated muscle. J of Appl Physiol 20(1):157-158, 1965.

16. Asmussen E, Bonde-Peterson F: Storage and elastic energy in skeletal muscle in man. Acta Physiol Scand 91:385-392, 1974.

17. Kamen G: Serial isometric contraction under imposed myostatic stretch conditions in high strength and low strength men. European J Applied Physiology 41:73-82, 1979.

18. Komi PV: Measurement of force-velocity relationship in human muscle under concentric and eccentric contractions. In Karger S (ed): Biomechanics III pp. 224-229, 1973.

19. Markos PD: Ipsilateral and contralateral effects of proprioceptive neuromuscular facililation technique on hip motion and electormyographic activity. Physical Therapy 59:1366-1373, 1979.

20. Sapega AA, Quedenfield TC, Mayer RA, Butler RA: Biophysical factors in range of motion exercises. The Physical and Sports Med 9:57-65, 1981.

21. Logan GA, Egstrom: Effects of slow and fast stretching on the sacro-femoral angle. J Assoc for Phys and Mental Rehab 15:85-89, 1961.

22. DeVries HA: Evaluation of static stretching procedures for improvement of flexibility. Res Quart 33:222-229, 1962.

23. Holt LE, Kaplin HM, Okita T, Hoshiko M: The influence of antagonistic contraction in hip position of the responses of agonistic muscle. Arch Physical Med Rehabil 50:279-283 passim, 1969.

24. Tanigawa MC: Comparison of hold relax procedure and passive mobilization on increasing muscle length. Phys Ther 52:725-735, 1972.

25. Hartley-O'Brien SJ: Six mobilization exercises for active range of hip flexion. Res Quart for Exercise and Sport 51:725-735, 1972.

26. Moore MA, Hutton RS: Electromyographic investigation of muscle stretching techniques. Med Sci in Sports and Exer 12:322-329, 1980.

27. Williford HN, Smith JF: A comparison of proprioceptive neuromuscular facilitation and static stretching techniques. Amer Corr Ther J 39(2):30-33, 1985.

28. Smith JL, Hutton RS, Eldred E: Post contraction changes in sensitivity of muscle afferents to static and dynamic stretch. Brain Res 78:193-202, 1974.

29. Suzuki S, Hutton RS: Postcontractile motoneuromal discharge produced by muscle afferent activation. Med Sci in Sports and Exerc 12:322-329, 1976.

30. Lehmann JF, Masock AJ, Warren CG, Koblanski IN: Effect of therapeutic temperatures on tendon extensibility. Arch Phys Med and Rehab 51:481-487, 1970.

31. Warren CG, Lehmann JF, Koblanski JN: Heat and stretch procedures: An evaluation using rat tail tendon. Arch Phys Med and Rehab 57:122-126, 1976.

32. Henricson AS, Fredricksson K, Persson I, Pereira R, Rostedt Y, Westlin NE: The effect of heat and stretching on the range of hip motion. JOSPT 6:110-115, 1984.

33. Wiktorsson-Moller M, Obert B, Ekstrand J, Gillquist J: Effects of warming up, massage and stretching on range of motion and muscle strength in the lower extremity. Am J Sport Med 11:249- 252, 1983.

34. Hubley CL, Kozey JW, Stanish WD: The effects of static stretching exercises and stationary cycling on range of motion of the hip joint. JOSPT 6:104-109, 1984.

35. Williford HN, East JB, Smith FH, Burry LA: Evaluation of warm-up for improvement in flexibility. Am J of Sport Med 14(4):316-319, 1986.

CHAPTER 13

Flexibility Conditioning for Running

Virginia B. Davis, MA, PT

Introduction

The sport of jogging can no longer be considered just a fad, as it has captured the fancy of hundreds of thousands of loyal enthusiasts over the past ten years. Persons who were previously uninterested in physical activity of sports have taken to the city sidewalks, parks, and country backroads. Some of these active participants were one-time high school or collegiate athletes, but the vast majority have never before participated in athletic endeavors to any great extent. They are encouraged in their sport by each other and by the proliferation of magazine "how-to" articles. Unfortunately, there seem to be as many different "how-to's" as there are authors, and the guidelines purported are often not founded on sound physiological principles.

It is no wonder, then, that physician offices and physical therapy clinics are filled with seemingly healthy persons with a variety of musculoskeletal complaints. It is the feeling of this writer that many runners' and joggers' injuries may be related to inadequate preparation for the sport, most significantly inadequate flexibility. In fact, we have found that 92% of the injured runners seen in our physical therapy clinic exhibited one or more muscle inflexibilities that may have been the cause of, or contributed to, the runner's injury. In a review of 140 injured runners referred by physicians for physical therapy, 90% were found to have hamstring muscle tightness, and 93% were found to have gastrocnemius muscle tightness. Combined tightness in both hamstring and gastrocnemius muscles was found in 86% of those referred, independent of referring diagnosis.

Types of Stretching

Traditionally, flexibility routines have centered around ballistic and static types of stretching, however, routines utilizing the principles of proprioceptive neuromuscular facilitation are receiving much attention by physical therapists.

Ballistic Stretching

This type of stretching is characterized by bouncing or quick, jerking movements in an attempt to produce maximum muscle lengthening. Physiologically, however, this method has been demonstrated sometimes to do more to impede motion than to improve it. The muscle to be lengthened is quickly stretched, thus invoking a stretch reflex that then produces a recoil, or shortening reaction, in the muscle, which actually reduces its overall length.

Static Stretching

This method of stretching emphasizes a gradual lengthening of a muscle group in an attempt to gain maximum length with as little accompanying muscle activity as possible, thus avoiding possible reflex stimulation of the involved muscle.

Neither of the above techniques use central mechanisms to achieve maximum muscle lengthening for improved flexibility. Types of stretching that are founded on neurophysiological principles are as follows.

Proprioceptive Neuromuscular Facilitation (PNF)

3-S Stretching: The muscles to be stretched are first contracted isometrically, in a lengthened position, followed by concentric contraction of the opposite muscle group, along with slight assistance from a partner. This method utilizes the reciprocal innervation and contraction inhibition described in detail by Holt in his monograph "Scientific Stretching for Sport."[1] Stretching exercises, as presented by Holt, require the assistance of a partner. A study conducted by Holt demonstrated that his 3-S approach is superior to both ballistic and static stretching methods.[1] Athletes rapidly increased flexibility when exercises were carried out exactly as described by Holt, with participants working in pairs.

Combo Stretching: This method combines the gradual lengthening of the muscle, along with simultaneous isometric contraction of the opposing muscle group, to produce relaxation in muscles being stretched, and further increase in muscle length. This method utilizes the neurological principle of reciprocal innervation, as described by Kabat[3] and further explained by Knott and Voss in their book "Proprioceptive Neuromuscular Facilitation."[4] Assistance of a partner is not necessary with this method. Certainly some muscles cannot be adequately stretched using PNF techniques without the assistance of a partner (hip flexors, low back extensors), but many runners or joggers prepare for their sport alone. The Combo stretching method has been developed out of the need for runners to be able to stretch independently, while taking advantage of central mechanisms to achieve maximum flexibility.

Gross Assessment of Flexibility for Running

The discussion of the importance of flexibility and stretching exercises for runners would be incomplete without mention of the simple tests that may be utilized by the clinician or athlete to determine muscle tightness. The following flexibility tests are utilized as a part of our runners' evaluation. Runners found to have muscular tightness are advised to follow a flexibility development program. Those runners who are already flexible are encouraged to maintain their flexibility by stretching before and after running. Inflexible runners who hesitate in embarking on a flexibility program while running increased distances and/or faster times will almost certainly incur injury at some point in their running career.

Flexibility Testing

1. CALF MUSCLES

A. Gastrocnemius Muscle: Runner is lying down with knee fully extended. The foot is placed by the examiner in a neutral talar position and then dorsiflexed maximally by the runner with assistance of the examiner (neutral position must be maintained). Goniometric measurement is taken with one arm of the goniometer along the fibula, the other along the fifth metatarsal (Figure 13-1). Normal dorsiflexion in this position is 8° or more. Less than 8° indicates gastrocnemius muscle tightness.

B. Soleus Muscle: This test is identical to test 1A with the following change: the runner's knee is flexed to approximately 45° (Figure 13-2). Normal dorsiflexion in this position is 15° or more. Less than 15° indicates soleus muscle tightness.

2. HAMSTRING MUSCLES

Runner is lying supine with one leg maintained in extension at hip and knee while the leg being tested is flexed to 90° at the hip and knee. The runner then maintains 90° hip flexion while the examiner passively extends the knee until full knee extension of 0° is achieved or until extension is limited by hamstring muscle length. Neutral hip rotation must be maintained throughout the test. The runner's foot may be in plantar-flexion. Goniometric measurement is taken with

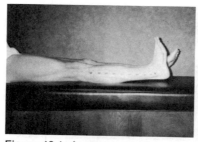

Figure 13-1. Assessment of gastrocnemius muscle.

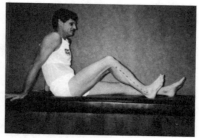

Figure 13-2. Assessment of soleus muscle flexibility.

one arm of the goniometer along the femur in line with the greater trochanter and the other along the fibula in line with the fibular head and the lateral malleolus (Figure 13-3). If the runner's knee is flexed more than 10° with the hip maintained at 90°, hamstring muscle tightness exists.

3. COMBINED HAMSTRING AND CALF MUSCLES

This test is identical to test 2 for the hamstring muscles with the following change: the runner is asked to maximally dorsiflex the foot before the examiner passively extends the knee (Figure 13-4). This maximal dorsiflexion is maintained throughout the test (Figure 13-4A). Goniometric measurement of more than 15° of knee flexion demonstrates combined hamstring and calf muscle tightness.

4. HIP FLEXOR MUSCLES

The runner is asked to lie supine with both knees flexed over the edge of the examining table. One hip and knee is flexed maximally to the runner's chest while the low back and opposite thigh are maintained flat on the table (Figure 13-5). Hip flexor tightness is measured with the low back maintained flat on the table and one arm of the goniometer in line with the lumbar spine and the other in line with the femur. Hip flexor tightness exists if the thigh flexes up from the table while the low back is maintained in the flattened position.

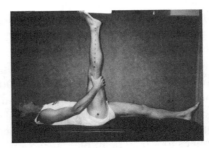

Figure 13-3. Assessment of hamstring muscle flexibility.

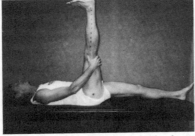 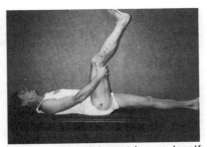

Figure 13-4 and Figure 13-4A. Assessment of combined hamstring and calf muscle flexibility.

5. ADDUCTOR MUSCLES

The runner sits on the floor, back supported flat against a wall. Both hips and knees are flexed and soles of feet are placed together. Heels to be placed approximately six inches from the body. Let knees fall apart toward floor as much as possible. Flexibility is normal if the distance between the outside of the knee and the floor is three inches or less (Figure 13-6).

Techniques of Stretching

One does not prepare for running simply by running, just as a football player would not take to the field for a season opener without benefit of off-season training. A person who does not prepare for running by a program designed to promote muscle balance for strength and flexibility may be asking for a great many aches and pains due to musculoskeletal imbalance.

Central mechanisms play a paramount role in the fundamental aspects of exercise. Physical therapists have long used neurological treatment techniques in their practices, but only recently have these techniques been espoused for use in athletic conditioning.

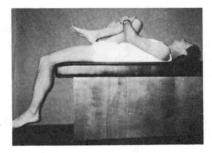

Figure 13-5 . Assessment of hip flexor tightness.

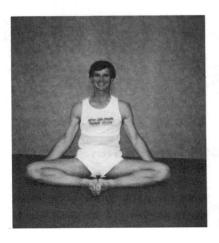

Figure 13-6. Assessment of adductor muscle flexibility.

The specific techniques of stretching to be illustrated in this text incorporate neurological principles to promote maximal muscle lengthening. Exercises have been designed specifically to meet the needs of runners. These exercises have been used in our physical therapy and running clinics in New Orleans as a part of our program to prepare individuals for running, by promoting the full range of motion necessary to prevent injury.

The limiting factor for flexibility is often the length of the muscles that are antagonistic to a specific movement. For example, if one first flexes the hip maximally with the knee fully extended and then flexes the knee, additional hip flexion may be appreciated. The initial hip flexion limitation was due to the limited length of the two-joint hamstring muscles.

The converse is also true and may be appreciated by the runner who flexes his hip after toe-off, with his knee simultaneously flexed. As the knee is extended towards heel strike, knee extension or length of stride may be inhibited by the amount of hip flexion when limited hamstring flexibility exists. Inadequate hamstring flexibility in this instance may prove to be a mechanism for injury to the hamstring itself, the low back, the hip, the knee, the lower leg, or even the foot. This illustrates the importance of examining joint motions occurring simultaneously during running when evaluating flexibility.

We have found that many running problems center around the low back, hip flexors and adductors, hamstrings, and foot plantar flexors.

Inflexibility in muscle groups may contribute not only to injury of the "tight" muscle or muscle group but also to injury of opposing or adjacent muscles and bony structures that may try to compensate for the inflexibilites. For example, inflexibility in the gastrocnemius muscle (a two-joint muscle) may promote plantar fasciatis, "shin splints" or medial knee pain while hamstring tightness may promote patello-femoral pain, medial or lateral knee pain, hip, or low back pain. Muscular inflexibility in one or more muscle groups may be a factor in the alteration of the biomechanics of the lower extremity in running and may be one of the causative factors in producing stress fractures.

The following exercises are presented as a means to promoting flexibility in specific areas. The exercises do not require special equipment and they may be done, in most instances, without the assistance of a partner.

Care should be taken that exercises are done as directed. Exercises may be used to gain flexibility as part of a conditioning program, a warm-up/cool-down routine, or as a part of a rehabilitation program. In addition, exercises may be combined with other treatment modalities, such as application of heat or cold.

The number of repetitions of each exercise may vary depending upon the purposes of the program: ten repetitions may be adequate to maintain flexibility before and after running, whereas 30-70 repetitions a day of the hamstring stretch is advocated to produce flexibility where severe limitation exists.

Flexibility Exercises for Runners

1. HAMSTRING STRETCHES

A. *Hamstring Stretch "A":* This stretch is only for people who have never experienced lower back pain or disability. Those who have experienced lower back pain or those with more than 25 degrees of hamstring tightness, as measured in Flexibility Test 2, should proceed to Hamstring Stretch "B."

Sit with the leg to be stretched fully extended and the opposite leg flexed at the hip and knee (Figure 13-7). 1) Tighten the quadriceps muscle (isometric contraction), 2) dorsiflex the foot maximally, and 3) then reach both hands toward the toes while maintaining full knee extension and keeping back straight (Figure 13-7A). Hold for ten seconds. Relax. Repeat, each time trying to reach the hands farther toward and then past the toes. Do not hold on to the toes. It is extremely important to hold the isometric contraction of the quadriceps while maintaining maximum dorsiflexion throughout the ten second stretch, thus allowing reciprocal relaxation of the hamstrings for maximal lengthening.

B. Hamstring Stretch "B": Lie in supine with one leg extended fully at the hip and knee. The leg to be stretched is flexed to 90° at the hip and knee (Figure 13-8). Maximally dorsiflex the foot and then extend knee as far as possible while maintaining 90° of hip flexion (Figure 13-8A). Hold this position for ten seconds. Relax, repeat. Care must be taken to do this exercise gently so that the opposite leg and pelvis are not moved during the stretch.

2. CALF STRETCHES

A. Gastrocnemius Muscle Stretch.:: Stand facing a wall with feet six inches apart, with one foot forward. Hands should be placed against a wall. The toes of both feet should point straight forward (Figure 13-9). Hold the back knee straight by

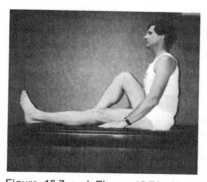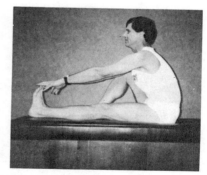

Figure 13-7 and Figure 13-7A. Hamstring stretch "A"

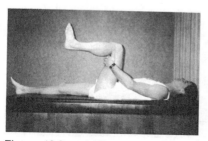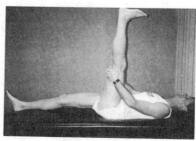

Figure 13-8 and Figure 13-8A. Hamstring stretch "B"

tightening the quadriceps muscle (isometric contraction) while lifting toes into maximal extension, thus forcing the heel to the floor while leaning the hips forward (Figure 13-9A). Hold for ten seconds. Relax, then repeat. NOTE: Persons with pronated feet may need to "toe in" slightly to insure adequate stretch of the gastrocnemius muscle. Additionally, persons with a moderate to severe forefoot varus may require a folded towel to be placed under the first metatarsal head to align the foot before stretching.

B. Soleus Muscle Stretch: This exercise is performed exactly like exercise 2A with the following change: the back knee is flexed to approximately 30° and held in this position while toes are extended and hips brought forward (Figure 13-10). The position is held for 10 seconds. Relax, then repeat.

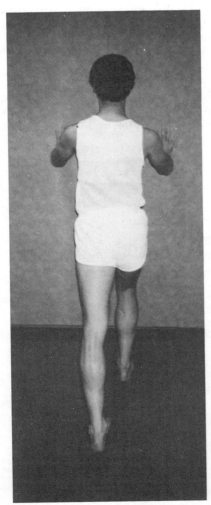
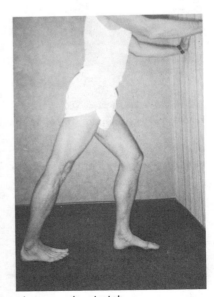

Figure 13-9 and Figure 13-9A. Gastrocnemius muscle stretch.

3. HIP ADDUCTOR AND INTERNAL ROTATOR STRETCH

Sit with the soles of the feet together. Let the knees fall apart as far as possible. Place the hands on the outside of the knees. Attempt to move knees apart while resisting movement with hands (isometric contraction) (Figure 13-11). Maintain resistence for ten seconds, then let the hands move outward with push of the knees, as the knees are actively moved apart as far as possible for six seconds (Figure 13-11A). Relax. Repeat, starting with knees in the new position farther apart and closer to the floor. As this exercise is repeated, the heels should be moved in closer to the body.

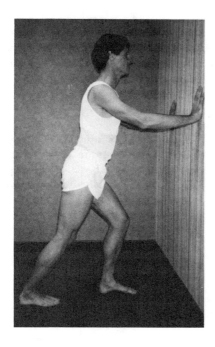

Figure 13-10. Soleus muscle stretch.

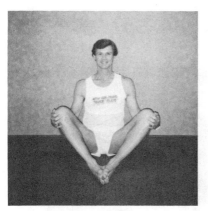
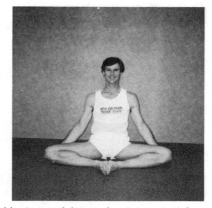

Figure 13-11 and Figure 13-11A. Hip adductor and internal rotator stretch.

4. HIP FLEXORS (HOLT's 3-S)[1]

Lie prone with the leg to be exercised in a flexed knee position and thigh raised as high as possible. A partner, positioned behind, rests on one knee with the opposite foot on the floor, one hand under the subject's knee, and the other slightly above the buttock (Figure 13-12). Attempt to pull the knee downward to the floor while the partner is resisting (isometric contraction). After a six-second isometric contraction, lift the bent leg higher with slight assistance of the partner (Figure 13-12A). Repeat three more times, each time beginning the procedure from the new lengthened position.

5. LOWER BACK STRETCH

Sit straight on the edge of a chair with feet supported on the floor, knees apart. Tuck your chin into chest and roll body slowly forward, one vertebrae at a time, hands moving toward the floor, until trunk is fully flexed (Figure 13-13). Then return immediately to the starting position by reversing the roll.

6. ABDOMINAL STRETCH

Lie on the floor in prone position. Place hands, palms down, on the floor next to your shoulders (Figure 13-14). Push with hands to straighten your elbows thus raising head, neck and shoulders. This will create a sag in your back as you keep your hips flat on the floor (Figure 13-14A). Return to starting position immediately by bending your elbows.

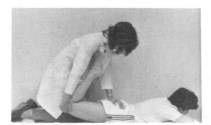 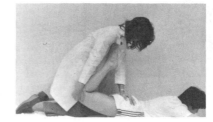

Figure 13-12 and Figure 13-12A. Hip flexor stretch.

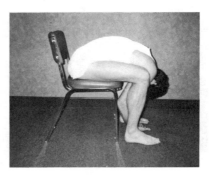

Figure 13-13. Lower back stretch.

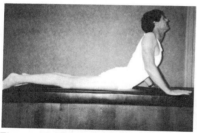 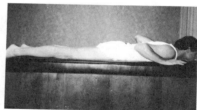

Figure 13-14 and Figure 13-14A. Abdominal stretch (pressup).

REFERENCES

1. Holt LE. Scientific Stretching for Sport (3-S). Biomechanics Laboratory, Dalhousie University, Halifax, Nova Scotia. 1979.
2. Holt, L.T. et al. A Comparative Study of Three Stretching Techniques. Perceptual Motor Skills 31:611-616, 1970.
3. Kabat H: Studies on Neuromuscular Dysfunction: XV. Arch Phys Med 33:521-533, 1952.
4. Knott M. Voss D: Proprioceptive Neuromuscular Facilitation. Harper and Row, New York, 1965.

CHAPTER 14

Eccentric Exercise for Chronic Tendinitis

Sandra Curwin PhD.

Introduction

The running athlete, competitive or recreational, is subject to a number of lower limb injuries. Considering the fact that one running mile involves hundreds of footstrikes of each lower limb, perhaps this is not entirely surprising. Knee problems are probably the runner's most common complaint, but tendon injuries such as posterior tibial syndrome and Achilles tendinitis are not uncommon. Indeed, they followed a close second and third to knee complaints in a survey of runners conducted by James et al[1]. Tendon injuries may follow a single traumatic event, or may develop insidiously as part of the runner's daily routine. One feature, however, is the persistence of tendon pain during running, and a gradual increase in pain with time. Because of the gradual onset, the runner may not seek medical attention until his or her tendinitis is well established. Hence the all-too-familiar appearance of the running athlete with a chronic tendinitis of six weeks' to six years' duration!

The magnitude of the tendinitis problem for competitive runners was shown by Welsh and Clodman[2] in their survey of 50 track and field athletes afflicted with Achilles tendinitis. Sixteen percent were forced to abandon sports participation permanently and 54% could compete only under duress, and then at a reduced level of performance. The lack of response of many forms of chronic tendinitis, especially Achilles tendinitis, to traditional forms of treatment is well known to any physician or therapist treating runners. This is plainly apparent in the plethora of treatment techniques on the market - ultrasound, ice, heat, flexibility exercises, strengthening exercise, anti-inflammatory drugs, corticosteroids, rest, immobilization, TENS, surgery - the list goes on. In our early experience, many runners with chronic Achilles tendinitis had experienced several of these treatment techniques, to no avail. This led us to rethink our approach to the non-surgical management of Achilles tendinitis. In this chapter we review some of the current knowledge concerning the physiology and pathology of the tendon, and present a rationale for the treatment of chronic tendinitis based on this knowledge.

Tendinitis and Tendon Structure

The bewildering variety of treatment techniques used to treat tendinitis is reflected in the lack of agreement on the exact pathology involved, or even on the structure of tendon. Indeed, it is likely that the fine structure of different tendons varies, although many features are common to all. The basic elements of all tendons are collagen, the main structural protein, and "ground substance," a glycosaminoglycan-water gel. Both are produced by fibroblasts, or tenocytes, the cells within the tendon. Collagen molecules aggregate, under the influence of the ground substance, into fibrils, once they are secreted from the fibroblast. Bundles of collagen fibrils, separated longitudinally by columns of fibroblasts and transversely by cytoplasmic extensions of the same cells, are called fibers (primary bundles). The fibrils, and thus the fibers, have a crimped or zig-zag appearance. Groups of these fibers, encased in a thin sheath called the endotenon, form a fascicle (secondary bundle). Presumably the fascicles are the tension-transmitting structures connecting muscle fibers to skeletal elements[3]. Individual fascicles are associated with discrete groups of muscle fibers or motor units and thus may be stressed independently of other fascicles. Several fascicles may form a larger group (tertiary bundle) also surrounded by endotenon, while the entire tendon is surrounded by a sheath, the epitenon, which is continuous with the endotenon. These two layers have a similar structure and have numerous blood vessels and fat cells embedded within them, forming a nutritional sheath [3-4]. Many small nerves are also found in these layers. These may extend down to the fibril level, with some unmyelinated fibers ending near collagen fibrils, others in the ground substance. Outside the epitenon is a further sheath, the peritenon, which is separate from the epitenon and apparently has the purpose of allowing smooth gliding of the tendon relative to other nearby structures [5]. Figure 14-1 illustrates the general features of tendon structure.

The result of this organization is that the tendon is somewhat elastic at low loads, the crimp of the fibers straightening under stress and recoiling when the load is removed. Loads above the safe limit (2% to 4% elongation) may result in damage to the tendon. Short-time x-ray diffraction techniques have recently shown that initially intrafibrillar slippage takes place, followed by interfibrillar slippage and finally gross disruption, if stress is continued [6]. The increase in severity of tendon injuries thus appears to be a progressive lack of lateral cohesion between various components, beginning at the fibrillar level. This collapse of lateral adhesion can result in a reduction of tensile strength that is greater than that suggested by the number of torn fibrils or fibers. Such damage can occur not only during loading but also during rapid unloading, which induces shearing within the tendon [6]. Fiber slippage and/or rupture may result in capillary hemorrhage within the tendon, and damaged collagen fibrils are susceptible to digestion by enzymes secreted by cells released from the capillaries. The resulting collagen peptide fragments may further encourage an inflammatory response, which may be responsible for the pain associated with chronic tendinitis [7]. The issue of whether tendon tissue per se can undergo this response, or if inflammatory changes are restricted to the peritenon remains unclear. The distribution of blood vessels, and the fact that such changes have been demonstrated in other species, makes it appear unlikely to the authors that inflammatory changes must necessarily be restricted to the tendon sheath.

Etiology of Tendinitis

Based on the description above, it appears that tendon injury (and thus tendinitis) should result from the application of loads that stretch the tendon more than 2% to 4% beyond its resting length. Whether this happens in vivo remains debatable. It has often been stated that the tendon is rarely elongated more than 2% during physiological activities, involving forces that seldom exceed 25% of the maximum possible [8]. This maximum is thought to be in the range of 5 to 10 kg/mm (50-100 N/mm, or MPa) for mammalian tendon [4]. Assuming the cross-sectional area of a human Achilles tendon to be 75 to 100 mm (based on cadaver estimates made by the authors), the maximum tensile strength should be roughly 4000-7000 N. The forces estimated to act on the Achilles tendon during various activities are listed in Table 14-1. Walking produces forces which are 30% to 60% of this maximum, while running produces forces up to 80% of maximum. While the amount of tendon elongation associated with these loads is unknown, it would appear that the tendon is loaded to near-maximum loads during running. Interestingly, in a comparison of three sport-related activities by one of the authors [9], running consistently produced larger Achilles tendon forces than either jumping or a motion intended to simulate the push-off motion in badminton that has been associated with Achilles tendon rupture [10]. The maximum Achilles tendon force coincided with the maximum length of the gastrocnemius and soleus muscles at midstance when the foot was flat and the knee extended, a time when elongation of the tendon should

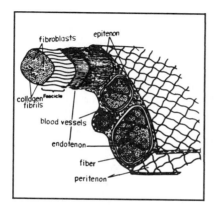

Figure 14-1. The hierarchial structure of tendon. See text for description.

be maximal (see Figure 14- 2). This may account for the fact that runners usually comprise the largest group of sufferers of Achilles tendinitis. A survey of 57 patients with Achilles tendinitis showed that 40% were runners, while 20% were involved in jumping sports and 25% participated in racquet sports[11].

The repetitive nature of running suggests that some type of additive microtrauma to the tendon may be occurring, analogous to the stress fractures which runners sometimes experience. This was termed "accumulated impact loading" by James et al[1]. Assuming that normal tendon is subjected to loads within the physiological range, it is difficult to see why this would occur. There are a number of ways, however, where loading conditions could change. If the tendon is subjected to near-maximum loads during running, even subtle changes may be sufficient to induce injury.

Factors Contributing to Tendinitis

Fatigue

Total elongation of the muscle-tendon unit requires deformation of both the muscle and tendon. After repeated contraction, the muscle becomes stiffer [12].

Table 14-1		
Activity	Tendon Force	Reference
walking	1100N	Morrison (1970)
walking	3200N	Pedotti et al. (1978)
running	4400N	Alexander and Vernon (1975)
running	5000N	Curwin (1984)
jumping	4400N	Smith (1975)
jumping	4500N	Curwin (1984)
push-off	4000N	Curwin (1984)

Table 14-1. Estimated forces acting on the Achilles tendon during various activities. Assuming a maximum stress of 7000 N (see text), the Achilles tendon may be subjected to loads greater than 80% of maximum during running.

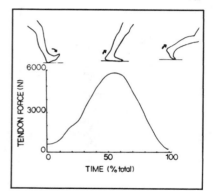

Figure 14-2. Maximum stress in the achilles tendon occurs at mid-stance. This is the end of the acentric phase of calf muscle contraction, just as the heel begins to lift from the ground.

This may cause increased deformation in the tendon and possible structural damage since the tendon will be forced to elongate more to allow the same total length change of the entire muscle-tendon unit. This situation can be avoided by increasing the endurance capability of the muscle with repeated, progressively increasing loads. This means the athlete should increase training gradually, especially after any period of inactivity, even if only a few days. The athlete should also monitor signs of fatigue carefully, since this is when injury may occur. Stinging, stabbing, or unusually localized pain (rather than the general discomfort of fatigue) may indicate a tendon injury.

External Sources

This includes friction from overlying shoes, tape, etc, or external blows to the tendon. Usually the outer sheath of the tendon (peritendon) is involved. It becomes inflamed and movement of the tendon within the sheath results in pain. Excessive movement, rather than increased loading, will reproduce the symptoms. The source of injury should be removed, and the treatment for acute tendinitis employed .

Load and Deformation Changes

The tendon may be subjected to larger loads than normal, due to a variety of causes:

1. Change in shoes - a new, stiffer sole increases the moment arm for force application to the foot, resulting in larger joint torques at the ankle, and thus larger tendon forces. A change to flat shoes, on the other hand, will cause greater elongation of the tendon than usual.

2. Change in training - this may involve a change in surface (increased load), a change in duration (repetitive microtrauma), or a change to uphill running (increased deformation). Ideally, the runner should introduce such changes gradually. Numerous studies have shown that connective tissues will adapt readily to the stresses imposed upon them, but like any form of training, these changes must be gradual [13,14,15,16,17,18] .

Unexpected events - sudden loads on the tendon may be the result of misplacing the foot, resulting in sudden contraction of the calf muscles. If the foot is misaligned at the time, some fascicles within the tendon may be stretched more than others, and also may be subjected to larger forces if different regions of the muscle are differently activated. This is due to the fact that individual fascicles are associated with different groups of muscle fibers, and thus some fascicles may be loaded, while others may not. This may lead to shear forces between adjacent regions in the tendon, reducing lateral cohesion.

Anatomical Factors

The runner with decreased calf muscle flexibility or strength is at increased risk for tendinitis: decreased flexibility because more stretch is demanded of the tendon to allow the entire muscle-tendon unit to elongate; decreased strength because it leads to fatigue. The alignment of the hindfoot and forefoot has been emphasized by other authors[19]. Excessive pronation of the forefoot can lead to increased stress on the inner portion of the tendon, causing it to deform more than the lateral side. This is compounded by the fact that the gastrocnemius and soleus tendons do not follow a straight course to the calcaneus but twist laterally as they descend (see Figure 14-3), as described initially by Cummins et al[20]. This twisting is increased by pronation of the forefoot, thus at each heel strike there is increased rotation and strain in the tendon. The result is a "sawing" action on the tendon [13]. Interestingly, the location of the twisting is in the region 2-6 cm above the calcaneus, where Achilles tendinitis most often occurs. This region has also been described as having a reduced blood flow, which may decrease the rate of healing [21].

Alignment problems of this type are usually the cause of posterior tibial syndrome, and it should immediately be considered in such cases. The situation is readily corrected by the use of the appropriate orthotic device, as illustrated in Figure 14-4. (See Orthotics Chapter 15.)

Treatment of Tendinitis

Acute Tendinitis

Acute tendinitis is ideally treated the same as a joint sprain. Ice should be applied immediately after injury and the athlete should refrain from stressing the tendon for 3 to 5 days. During this time the initial inflammatory response will have subsided and collagen production will be increasing. As soon as pain permits the athlete can begin stretching exercises and later combine this with loading on the tendon around three weeks post- injury. Application of force is essential after this time to ensure correct alignment of newly-formed collagen fibers. A general scheme of progression is outlined in Figure 14-5. By 6 to 8 weeks the athlete is ready to resume training at a reduced level. The runner must realize that because

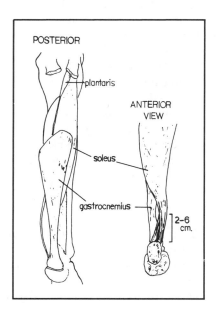

Figure 14-3. Note the lateral twisting of both portions of the Achilles tendon. This can lead to areas of stress concentration, particularly if any rotary abnormality is present in the lower limb. The location of maximum twist coincides with the most common site of Achilles tendinitis.

of the large tendon forces created in running this activity must be approached cautiously after an injury. For example, a distance of one-half or one mile may be chosen to begin with. This can be increased one-half to one mile weekly if no discomfort ensues. Once the athlete can run five miles without discomfort he can readily monitor his own progress (this may be a total of 12 weeks from the time of the initial injury). Less severe injuries can be progressed more rapidly, and athletes in sports other than running may be capable of returning to full activity sooner. It is, of course, essential to determine the cause of the tendinitis and correct it if necessary, ie, look for the factors described above. Unfortunately, most tendinitis is not acute and has not been treated this way.

Chronic Tendinitis

Ljungqvist[10] (1968), in a review of 92 cases of partial Achilles tendon rupture, lists the following situations as most likely to cause injury to the Achilles tendon:

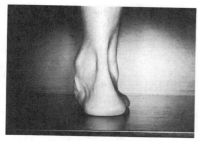

Figure 14-4. This figure illustrates the effect of hidfoot valgus and forefoot pronation on the tendons of the leg.
Note the valgus hindfoot, leading to medial displacement of the medial malleolus and over-stretching of the medial side of the Achilles tendon and posterior tibial tendon.

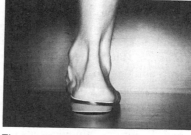

Figure 14-4A. After orthotic correction, hindfoot valgus has been reduced and the Achilles tendon restored to its central position. Arch support decreases excess stress on the posterior tibial tendon.

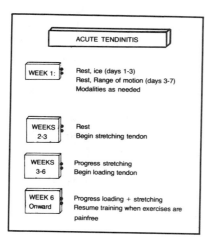

Figure 14-5. Flow chart illustrating principles of treatment of acute tendinitis.

1. Pushing off with the weight-bearing foot while simultaneously extending the knee, common in sprinting or running uphill. The calf muscles are maximally contracted. This situation also occurs at midstance in level running (illustrated in Figure 14-2).

2. Sudden and unexpected dorsiflexion of the ankle, such as slipping on a stair or stumbling into a hole, where the heel drops suddenly. The calf muscles contract maximally in reflex to the sudden stretch.

3. Violent dorsiflexion while the foot is plantar flexed, such as in jumping and falling. The calf muscles are maximally contracted and sudden movement leads to marked stretching of the muscle-tendon unit, especially the tendon.

All of these examples involve eccentric loading of the muscle. Athletes suffering from Achilles tendinitis often feel more pain during eccentric movement. This is easily tested by having the athlete hop on one foot or drop the heel rapidly over the edge of a step. In fact, these types of movements are frequently the only ones that are painful, concentric or isometric contractions being painfree in many cases. This observation led us to the development of a specific "eccentric exercise program" to treat such cases of chronic tendinitis.

The concept of using exercise as part of the treatment of chronic tendinitis is not new. It has been advocated for tennis elbow [22], jumper's knee [23] and Achilles tendinitis [19]. The beneficial effects of exercise on connective tissues, such as ligaments and tendons, are well known, as are the detrimental effects of disuse [14]. The use of prolonged rest, and particularly immobilization, therefore appear to have very little place in the treatment of tendinitis. In fact, a vicious cycle begins with rest weakening the tendon so that symptoms recur as soon as activity is resumed. Eventually any vigorous physical activity provokes symptoms. Only in cases of acute tendinitis, where pain is intense, should complete rest be enforced, and then only until the acute symptoms subside. Immobilization is indicated only in cases of complete tendon rupture, where apposition of sutured tendon ends must be maintained.

The use of exercise in treating chronic tendinitis must follow the same principles involved in muscle strength training, or any other exercise program: maximal loading, progressive loading, and specificity. The eccentric exercise program was designed to meet these criteria. The maximal load is determined by the discomfort experienced by the patient (some pain at the end of 30 repetitions). Progression is made by increasing the speed of movement or increasing the external resistance (increasing weight). It has been shown that increasing the speed of eccentric exercise increases muscle force output, while the opposite is truce for concentric loading[24]. Specificity is achieved by duplicating the movement associated with maximal tendon forces, ie, a lengthening of the muscle-tendon unit, immediately followed by shortening. This is accomplished for the Achilles tendon by having the athlete stand on the edge of a step. The body weight is supported on the ball of the foot so the heel is free. The heel is then allowed to drop downward with gravity, below the level of the step, as shown in Figure 14-6.

Progression is made by increasing the speed of movement or increasing the resistance. The daily program proceeds as follows:

1. General body warm-up (pushups, situps, etc.)

2. Stretch calf muscles with knee bent (soleus) and straight (gastrocnemius). Hold 30 seconds, repeat 3 times.

3. Perform 3 sets of 10 repetitions of exercise program.

4. Repeat stretching exercise (3).

5. Apply ice to areas of discomfort.

Within each level of resistance, the speed is increased from slow (days 1, 2) to moderate (days 3, 4) to fast (days 5, 6). The flow chart in Figure 14-7 illustrates the general outline. The starting point is determined by the severity of the initial symptoms. No progression is made until 30 repetitions can be performed without pain, then the patient progresses to the level that produces some discomfort near the end of the 30 repetitions. Typically, by the end of 6 to 8 weeks the athlete experiences a marked reduction in symptoms. We reviewed our first 57 patients on this program and found that by the end of 6 weeks, 31 had complete relief of symptoms, while 26 had a marked decrease in symptoms. None were hampered in their athletic activities, while all had been performing at reduced levels prior to the exercise program. All had continued to participate in sports while carrying out the program. In many cases, the program was carried out independently by the athlete, with weekly checks by the therapist.

Summary

Chronic tendinitis is a problem for both those giving and receiving treatment. Unfortunately, our knowledge about tendinitis and its treatment remains

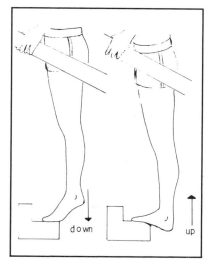

Figure 14-6. How to perform the eccentric exercise program for Achilles tendinitis. The patient allows the body weight to drop as rapidly as possible, then immediately returns to the toe-raise position.

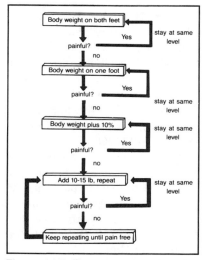

Figure 14-7. The general outline for progression of the eccentric exercise program for Achilles tendinitis.

limited. It would appear, however, that much treatment is empirically based rather than being based on the patient history and existing scientific knowledge concerning the response of tendon to increased and decreased stress levels. Using the latter, we have designed an exercise program that aims to both stretch and increasingly load the affected tendon. The result is a decrease in pain and return to full participation in activities. To achieve success with this program the role of eccentric muscle contraction must be firmly established prior to commencing treatment, and any anatomical or predisposing factors must be dealt with concurrently. These principles have proved successful in the treatment of many forms of chronic tendinitis, and allow the athlete to rehabilitate the injury while continuing to train.

REFERENCES

1. James, S.L., B.T., Bates and L.R. Osternig, Injuries to runners, Am J Sports Med, 6:40-50, 1978.
2. Welsh, R.P. and J. Clodman, Clinical survey of Achilles tendinitis in athletes, Can Med Assoc J, 122:193-196, 1980.
3. Rowe, R.W.D., The structure of rat tail tendon, Conn Tiss Res, 14:9-20, 1985.
4. Elliott, D.H., Structure and function of mammalian tendon, Biol Rev, 40:392-421, 1965.
5. Clancy, W.G., Tendinitis and plantar fasciitis in runners, in D'Ambrosia, R. and Drez, D., Jr. (eds.), Prevention and Treatment of Running Injuries, Thorofare, N.J., Charles B. Slack, pp. 77-88, 1982.
6. Knorzer, E., W. Folkhard, W. Geercken, C. Boschert, M.H.J. Koch, B. Hilbert, H. Krahl, E. Mosler, H. Nemetschek- Gansler and T. Nemetschek, New aspects of the etiology of tendon rupture, Arch Orthop Trauma Surg, 105:113-120, 1986.
7. Perugia, L., E. Ippolito and F. Postacchini, A new approach to the pathology, clinical features and treatment of stress tendinopathy of the Achilles tendon, Ital J Orthop Traumatol, 2:5-21, 1976.
8. Harkness, R.D., Mechanical properties of collagenous tissues. In Gould, B.S. (ed.), Treatise on Collagen, Vol. 2, Pt. A, New York, Academic Press, pp. 248-310, 1968.
9. Curwin, S., Force and length changes of the gastrocnemius and soleus muscle-tendon units during a therapeutic exercise program and three selected activities, unpublished M.Sc. thesis, Dalhousie University, 1984.
10. Ljungqvist, R., Subcutaneous partial rupture of the Achilles tendon, Acta Orthop Scand (Suppl), 113:1-86, 1968.
11. Curwin, S. and W.D. Stanish, Tendinitis: Its etiology and treatment, D.C. Health and Company, Lexington, MA, 1984.
12. Komi, P.V., Neuromuscular performance: factors influencing force and speed production, Scand J Sports Sci, 1:2- 15, 1979.
13. Barfred, T., Experimental rupture of the Achilles tendon: Comparison of various types of experimental rupture in rats, Acta Orthop Scand, 42:528-543, 1971.
14. Booth. F.W. and E.W. Gould, Effects of training and disusue on connective tissue, Exer Sport Sci Rev, 3:83-107, 1975.

15. Noyes, F.R., P.J. Torvik, W.B. Hyde and J.L. DeLucas, Biomechanics of ligament failure. II. An analysis of immobilization, exercise and reconditioning effects in primates, J Bone Joint Surg, 56A:1406-1418, 1974.
16. Tipton, C.M., R.D. Matthes, J.A. Maynard and R.A. Carey, The influence of physical activity on ligaments and tendons, Med Sci Sports, 7:165-175, 1975.
17. Woo, S.L.-Y, J.V. Matthews, W.H. Akeson et al., Connective tissue response to immobility: A correlative study of biochemical and biomechanical measurements of normal and immobilized rabbit knees, Arthritis Rheum, 18:257-264, 1975.
18. Zuckerman, J. and G.A. Stull, Ligamentous separation force in rats as influenced by training, detraining and cage restriction, Med Sci Sports, 5:44-49, 1973.
19. Smart, G.W., J.E. Taunton and D.B. Clement, Achilles tendon disorders in runners - a review, Med Sci Sports Exer, 12:231-243, 1980.
20. Cummins, E.J., Anson, B.J., Carr, B.W. et al., The structure of the calcaneal tendon (of Achilles) in relation to orthopaedic surgery, Surg Gynecol Obstet, 83:107-116, 1946.
21. Lagergren, C. and a. Lindholm, Vascular distribution in the Achilles tendon, Acta Chir Scand, 116:491-495, 1958.
22. Nirschl, R.P., The etiology and treatment of tennis elbow, J Sports Med, 2:308-319, 1974.
23. Blazina, M., Jumper's knee, Orthop Clin North Am, 2:665-678, 1973.
24. Komi, P.V., Measurement of the force-velocity relationship in human muscle under concentric and eccentric contractions, Med Sport, 8:224-229, 1973.

CHAPTER 15

Orthotics

Robert D. D'Ambrosia, M.D.
Nicholas Rightor, C.O., Roy Douglas, C.P.

Introduction

An orthotic is used to bring the foot into proper alignment when it strikes the ground. The use of orthotics has become popular as a means of preventing and curing the stress-related injuries found in long-distance runners whose malalignment problems become manifested as injuries because of the high forces generated in running. Advocates of orthotics speculate that excessive foot pronation (Figure 15-1) is the cause of most leg and foot problems among runners. They maintain that proper leg-foot alignment is critically important in running because the force on the foot is much greater in running than in walking; malalignment problems that may have been asymptomatic earlier are believed to be greatly magnified by the increased force. The use of orthotics is therefore espoused as a means of preventing excessive or abnormal pronation while preserving normal resupination.

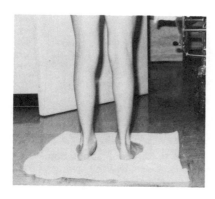

Figure 15-1. Excessive foot pronation causing symptomatic plantar fasciitis.

To understand why some physicians use orthotics and why they are prescribed requires an understanding of the biomechanics of the subtalar joint, the joint the orthotic attempts to control. We shall briefly discuss biomechanics in this chapter, but the reader is referred to Chapter 1 and The "Joints of the Ankle" for more detailed information on the subtalar joint.

Biomechanics of Orthotics

During running, the lower extremity joints not only go through flexion and extension, but also undergo considerable rotation.[1] Such rotation occurs at both the knee and the subtalar joint, not just at the hip (Figure 15-2). The subtalar joint is an oblique hinge aligned 42° to the horizontal and deviating 16° medially to laterally.[2,3] Inward rotary motion of the tibia at the subtalar joint is pronation (Figure 15-3) and outward rotation of the tibia is supination (Figure 15-3A).

Just before initial ground contact, the tibia is in slight outward rotation and the calcaneus is usually inverted, with the foot in slight supination. On ground contact, internal rotation of the tibia occurs, and as the foot becomes loaded the heel goes into eversion through an inward rotatory motion of the tibia at the

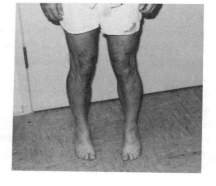

Figure 15-2. Excessive femoral internal rotation (femoral anteversion) causing intoeing. Note the inward rotation of both patellae, implicating the femur as the cause of intoeing.

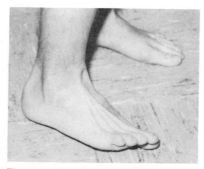

Figure 15-3. Foot pronation. The heel (calcaneus) is everted (valgus). The arch is depressed.

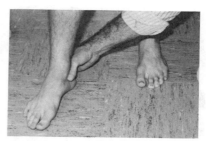

Figure 15-3A. Foot supination. The calceneus is inverted (varus). the arch is elevated.

subtalar joint. The subtalar joint, acting as an oblique hinge, translates the internal rotation of the lower extremity into eversion of the calcaneus. As the calcaneus is everted at ground contact, the rest of the foot becomes pronated due to the inward rotatory motion occurring at the subtalar joint. This pronation of the foot unlocks the midtarsal joint, making the foot more flexible so that it can adapt to the underlying surface.

It is this pronation that an orthotic attempts to control. However, if the pronation is controlled completely, the foot becomes rigid and absorbs shock poorly. Therefore, an orthotic attempts to control only an excessive amount of pronation. Pronation is normal and an important factor in enabling the foot and body to absorb the force and shock of impact while running. Pronation results in a flexible transverse tarsal joint, allowing collapse of the longitudinal arch as the foot comes in contact with the ground. The normal factors limiting pronation are largely passive and controlled by supporting ligaments and bone contours in the joints. If pronation is excessive (Figure 15-4 and 15-4A), characterized by a falling over on the medial side of the foot, then supporting ligaments and connective tissue may become strained as excessive stress is placed on them.

In the remaining part of the cycle, once the foot is firmly on the ground, another series of events occurs, beginning with external rotation of the lower extremity. As the tibia rotates externally, the talus at the subtalar joint rotates in the opposite direction so that inversion of the calcaneus occurs concomitantly with supination of the remainder of the foot. Supination stabilizes the transverse tarsal joint, helping to create a rigid longitudinal arch. This stabilization creates a more rigid lever for push-off. Several factors work to help this outward external rotation at the subtalar joint to take place. The metatarsal break, which has an oblique axis, causes calcaneus inversion and lower extremity external rotation. With toe dorsiflexion during the latter part of stance phase, the attachment of the plantar aponeurosis around the metatarsal heads elevates the longitudinal arch. Active firing of the intrinsic flexor musculature also helps stabilize the arch.

The mechanisms involved with supination are more active than the process of pronation. The resupination process, which begins in midstance and terminates with the foot acting as a rigid level at toe-off, is also important in preventing

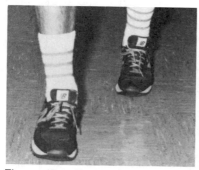

Figure 15-4. Excessive foot pronation from front.

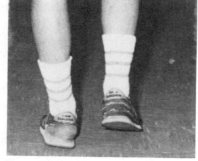

Figure 15-4A. Excessive foot pronation from back.

overuse syndromes. If it does not occur normally, it places undue stress on the surrounding ligaments, capsule, and bone.

The advocates of orthotics theorize that over-pronation or prolonged pronation greatly increases, both actively and passively, stresses to the supporting structures of the foot. Theoretically, abnormal rotation at the subtalar joint can cause injuries to the posterior tibial tendons, plantar fascia, tendoachilles, and iliotibial band, from stress translated to these structures. Thus by controlling and partially restricting the rotatory motion of the subtalar joint, orthotics can prevent undue stress to the active and passive supporting structures of the foot, ankle, and, indirectly, the knee.

If worn constantly, foot orthotics may cause the muscles and ligaments around the joints to weaken through disuse to the point that the orthotic device could become a detriment rather than an aid to better foot alignment. If worn temporarily, however, during periods of severe or repeated stress such as long-distance running, and if properly fitted, they can help prevent arch breakdown and excessive pronation.

Many contemporary foot orthotics for runners cannot hold the calcaneus in alignment to stabilize the subtalar joint adequately. Not until Henderson and Campbell's device, designed at the University of California Biomechanical Laboratory (UCBL), has there been an effective orthotic designed to control the subtalar joint.[4] An orthotic becomes effective when it creates an inner contour that is capable of giving the architecture of the foot maximum passive support. The orthosis must also be adequately stabilized in the shoe so that it cannot roll into varus or valgus. The UCBL design lends itself well to solving a wide range of malalignment and pressure distribution problems of the foot.[5,6]

Our orthotic design embodies the UCBL concept of firmly gripping the heel (Figure 15-5) as the only effective way of controlling the subtalar joint.

Orthotic Casting Technique

To fabricate a proper orthotic, the physician/orthotist must know how to place the foot and subtalar joint in the "neutral position ",the position in which the foot functions in its most efficient manner, thereby receiving the least amount of stress from the surrounding joints, ligaments, and tendons. The foot should be positioned so that, with weight bearing, the vertical axis of the heel is parallel to

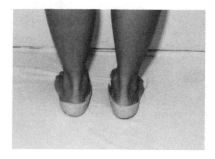

Figure 15-5. Orthotic firmly gripping the heel of a runner with posterior tibial tendonitis secondary to excessive pronation.

the longitudinal axis of the distal tibia and the plane of the metatarsal heads is perpendicular to the heel. To obtain the neutral position, from which the casting of the foot is made, the person taking the mold of the foot must accurately align the foreleg, heel, and heel- forefoot, which may be done by several techniques. This may be obtained with the patient standing, prone or supine (Figure 15-6, 15-7 and 15-8).

Neutral Position With Patient Standing

With the patient standing and looking straight ahead, grasp the head of the talus between the thumb and index finger (Figure 15- 6). Instruct the patient to look behind him by rotating his pelvis as far as he can laterally while keeping his foot planted on the floor (Figure 15-9). With the patient's upper torso rotated laterally and his feet and extremities straight ahead, his foot will supinate and the head of the talus will protrude laterally (Figure 15-10). The patient is then told to look forward and to bring his upper torso back in level with his lower extremity. As he rotates his pelvis back over the fixed heel, the forefoot will

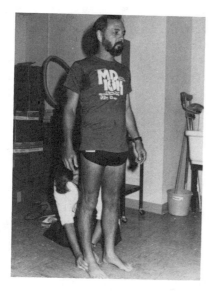

Figure 15-6. Neutral position standing.

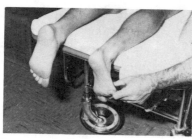

Figure 15-7. Neutral position prone.

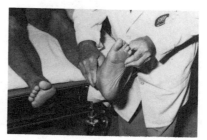

Figure 15-8. Neutral position supine.

pronate and the head of the talus will protrude medially. The point at which the foot seems to fall to one side or the other (Figure 15-11) is the neutral position of the subtalar joint.

Neutral Position With Patient Prone

Have the patient lie prone on the examining table with his feet extending over the end. With index finger and thumb, grasp his foot at the fourth and fifth metarsal heads and gently dorsiflex it until some resistance is felt (Figure 15-7). Then move the subtalar joint through an arc of pronation and supination; at one point during this rotatory arc, the foot will tend to fall more easily to one side or the other. The point where the talar head does not protrude medially or laterally is the neutral position.

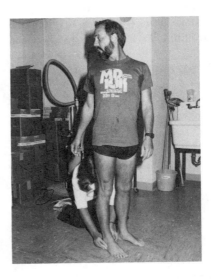

Figure 15-9. Patient looks backward causing supination, higher arch, and heel varus.

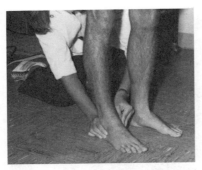

Figure 15-10. Looking backward causes foot supination and head of talus protrudes laterally.

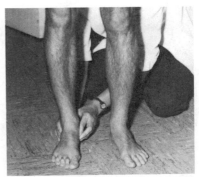

Figure 15-11. Neutral position of subtalar joint. The talus is neither medial nor lateral.

Neutral Position With Patient Supine

With the patient supine, palpate the head of the talus with the index finger and thumb while pronating and supinating the foot back and forth through a rotatory arc (Figure 15-8). With inversion of the calcaneus, the head of the talus will be felt as a bulge laterally (Figure 15-12). With eversion of the calcaneus, the bulge will be medial (Figure 15-13). The neutral position is that point at which the foot is positioned so that the talar head does not bulge either medially or laterally (Figure 15-8). At that point the talus is anatomically aligned with the navicular and does not protrude in any direction.

Neutral Position Cast

The neutral position cast is best obtained with the patient lying supine, as described above. The patient is instructed to relax completely and to refrain from actively dorsiflexing his foot during the procedure. The neutral position cast is obtained by making a plaster mold of the patient's foot, while exerting passive dorsiflexion force on the lateral column of the foot (basically the fourth and fifth metatarsals). This produces a locking position of bone against bone with the foot in its best functional position. If dealing with a patient who has a severely pronated flatfoot, the head of the talus will protrude markedly on the medial side and will not be palpable laterally. On the other hand, if dealing with a cavus or a highly arched foot, the head of the talus will protrude prominently on the lateral side and will not be easily palpable on the medial aspect.

To make the mold, have the patient lie supine on the casting table. A towel or pillow under the hip corresponding to the affected foot helps bring the foot up to a vertical position (Figure 15-14), and is the best position for obtaining a neutral cast. The mold is made with two 4 × 20 inch plaster-of-paris splints (Figure 15-14A). If a 4 × 30 inch splint is wrapped around the foot it can be cut to the exact size needed. The splints are immersed in tepid water and placed on the foot so that they extend from the fifth metatarsal head around the heel (Figure 15-14B) and up the medial aspect of the first metatarsal head (Figure 15-14C). Next, one side of the plaster is folded over the sole of the foot (Figure 15-14D) and the opposite side is folded over it as well (Figure 15-14E). Then, with a gloved hand, smooth the plaster over the contours of the foot until the plaster is

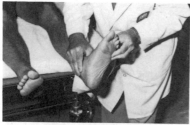

Figure 15-12. The talar head bulges laterally with heel inversion and forefoot supination.

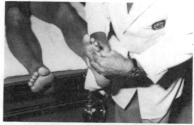

Figure 15-13. The talar head bulges medially with heel eversion and forefoot pronation.

free of irregularities (Figure 15-14F). Then, grip the fourth and fifth metatarsal heads with the thumb on the plantar surface and the index finger on the dorsal surface of the metatarsals (Figure 15-14G), and with the opposite thumb and index finger for the head of the talus. With the head of the talus in the neutral position, pressure is maintained on the fourth and fifth metatarsal heads. The foot must not slip out of the neutral position while the cast is setting. The position of the cast must be maintained until the drying plaster is no longer pliable.

To remove the cast, pull it away from the dorsal aspect of the foot (Figure 15-14h). Then grasp the cast on the medial and lateral sides of the heel and pull straight down; the cast will separate from the heel. As soon as the cast is off the heel, pull it forward, and it will slide off the plantar surface of the foot (Figure 15-14I). The completed plaster molds of the foot are shown in Figure 15-14J).

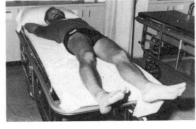

Figure 15-14. Folded towel under hip brings the foot to a more vertical position.

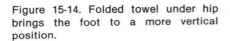

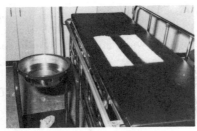

Figure 15-14A. Materials necessary to obtain a neutral cast of the foot.

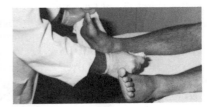

Figure 15-14B. Beginning application of plaster.

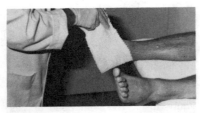

Figure 15-14C. Plaster splint applied around foot.

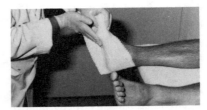

Figure 15-14D. Plaster splint folded on medial side.

Orthotic Fabrication

A positive mold is then made from the plaster mold of the foot. The modeling plaster is poured in and allowed to dry, and the plaster bandages are removed (Figure 15-15). The positive model is then smoothed, and the plantar surface at and just proximal to the metatarsal heads and at the heel is flattened precisely perpendicular to the vertical. If the deformity is especially severe it is advisable to flatten the heel at a slight angle of 5° to 10°, depending on the amount of correction needed, by removing more plaster from the medial or lateral side to correct for supination or pronation, respectively. The forefoot is left alone.

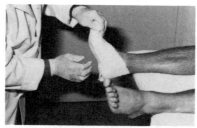

Figure 15-14E. Lateral side folded over medial side.

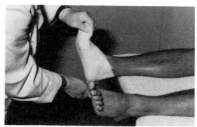

Figure 15-14F. Plaster is smoothed of irregularities.

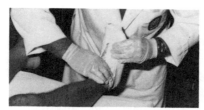

Figure 15-14G. Grip the fourth and fifth metatarsal heads with thumbs on plantar surface and index and long fingers on the dorsal surfaces of the metatarsal. With the opposite thumb and index finger, feel for the head of talus.

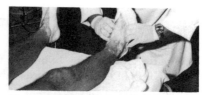

Figure 15-14H. Cast pulled from the foot of the patient.

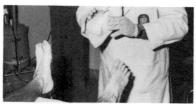

Figure 15-14I. Plaster cast pulled from the foot of the patient.

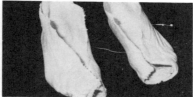

Figure 15-14J. Completed plaster molds of both feet.

Perhaps the most important phase in modification of the positive model is the exaggeration of the posterior aspect of the longitudinal arch and its blending with the medial support area above the calcaneal tuberosity. Locating the navicular and the calcaneal tuberosity are important because as much plaster as necessary must be removed from between these two positions to create the pressure needed for direct support of the calcaneus in the area of the sustentaculum tali.

The effectiveness of a good supporting inner contour of an orthosis should never be compromised by inadequate trimming of the model. Trim lines should be left as high as comfort will allow. This rule is important in order to obtain effective support around the subtalar joint.[6]

The mold is now ready for orthotic construction. Selection of material depends on the prescription (Figure 15-16). For correction of supination, pronation, pes cavus, heel spurs, or any deformity that needs solid support, a polyethylene material called streyfylast is used. This material is nontoxic, highly compressible, and easily reshaped with the use of a heat gun. After a blank is cut it is then placed in an oven on a piece of aluminum coated with a parting agent at 177°C, for 10 to 15 minutes to achieve optimal working temperature (Figure 15-16A). The streifylast is then removed from the oven, draped over the mold, and then placed in a vacuum-forming machine (Figure 15- 16B). Pressure of 25 lbs. per square inch is applied, and the material is then left to cool for ten minutes under that pressure (Figure 15-16C). Finally, the form is released from the mold, (Fig.15-16D), trimmed (Figure 15-16E), and the surfaces sanded (Figure 15-16F). The orthotic is now ready for fitting to the patient's foot (Figure 15-16G).

Patient Results

During the ten years the Louisiana State University Medical Center Runner's Clinic has been in existence, more than 1500 runners with stress-related injuries have been examined and treated in a team approach that includes an orthopedist, a physical therapist, and an orthotist. Ten percent of these runners received orthotics for stress syndromes that we were unable to relieve through modification of training techniques. Before an orthotic was prescribed, we first altered training techniques to avoid sudden increases in mileage and to see whether a more cushioned surface or shoe could be fitted to alter the stress pattern. Training techniques were modified to discourage rapid changes in mileage, avoid hill-running and hard-surface running, practice proper stretching techniques, and to encourage shoe modifications. The most common problem in

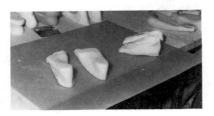

Figure 15-15. Positive models made from the plaster molds of both feet.

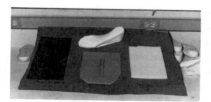

Figure 15-16. Three materials most commonly used for orthotic fabrication. streifylast, Plastozote #2, and Plastozote #3.

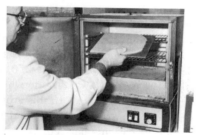

Figure 15-16A. Blank cut of streify-last placed in oven on aluminum slab coated with a parting agent.

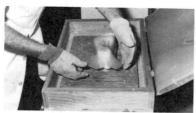

Figure 15-16B. Streifylast removed from oven and placed over the mold.

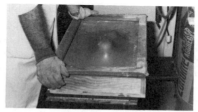

Figure 15-16C. Streifylast mold left in the vacuum-forming machine for ten minutes until cool.

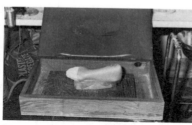

Figure 15-16D. Completed mold after release from the vacuum-forming machine.

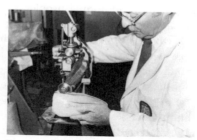

Figure 15-16E. Trimming of the orthotic.

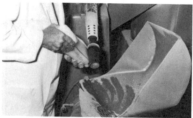

Figure 15-16F. Sanding of the orthotic.

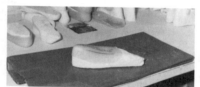

Figure 15-16G. Orthotic ready for patient fitting.

runners is, of course, inadequate stretching, which is dealt with in Chapters 12, 13 and 14. Only after we have carefully evaluated the patient's running techniques and stretched out controlled muscle groups will we resort to an orthotic to help the runner with his stress problem.

Seven years ago we evaluated 50 runners who had been given orthotics over a three year period to determine whether their pain and discomfort from stress syndromes had improved. In this group of patients, 22 (44%) had flat arches, 16 (32%) had high arches (cavus), and 12 (24%) had normal arches (Table 15-1). This ratio of patients has remained approximately the same through the years.

No specific diagnosis was associated with a particular type of arch. Diagnoses have varied, depending on which part of the body was acting as the shock absorber when the foot stikes the ground. It was usually in the tendons, fascia, and, less frequently, the bone. The diagnoses have included iliotibial band tendonitis, posterior tibial tendinitis, tendoachilles tendinitis, plantar fasciitis, tarsal tunnel syndrome, metatarsalgia, heel spur, and chondromalacia patellae. The tendon conditions usually helped have been for posterior tibial tendinitis, plantar fascitis, and iliotibial band tendinitis (when genu varus at the knee is associated with iliotibial band tendonitis and the patient has to excessively pronate to compensate for the genu varus). Metatarsalgia and heel spur respond to a metatarsal bar built directly into the orthotic for the former and relief built in the orthotic for the latter. Approximately 72% of our patients have reported improvement after the use of the orthotic. An improvement was defined as a decrease or elimination of the pain associated with running. Our original failure rate of 28% has decreased to 10% because of more careful decisions based on past failures. A failure is no improvement, a worsening of symptoms, or the development of additional problems.

The flat or pronated foot is more apt to be helped by an orthotic than the high arch or cavus foot. The cavus foot, which is by far the most difficult problem to manage with an orthotic, is usually intractable, rigid, and poorly adapted to absorb the accumulated forces generated on impact with distance running. Since 42% of the patients in our original group with cavus feet were unimproved with the use of an orthotic, we recommend caution in prescribing an orthotic for this condition. The best results for cavus feet were obtained with the more cushioned orthotic materials, which, unfortunately, hold their contour poorly.

We evaluated the improved versus the unimproved groups in relation to several factors: age, sex, distance run, duration of participation in the sport, and type of running surface. The average age of both the improved and unimproved groups was 33.7 years (range: 14-52 years and 24-45 years, respectively).

Table 15-1
Type of Arch Related to Improvement

	Total	Improved	Unimproved
Flat arch	22	18	4
Normal arch	12	8	4
High arch	16	10	6
Total patients	50	36	14

Seventy eight percent of our improved group were men and 22% were women. The unimproved group had 86% men and 14% women Overall, 80% of the women and 70% of the men showed improvement. The improved group of runners ran slightly less than did the unimproved runners. The runners in the improved group ran an average of 23.6 miles per week; 89% ran less than 40 miles per week. The unimproved runners ran an average of 30 miles per week; half of these runners ran less than 20 miles per week (Figure 15-17).

The running surfaces used by the two groups differed considerably. Seventy two percent of the improved patients ran on paved surfaces only part of the time or not at all. Seventy one percent of the unimproved group ran on paved surfaces only. Thirty six percent of the runners who showed improvement also decreased their speed and/or distance run. One runner changed completely from a paved to a clay surface. Thirty six percent of the patients who showed no improvement had extreme difficulty adjusting to the orthotic. This difficulty probably led to decreased usage of the orthotic device.

From our experience with prescribing orthotics for runners, we cautiously state that orthotics are a legitimate part of the runner's treatment program. Although we found no significant differences in many of the factors examined, the overall improvement was 72%, which probably justifies the use of orthotics. In analyzing our runners with orthotics, however, we have determined that the conditions most often helped by orthotics are: posterior tibial tendonitis, plantar faciitis, iliotibial band tendinitis (when associated with genu varus and pronation), metatarsalgia, and heel spur. Runners with flat feet and excessive pronation do much better than patients with rigid cavus feet. Almost half of the unimproved runners in our original group had cavus feet. The use of an orthotic seems certainly more appropriate in the flat-footed or normal-arched runner than in the runner with cavus feet.

The physician seeing running problems should be aware that the orthotics are just one factor in the treatment of stress syndromes. Most stress syndromes are related to training errors and are improved with rest, reduced mileage, and a change to a more cushioned surface, or to a modified or more cushioned shoe. The next most useful therapy is instituting proper stretching techniques, both in prophylaxis and in the treatment of specific injuries. It is only after the above treatments fail that an orthotic should be used to correct malalignment problems. Although the science of orthotics is inexact, when it is correlated with the biomechanics of the lower extremity, orthotics may be effective in training recalcitrant problems that have not been helped by improved techniques, stretching, surface changes, or shoe modifications.

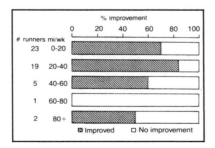

Figure 15-17. Graph showing relationship of miles run with improvement or lack of improvement.

REFERENCES

1. Inman VT: The Joints of the Ankle. Baltimore, Williams and Wilkins, 1976.
2. Manter JT: Movements of the subtalar and transverse Tarsal joints. Anatomical Record 80:397-410, 1941.
3. Hicks JH: The mechanics of the foot. I. The joints. J Anat 87:345-357, 1953.
4. Henderson WH, Campbell JW: UC-BL shoe insert: Casting and fabrication. Biomechanics Laboratory, University of California, San Francisco, Laboratory, 1967. Reprinted in Bull Pres Thet Res 10-11:215, 1969.
5. Campbell JW, Inman VT: Treatment of Plantar Fasciitis and Calcaneal Spurs with the UC-BL shoe insert. Clin Orthop 103:57-67, 1974.
6. Colson JW, Berglund G: An effective orthotic design for controlling the unstable subtalar joint. Orthotics and Prosthetics 33:39-49, 1979.

CHAPTER 16

Nutritional Needs of the Runner

Diane M. Huse, RD, MS

Introduction

Interest in the relationship between the athlete's diet and his performance is probably older than organized sports. Many of the dietary superstitions of primitive tribes are based on the idea that certain foods-in particular the meat of certain animals- endowed the consumer with the qualities of strength, endurance, and courage with which his prey was identified.[1] Perusal of the daily press leads one to believe that some special nutritional factors are responsible for the preparation and success of members of professional or Olympic teams. Proper nutrition all too often loses out to food fads, quackery, and superstition among athletes. Special properties are ascribed to specific foods and food supplements that have little scientific merit. Evaluating the effect of a single food on performance is extremely difficult because of the interference of such variables as motivation, differences in experimental conditions, types of work performed, and the wide range of individual response. The practices being followed may have potentially harmful effects (eg, megavitamin treatment) or may reinforce eating habits or attitudes about food that may be detrimental in later life (e.g., inappropriate high calorie intake leading to obesity). The implications of dietary practices for future health should be carefully considered, especially when dealing with the young athlete whose growth and development must be protected.

The athlete's nutritional needs are similar to those of nonathlete; he requires calories, protein, water, vitamins, and minerals in quantities determined by his age, body size, and activity level. These requirements can be met by a basic, well- balanced diet.

Calorie Needs

The calorie or energy requirement of a person is determined by his basal energy expenditure and the energy expended in physical activity. Basal energy expenditure is relatively constant and includes energy required for maintenance of muscle tone, body temperature, circulation, respiration, and other glandular and cellular activities, including those related to growth. The primary determinants of basal metabolic energy requirement are body size, age, and sex. With these determinants, basal energy requirement can be determined from a nomogram,[2] or can be estimated from the formula: basal enrgy needs equals one kilocalorie per kilogram of body weight per hour.[3] In general, the basal energy requirement increases as body size or surface area increases, is higher in young people than in older persons, and is higher in males than in females.

Physical activity is the major determinant of variation in energy expenditure among individuals. Whenever muscular work is done, energy is used, and the amount required is proportional to the work done. Estimates of energy needs are: for extremely light or sedentary activity, such as writing at a desk or standing in one place, add 30% of the basal metabolic energy needs; for light activity, such as filing or other office work, 50%; for moderative activity, such as that allowing for little sitting, 75%; and for strenuous activity, such as construction work or athletics, 100% or more.[4]

The nonathlete can, therefore, estimate his daily energy requirement by determining his daily basal energy requirement using 24 kilocalories per kilogram of body weight and adding to that the appropriate percent of the basal calorie needs for the level of activity selected by the person as most typical of his daily routine. The athlete also uses this method of determining calorie needs but must determine the additional calories required for his athletic activity by considering the frequency and duration of his participation in the activity. The amount can be approximated by knowing the caloric cost per minute of the activity. The athlete's daily energy requirement will change depending on whether the day is the day of competition, a training day, or a day during off-season. The duration of activity will differ in each of these situations. For the runner, the approximate calorie cost of cross-country running is 10.6 kilocalories per minute;[1] of long distance running 15.0 kilocalories per minute;[5] and of marathon running, 20.7 kilocalories per minute.[6]

Estimates of energy expenditure in running are made more difficult by variations in terrain and air resistance. Various investigators have shown that the total energy expenditure in running on a level surface is constant and independent of velocity for a given person; pace has little effect on the caloric cost of running. Running up a hill with an incline of 6% requires 35% more energy than running on level ground. Running down a similar grade reduces the effort by only 24%. Studies of running in still air and against the wind suggest that in distance running about 5% to 8% of the energy spent is needed to overcome air resistance.[6] Of more importance, perhaps, is the energy cost based on the weight of the runner.

Because the work of exercise, as measured by oxygen consumption, increases as body weight increases, it is easy to understand the advantage attributed the runner who has small bones and minimal body fat. The less nonpropulsive weight or fat, the greater the efficiency of movement. Anatomically, marathoners are usually small and thin. The average height and weight of all the Boston Marathon Champions from 1897 to 1965 was 170 cm (range 155-188 cm) and 61 kg (48.8-78.2 kg).[6] An estimate of excess weight can be made by comparing the athlete's weight to a standard weight chart for height and age. A weight chart may give a false impression of overweight for the muscular athlete, however, because muscle tissue is heavier than fat tissue. A more accurate method to assess an athlete's excess weight is to measure the percent of body fat by use of calipers designed to measure the thickness of a fold of skin. Buskirk[7] advocated measuring the skin over the triceps muscle and advised that a skinfold less than eight millimeters thickness indicates a "lean" body build, eight to fifteen millimeters is "acceptable",and greater than fifteen millimeters (about one-half inch) is "over-fat." These measurements apply to highly trained athletes in top condition whose ideal fat content is 5% to 8%, the figures must not be broadly applied. When skinfold estimates of body fat were made on 114 competitors at the 1968 U.S. Olympic Marathon Trial, they showed that the marathon runners had about 7.5% fat or about 9% less than normally active men of comparable age.[8] Several of the top finishes were found to have less than 5% body fat.[6]

Cureton and co-workers investigated the effect of experimental alterations in excess weight on aerobic capacity and distance running performance.[9] Additional weight was found to decrease significantly maximal oxygen uptake (expressed relative to total weight carried), maximal treadmill run time, and 12-minute run distance. An increase of 5% additional weight was found, on the average, to decrease maximal oxygen uptake by 2.4 ml, the treadmill run time by 35 seconds, and the 12-minute run distance by 89 meters. These decreases were direct consequences of the increased energy cost of running at submaximal speeds.

The determination of and adherence to a daily caloric intake appropriate for body size and activity needs are, therefore, of great importance, because if the runner's caloric intake exceeds his needs, his total body fat will increase. The increase in body fat resulting from caloric intake exceeding caloric needs will not only decrease the runner's performance by increasing the work of his exercise but also may create eating habits and attitudes about food that may contribute to the development of obesity in later life.

Caloric balance is especially important for athletes during the off-season and in the post-competitive years. Many athletes develop weight problems at these times because they fail to realize that when competition and training stops, habitually high calorie intakes must be lowered for adaptation to decreased energy demands.

Protein

Proteins are more complex molecules than either fats or carbohydrates. The molecules are similar in that they all contain oxygen, hydrogen, and carbon, but proteins (unlike fats or carbohydrates) also contain nitrogen; many contain sulfur, phosphorus, iron, and other minerals as well. Proteins are made up of great numbers of relatively simple units, the nitrogen- containing compounds called amino acids.

The major roles of proteins in the body are for building new tissues in growing children, in athletic training, and after injury; for maintaining tissues already built and replacement of regular losses; as regulatory substances for internal water and acid-base balance; as a precursor for enzymes, antibodies, and some hormones; and as energy. If more protein is eaten than is needed for essential functions, the extra protein is oxidized to supply energy or is converted to body fat if the total energy intake is excessive. If the content of the diet is inadequate (ie, if sufficient carbohydrates and fats are not supplied to meet the energy needs of the body), proteins are burned for energy because energy needs have a higher priority than does maintenance of some of the tissue proteins. In this event, building or repair processes will suffer. Nitrogen, which is indispensable as long as protein is used for tissue building, becomes a liability when protein must be used for energy. The nitrogen-containing substances (primarily urea) that result from amino acid oxidation must be excreted by the kidneys. Because energy is more economically supplied by carbohydrates and fats, the consumption of protein greatly in excess of body needs is usually disadvantageous.

The requirement for protein in the diet has been set at 0.8 grams per kilogram body weight per day for adults. Because of the additional need for protein for growth in children, the requirement decreases gradually from 2.0 grams per kilogram at ages 0.5 to 1 year to 0.8 gram per kilogram at age 18 years.

Increases in lean body mass, enzymatic proteins, and hemoglobin, all typical effects of training, may temporarily require greater than normal intakes of protein. Athletes who develop proteinuria, hemoglobinuria, or myoglobinuria as a result of high-intensity exercise may also require greater than normal levels of protein until these conditions subside. One recommendation has been that during training and competitions the mature athlete needs 1 gram protein per kilogram body weight per day, and the growing athlete may require up to 1.5 grams protein per kilogram per day to meet his greater demand for amino acid retention and protein synthesis.[10] The recommendations for increased protein intake during athletic training vary, however. Consolazio and Johnson believe than an increased dietary protein above normal intake for men in athletic training is not necessary.[11]

Although early workers thought that protein was the primary source of muscular energy, the work of Voit and Pettenkofer, as Mayer and Bullen[1] pointed out, refuted this theory, and this refutation has been well confirmed. Nitrogen excretion has been shown repeatedly not to increase during muscular work. As Consolazio and co-workers[5] mentioned, Atwater showed that nitrogen excretion was not above that in the resting conditions, even when metabolic rate was nearly doubled by physical work. Astrand cited data showing the combustion of protein was not higher during heavy exercise than during rest, even after glycogen depots have been depleted.[12] Pitts, Consolazio, and Johnson[13] examined the effect of variation in the level of dietary protein on the physical fitness (ie, treadmill runs of various speeds and grades, followed by pulse counts, of three subjects studied under both temperate and tropical conditions while reclining, standing, and marching). There was no change in performance attributable to dietary protein level under any of these environmental conditions, although improvements due to training and acclimatization were observed.

More recently, it has been proposed by Evans and co-workers[14] that, in addition to carbohydrates and fats, amino acids can contribute to whole body energy metabolism. The availability of amino acids results from a substantial decrease in the rate of protein synthesis during exercise. These researchers estimate that protein can provide up to 5.5% of the total calorie cost of the exercise. According to this study, estimates of the extent of amino acid oxidation indicate that current recommendations for maximal protein requirements may not be adequate for physically active individuals.

Excess protein intake increases water requirements of the body because additional fluid is required to eliminate nitrogen by-products in the urine. Not only is excess protein unnecessary, it can be harmful, particularly when ingested during times of intense athletic competition, when it can compromise body hydration.

Vitamins

Vitamins are organic compounds that occur in small concentrations in foods; they are necessary in small amounts in the diet for normal growth, maintenance, and reproduction. Their absence in the diet or improper absorption results in specific deficiency diseases. They differ from each other in physiologic function, in chemical structure, and in distribution in food. The vitamins are classified into two groups based on their solubility. The solubility characteristic is important in determining whether the body can store the vitamin or whether the supply must be replenished daily. Solubility also has implications for the vitamin's toxic potential when taken in excess of body needs. The four vitamins A, D, E, and K are soluble in fat and fat solvents and are therefore known as the fat-soluble vitamins. They can be stored in the body to some extent, mostly in the liver, and as a result manifestations of deficiencies are likely to be slow. The water-soluble vitamins include vitamin C and the B complex vitamins. The body has limited ability to store water-soluble vitamins, except water-soluble vitamin B12, which is stored extensively in the liver. Tissues are depleted of their normal content of these vitamins in a relatively short period if the diet is deficient, so supplies are needed regularly to maintain tissues levels. The tissues take up only as much as is needed, and because water-soluble vitamins are freely soluble in water, most of the intake of these vitamins not required for day-to-day use is excreted in the urine. However, excessive intakes of some of the B complex vitamins may cause side effects.

Most B complex vitamins act as an organic catalyst or as a part of a catalyst. A catalyst is a substance that speeds up a chemical reaction without itself taking part in it. The special types of organic catalysts that promote these reactions in living tissues are known as enzymes and coenzymes, which aid enzymes in their tasks. Many of the vitamins occur in the body as coenzymes responsible for promoting some essential chemical reaction. For example, the cell gets much of the energy it requires through oxidation of the carbohydrate glucose. This oxidation takes place in many intermediate steps, so that energy is gradually set free. Several of the B complex vitamins are coenzymes that catalyze specific steps in the oxidation of carbohydrates. The absence of any of these enzymes means a failure of some link in the chain of tissue oxidations. Therefore, the lack of a vitamin that is an essential part of such an enzyme can inhibit oxidative processes in cells.

As in the case of caloric undernutrition, the impairment of the ability to perform work efficiently in cases of frank vitamin deficiency is well known. No conclusive evidence, however, supports the theory that once vitamin requirements are met, supplementation will enhance athletic performance. Greater attention should be directed to the possible detrimental effects of their indiscriminate use.

Easy fatigability, loss of appetite, irritability, and apathy are signs of vitamin B complex deficiency; the ability to perform work efficiently is impaired in this state. Review of the studies done on work efficiency of persons receiving diets adequate in B complex vitamin versus B complex vitamin supplements indicate that supplementation does not enhance performance. In normal young men, in experiments lasting 10 to 12 weeks, intakes of the B-complex vitamin thiamine at four different levels, from 0.23 mg per 1,000 kcal daily up to 0.63 mg per 1,000 kcal, exerted no beneficial effect on diets otherwise considered adequate. Muscular, neuromuscular, cardiovascular, psychomotor, and metabolic functions tested were in no way limited. Clinical signs, subjective sensations, and state of mind and behavior were likewise unaffected.[15]

Nicotinic acid, or niacin, is another of the B complex vitamins. It has been shown, in exercising men, to decrease mobilization of fatty acids from adipose tissue, resulting in increased utilization of muscle glycogen stores for energy.[16] The effects of large doses of niacin on myocardial metabolism in men, either at rest or during exercise, have been documented as undesirable on the metabolism of heart muscle.[17] Because fatty acids are important fuels for the heart, excessive consumption of niacin is contraindicated before endurance events.

Vitamin C supplementation is especially popular among athletes, because of its known role in collagen synthesis and the poor quality of tissue repair associated with vitamin C deficiency. The reasoning is that the athlete has perhaps a greater need for collagen synthesis and tissue repair, and thus athletic performance would benefit from supplementation. It has been found that vitamin C supplementation has a negligible effect on endurance performance, or on severity or duration of athletic injury.[18]

Excessive vitamin C supplementation increases vitamin C destruction in the body. Scurvy has been noted in persons who have had a history of taking excessive amounts of vitamin C and who returned to a diet containing normal amounts.[19] Seventeen subjects consuming 1 to 3 grams of vitamin C per day over a period of three to 36 months were studied to determine the serum ascorbic acid levels. The subjects' intake was first standardized to 2 grams vitamin C supplement per day for ten days. The serum ascorbic acid level was found to be 1.45 mg per 100 ml. The serum ascorbic acid level of 16 normal controls not receiving supplemental vitamin C was 1.20 per 100 ml, and increased to 2.75 mg per 100 ml after the administration of 2 grams vitamin C supplement daily for eight days. Therefore, the serum ascorbic acid levels initially increase, reaching a maximum value after about eight days of supplementation. The continued use of supplemental vitamin C leads to a gradual decline of the serum levels that cannot be compensated by increasing the dosage.[19]

Because adequate saturation levels of ascorbic acid may be maintained on recommended dietary sources of vitamin C, the habitual intake of larger amounts is not advantageous, while posing the risks of causing the ascorbic acid deficiency on termination of the regimen.

On the basis of these data, one can no longer presume that excessive intake of a water-soluable vitamin will simply result in excess quantities being excreted in the urine with no possibility for toxic effects. At high does, vitamins stop acting as vitamins and act instead as pharmacological agents. While nontoxic at recommended allowances for vitamins, impurities in vitamin preparation when vitamins are taken in megadoses can far exceed the limits of safety.

Vitamin E is a fat-soluable vitamin. There is no evidence that the healthy human is susceptible to vitamin E deficiency; supplementation has, likewise, not proved to be advantageous. Vitamin E toxicity in humans has not been confirmed. An oxidation product of vitamin E has been thought to be an inhibitor of vitamin K and, therefore, responsible for a prolongation in blood clotting time. Large doses of vitamin E potentiate the affect of warfarin. A study conducted by the National Institutes of Health on persons who had been ingesting up to 800 IU of vitamin E for more than 3 years did not find evidence of toxicity.[20] Although some athletes have taken vitamin E in hopes of improving athletic performance, vitamin E taken at a level of 900 IU daily for six months did not improve athletic performance in well-trained swimmers.[21]

Minerals

Sodium, potassium, and iron are the minerals most often affected by heavy exercise. While mineral losses may be incurred during strenuous exercise, athletes must be aware of the potentially toxic side effects of the inappropriate use of minerals. Because sodium and potassium are intimately related to the athlete's state of hydration, these minerals will be part of the discussion of water requirement.

Iron is distributed through the body as a component of essential metabolic enzymes in every cell. About 65% to 70% of the iron in the body is present in the blood as hemoglobin in the red blood cells. Hemoglobin is essential for oxygen transport in the blood. The remainder of the iron stored in the body is found in combination with protein in the liver, bone, and bone marrow or found in other tissues such as myoglobin in muscles. In all sites, the iron-containing compounds are involved in the vital processes of cells and tissues. The body guards its iron stores carefully and reuses any iron that is broken down in the body over and over again. Only small amounts of iron lost in the urine, sweat, hair, sloughed-off skin, and nails and by menstruation needs to be replaced normally only about 1 or 1.5 mg a day. About one-tenth of the iron in the diet is absorbed, which means that about 10 times the amount of iron must be eaten than the 1 or 1.5 mg a day that the body actually uses in its tissues. The 1980

National Research Council's recommended dietary allowances are 18 mg of iron per day for women and 10 mg per day for men.

Iron needs are greater during periods of growth, including pregnancy, lactation, and infancy through adolescence. Iron deficiency is the most common nutritional deficiency in the United States.[22]

Bunch states that the low or low-normal hemoglobin or hematocrit values commonly found in runners or other endurance-trained persons seldom reflect true anemia and do not indicate a need for folate or vitamin B12.[23]

In the past decade, interest has increased among athletes in the use of iron to improve performance. Low serum iron values and subnormal hemoglobin values have been demonstrated among athletes who are involved in intense physical activity. That finding has been looked on as a possible factor responsible for suboptimal oxygen transport and hence lower capacity for physical performance. The relationship between performance and serum ferritin was evaluated by Martin et al.[24] In the nine elite male distance runners studied, this relationship suggested that the iron depletion state may be significant in these runners, even in the absence of anemia.

The iron status and the possible effect of training on iron metabolism of a group of extremely hard-training long-distance runners has been reported from Sweden. A depressed absorption combined with an increased elimination were thought to explain these runners' suboptimal iron state.[25] Reports of anemia and suboptimal hemoglobin levels in athletes have generated much speculation regarding the possible causes of sports anemia. One or more of the three mechanisms could result in the development of anemia.[26] First, a relative anemia could develop through a hemodilution effect of an expanded plasma volume. This increase in total blood volume is thought to be a positive adaptation to increase stroke volume of the heart and maximal cardiac output.

Second, reduced hemoglobin synthesis and/or erythropoiesis could result in an actual decrease in total hemoglobin. Since endurance trained athletes tend to manifest a high total hemoglobin it seems unlikely that the rate of hemoglobin synthesis and red blood cell production are depressed in athletes as a group. However, it is possible that sports anemia could result from reduced or inadequate rates of hemoglobin and/or red blood cells synthesis in affected athletes.

Third, an increased rate of destruction of red blood cells and degradation of hemoglobin could decrease the concentration of hemoglobin in circulating blood. Ehn et al [27] have reported a high rate of iron loss, which was not explained by intravascular hemolysis or hemoglobinuria. It was suggested, however, that loss of iron through heavy sweating could have been a factor. Iron loss via sweat is usually considered to be negligible in humans. Vellar showed, however, that in cases of extreme sweating as much as 40 mg of iron per 100 ml sweat, resulting in perhaps an extra iron loss of 0.4mg to 1.0 mg per day. The increased elimination rate of iron found in the runner could be explained by the profuse sweating that occurs.

It has been suggested that hemolysis is a possible cause of low iron storage and sports anemia. A high rate of intravascular hemolysis may be a transient condition resulting from the breakdown of fragile red blood cells at the onset of heavy training. Runners and joggers may inflict trauma on red blood cells circulating through the capillaries in the feet. This may be manifested as hemoglobinuria, the presence of free hemoglobin in the urine. This condition has been reported in some athletes, but its incidence does not appear to be high.

Heavy menstrual blood losses may combine with other previously mentioned factors to increase the female athlete's risk of developing iron deficiency and/or anemia.

Many possible causes of sports anemia and suboptimal hemoglobin have been suggested, but few have been studied in depth. Sports anemia, as distinct from suboptimal hemoglobin, seems more likely to be associated with dietary deficiencies and/or high rates of iron loss through menstruation, sweating, and hemoglobinuria.

From the physical standpoint, the runner should be advised to include adequate quantities of iron in his diet. To advise oral iron therapy for women runners is appropriate because of menstrual loss. As recommendation for individuals in the general population, greater attention to good sources of iron in the diet seems reasonable. The best dietary sources of iron are meat, especially organ meats, fish, poultry, and eggs. Green leafy vegetables, potatoes, dried fruits, and enriched bread and cereal products are the best plant sources.

Water

Humans can live for about 30 days without food, but will die in 5 to 6 days if deprived of water. Water is lost from the body constantly from the skin as perspiration; from the lungs as water vapor in expired air; from the kidneys as urine; and from the intestines in feces. A minimum of 800 ml of water is lost daily through the skin and lungs and this amount may increase in hot, dry environments. The kidneys eliminate about 1,000 to 1,500 ml of water in urine; fecal losses approximate 200 ml daily.

Fluids are replaced by the ingestion of liquids and foods containing water. To ensure sufficient water, adults should drink 2,000 to 2,500 ml of water or other liquids daily.

Body water serves many functions. Nutrients, hormones, waste products, and antibodies are all transported in the water of the blood plasma. All of the body's chemical reactions are carried out in water and are significantly less efficient when an adequate amount of body water is not available.

The role of water in regulating body temperature is of particular importance to the athlete. The excessive heat generated by exercise must be dissipated, and the most effective way is through evaporation of sweat. This mechanism fails to function effectively, however, if the water supply is inadequate to meet the needs of the sweat glands.

When fluid losses exceed supply, dehydration follows. Dehydration is characterized by loss of appetite and limited capacity for work. Physiological changes that impair performance are detectable with losses no greater than 3% of body weight. When losses are 5%, evidence of heat exhaustion becomes apparent and at 7% hallucinations occur. Losses totaling 10% are hazardous and lead to heat stroke, sudden collapse, and loss of consciousness. Persons in excellent physical condition can perform adequately until body water equal to 4% to 5% of body weight is lost.[29] Generally, with the loss of water amounting to 4% to 5% of body weight, the capacity for hard muscular work declines by 20% to 30%.[30] For the most satisfactory fluid maintenance, no more than 2% of body weight should be lost.

During exercise and muscular work, changes take place in the distribution of body water. When exercise begins, water is immediately transferred from the extracellular fluid space to the intracellular space within cells. This transfer facilitates the utilization of energy. The extracellular fluid that moves into the muscle cells is rapidly replaced by water from blood plasma, thereby reducing the volume of circulating blood. The amount of blood plasma that is available to flow to the kidneys is thus reduced, and urine production is decreased.

Once exercise begins, the water is lost through sweating and increased breathing, this reduced excretion of urinary water provides a control mechanism that helps to conserve body water. Mechanisms for increased water intake are not nearly as effective. After a period of exercise and resulting dehydration, the average thirst response will not in itself call for complete replacement of body water for a considerable time, often up to several days. The need for a prescribed schedule for water intake to maintain hydration is important for the athlete.

The athlete who is well conditioned will voluntarily drink more often than one who is not well trained. The well conditioned athlete will also sweat more profusely and will thus more effectively dissipate his body heat. The athlete who is well acclimated replaces water and salt losses in sweat and urine by diet. There should be no need for an increased salt intake, just greater amounts of drinking water. Non-acclimatized athletes may sweat excessively and have salt losses that greatly exceed dietary intake. Graduated physical activity should be scheduled for one week to allow for acclimatization and permit the kidney and endocrine glands to adjust to sodium conservation.[31] Even the well-conditioned athlete, who drinks more and more nearly compensates for his water losses, may spontaneously replace the one-half to one-third of his sweat losses within 24 hours of a vigorous workout or competition if weight loss is not considered, along with thirst, in water needs.

Distance runners may lose 8 to 13 pounds of water during a marathon run. That loss causes dehydration of 13% to 21% of plasma water and 11% of muscle water.[32] All athletes should weigh-in before and after each event or practice. The difference in weights before and after the event or competition represents water loss, and the proper amount of water replacement required can be determined.[29] Weight loss should be a guide to water replacement. The athlete should take 2 to 3 cups of water or liquid supplement for each pound of weight loss.

In addition to their role in maintaining acid-base balance, sodium and potassium exert a primary influence on the distribution of body water. Sodium is concentrated primarily in the extracellular fluid, whereas potassium is concentrated in the intracellular fluid. Any salt ingested in excess of salt losses will cause a trapping of water between cells and deplete the intracellular supply. When water is in short supply in the body, the most critical need is to maintain the metabolically active water within cells.

Sweat is hypotonic compared with the body fluid, so that relatively more fluid than salts, such as sodium and potassium, is lost from the body during sweating. Athletes in training do not require electrolyte supplements to replace perspiration losses because healthy kidneys automatically compensate by conserving sodium and potassium. Clearly, the body has highly effective mechanisms for regulating its supply of sodium and potassium.

Specific salt replacement is rarely needed during athletic activity, even if excessive sweat loss occurs. About 20 to 30 milliequivalents of sodium are lost per 1,000 ml of perspiration. Excessive sweating can lead to sodium losses of 350 milliequivalents (8 grams) per day in the acclimated person.[33] The usual dietary sodium intake of the adult is 100 to 300 milliequivalents (2 to 7 grams) per day.[33] Americans eating a varied diet generally get more than enough sodium in their daily foods to meet even the extraordinary needs of vigorous athletic activity. As a general guideline, however, Smith[29] recommends that, if water loss exceeds 5 to 10 pounds in a given workout, some consideration may be given to specific salt replacement. This replacement can be made by liberally salting a normal diet or it can be provided by a highly dilute salt-containing fluid, whose concentration should not exceed 1.5 grams of salt per liter of water (or ⅓ of a teaspoon per quart). Smith states that the use of salt tablets is inappropriate because they provide a high concentration of salt and may complicate the state of dehydration.

Williams believes that salt tablets may not be necessary to restore lost electrolytes if the weight loss is less than 6 pounds per day.[32] The person who is not acclimatized to heat will lose about 4 to 5 grams sodium with a 6 pound loss; the acclimatized person will lose only about 3 grams. Because the average meal contains as much as 3 grams of sodium, normal food intake should suffice. Williams recommends that one salt tablet should be taken per pound of weight loss over 6 pounds and that a pint of water be taken with each 7 gram tablet (200 mg sodium). This dosage is consistent with the Food and Nutrition Board of the National Research Council recommendation of a 2-gram salt (800 mg sodium) replacement per liter of extra water lost in sweating.[33]

Potassium losses in sweat are negligible under any but the most extreme conditions, and potassium depletion is not a primary concern. The need for potassium has been suggested because of the low serum levels found in some athletes after exercise. Now, however, it is thought to be due to hemodilution rather than actual depletion of body potassium. Muscle weakness could result from excessive potassium losses. If additional needs do exist because of exercise losses, potassium may be increased in the normal diet by the inclusion of foods high in potassium, such as oranges, grapefruit, pineapples, apricots, bananas, and dried fruit.

Basic Diet

Optimal nutrition is one of the basic conditions necessary to maintain top performance for the athlete and nonathlete alike. As the previous review indicates, the athlete, aside from possible increases in caloric intake necessitated by increased energy expenditure and in water intake to ensure adequate hydration, does not need additional nutrients beyond those found in a balanced diet.

The diet recommendation for the athlete, and for the population in general, is one in which about 15% of calories are derived from protein, 30% to 35%

from fat, and 50% to 55% from carbohydrats. This distribution of nutrients will allow for a moderate intake of protein, which easily meets requirements during training and is reasonable in terms of the athlete's appetite for meat. It provides a fat intake that is less than that currently consumed in this country but meets the recommendations of the American Heart Association.

No single food or category of foods contains all of the nutrients in amounts sufficient to maintain life. The key to balancing the diet is combining different foods so that nutrient deficiencies in some foods are made up for by nutrient surpluses in others. Each nutrient performs specific functions in the body and each needs to be present for the body to be in peak condition. Eating a proper variety of foods at each meal is the secret.

An adequate guide on which an athlete should base his food selection is the use of food groups. These food groups include milk and milk products; meat and meat substitutes; fruit and vegetables; and cereals and grains-the Basic Four Food Groups as established by the United States Department of Agriculture in 1956. For a diet selected to meet high energy needs, such as the athlete's diet, additional groups such as fats and oils, desserts, and sugars and sweets are also appropriate. Foods included in each of these groups, the major nutrients supplied in each group, and the quantity of each food constituting a serving size are illustrated in Table 16-1.

Foods are classified into groups on the basis of similarities in nutrient composition; foods in a group are comparable in calories, protein, minerals, and vitamins, and can be interchanged if taken in the suggested serving sizes. There is a vast leeway in the choice of the foods within each of the groups. The diet is flexible enough to adapt to an almost unlimited range of conditions and circumstances.

A reference runner, male, 29 years old, 170 cm in height and 61 kg in weight, would require about 1,500 kcal for daily basal needs (24 kcal/kg see page 166). Calorie needs on a day when he is engaged in light activity would be met by the addition of 50%of basal needs or about 2,200 calories. A sample menu illustrating this calorie level with a nutrient distribution of 15% of calories as protein, 35% as fat, and 50% as carbohydrate is shown in Table 16-2, an additional 900 calories would be required by the athlete if he ran 60 minutes at a calorie cost of 15 calories per minute, increasing his calories needs to 3,100 on that day.

As the calorie level of the diet is adjusted depending on the daily calorie demands for activity, the distribution of protein, fat, and carbohydrate should remain relatively constant so that the diet remains well balanced, nutritionally. That is, the intake of calories should not be increased by merely adding more meat or decreased by eliminating bread or potatoes (Tables 16-3 and 16- 4).

Optimum body weight is important for the runner. If the reference runner weighs 70 kg and wishes to reduce to 61 kg at a comfortable rate of about 1 kg per week, he must reduce his daily calorie intake by 1,000. Because 0.5 kg body fat equals 3,500 calories, a deficit of 7,000 calories a week would result in 1 kg of body fat. To maintain this rate of weight loss, on light activity days, the reference runner's calorie intake should be about 1,200, and 2,100 on days when he runs about 60 minutes. In the weight-reduction diet plan, less emphasis is placed on foods from the desserts and sugars and sweet food groups, because they

Table 16-1
Food Guide

Food Group	Foods Included	Major Nutrients Supplied	Serving Size
Milk Group	Milk (skim, buttermilk, 2%,* whole*), yogurt	Calcium, protein, riboflavin, vitamin A and D (all milk should be fortified with vitamins A and D)	1 serving is 1 cup (8 ounces)
Meat Group	Beef, pork, lamb, veal, organ meats,* poultry, fish, shellfish, egg,* cheese,* cottage cheese. As alternates—dry peas, dry beans, lentils, peanuts,* peanut butter*	Protein, thiamin, riboflavin, niacin and iron	1 serving is —1 ounce lean cooked meat, fish, poultry —1 egg —½ cup cooked dry peas, beans or lentils —2 tablespoons peanut butter (25 peanuts) —1 ounce cheese or ¼ cup cottage cheese
Bread-Cereal Group	All whole grain or enriched breads and cereals, macaroni, grits, spaghetti, crackers, noodles and rice	Food energy (kilocalories), protein, B complex vitamins	1 serving is —1 slice bread —½ cup cooked cereal, rice, macaroni, grits, noodles, spaghetti —1 ounce ready-to-eat cereal —4-6 crackers
Vegetable Group	Vegetables, cooked or raw	Vitamins A and C primarily as well as other vitamins and minerals Good sources of vitamin C are broccoli, brussels sprouts, green peppers Good sources of vitamin D are deep yellow or dark green vegetables such as carrots, pumpkin, spinach, sweet potato, winter squash, broccoli, beets, collards, turnip and mustard greens, kale	1 serving is —½ cup cooked —1 cup raw Each day have one serving high in vitamin C; at least every other day have 1 serving high in vitamin A

(Table Continued)

Table 16-1 continued

Group	Food	Nutrients	Serving
Fruit Group	Fruits Fresh or cooked Fruit juice	Vitamins A and C primarily as well as other vitamin and minerals Good sources of vitamin C are cantaloupe, strawberries, grapefruit, lemon, oranges Good sources of vitamin A are cantaloupe and apricots	1 serving is —½ cup juice —1 medium piece fruit —½ cup cooked
Fat Group	Butter,* margarine, cooking fats* and oils, salad dressing, mayonnaise, sour cream,* gravy,* cream sauce,* cream*	Food energy (kilocalories) Carries of fat-soluble vitamins A, D, E	1 serving size is —1 teaspoon butter, margarine, oil, mayonnaise —2 tablespoons gravy, cream, sour cream, cream sauce —2 teaspoons salad dressing
Desserts	Ice cream,* frosted cake,* cookies,* pie,* sweet roll,* chocolate*	Food energy (kilocalories)	1 serving is —1/12 of 9-inch fruit pie —¾ cup ice cream —2" x 3" x 2" piece frosted cake —1½ ounces chocolate —2 - 2" cookies
Sugars and Sweets	Sugar, jelly, syrup, honey, hard candy, carbonated beverage	Food energy (kilocalories)	1 serving is —1 tablespoon sugar, jelly, syrup, honey —3 pieces hard candy —4 ounces carbonated beverage

*Omit to reduce cholesterol and/or saturated fat content of diet.

tend to be higher in calories and lower in essential nutrients than are appropriate at low calorie intakes. The percent of calories derived from protein is likely to be greater to meet the person's protein requirement of 0.8 gram per kilogram body weight (Tables 16-3 and 16-4).

Weight reduction efforts by means of starvation or fad diets that emphasize the omission or encourage the increased use of a particular group of foods are never appropriate. Fad diets are usually nutritionally inadequate and will compromise not only athletic performance but general health. Weight loss from starvation involves loss of protein, glycogen, potassium, sodium, phosphorus, sulfur, enzymes, and other important cell constituents. Fifty percent or more of weight loss induced by total starvation involves fat-free protoplasm. The result of these responses is diminished body reserves for athletic demands. Weight reduction efforts should include increased physical activity and a calorie-controlled, nutritionally well-balanced diet.

Table 16-2
Sample Menu
2200 Calories

Breakfast
Orange Juice	1 cup
Ready-to-Eat Cereal	2 ounces (about 1½ cups)
Milk	1 cup
Sugar	1 teaspoon
Ham	1 ounce
Toast	2 slices
Margarine or Butter	2 teaspoons
Jelly	2 teaspoons

Lunch
Roast Beef Sandwiches	2
Bread	4 slices
Roast Beef	4 ounces
Mayonnaise	2 teaspoons
Lettuce	
Celery and Carrot Sticks	
Fresh Pear	

Dinner
Baked Chicken	3 ounces
Rice	½ cup
Dinner Roll	1
Margarine or Butter	1 teaspoon
Broccoli	
Green Salad	
Salad Dressing	4 teaspoons
Ice Cream	3/4 cup

Evening Snack
Peanut Butter	2 tablespoons
Toast	2 slices
Margarine or Butter	2 teaspoons
Apple	1

Table 16-2. Sample Menu — 2200 calories.

If the athlete eats a varied diet that meets but does not exceed his calorie, protein, vitamin, and mineral requirements, he need not take protein, vitamin, or mineral supplements; his nutrient requirements will be met by food. A dietitian should be consulted if there are questions about the formulation of the diet.

Carbohydrate Loading

The key role of carbohydrate in exercise performance has been emphasized for several decades. The main source of carbohydrate was thought to be local glycogen stores in muscle tissue, which was confirmed by Bergstrom and co-workers[34] by direct determinations of glycogen content in human muscle tissue during exercise. In 1967, Bergstrom and co-workers[34] and Hermansen et al[35] reported studies in young men of the effect of muscle glycogen levels on physical performance and endurance. The results indicated that performance time to exhaustion averaged 59, 126, and 189 minutes after three days on a high

	Protein		Fat		Carbohydrate	
Calories	grams	% of kcal	grams	% of kcal	grams	% of kcal
1200	60	20	40	30	150	50
2200	80	15	85	35	275	50
3100	115	15	120	35	390	50

Table 16-3
Nutrient Content of Meal Plans at
Sample Calorie Levels

Table 16-3. Nutrient Content of Sample Meal Plans

Table 16-4
Number of Servings of Food
at Sample Calorie Levels

Food Group	1200 Calorie	2200 Calorie	3100 Calorie
Milk	1	1	3
Meat	7	7	9
Bread-Cereal	4	12	12
Vegetable	2-3	2-3	2-3
Fruit	8	4	9
Fat	1	9	14
Dessert	0	1	1
Sugar-Sweet	0	1	4

Table 16-4. Meal Plans for Sample Calorie Levels

fat-high protein diet, a mixed diet, and a high carbohydrate diet, respectively. Muscle biopsy measurements indicated that the nutrient composition of the diet could affect the muscle glycogen stores. These stores were observed to be reduced during strenuous exercise, and when the muscle glycogen drops to a critical level, work usually stops or the physical activity rate is decreased. In this instance, an increased energy yield from free fatty acids results. These studies show that the working muscles have a requirement for carbohydrate as an energy source and that carbohydrate is obtained directly from the muscle stores of glycogen.

In the well-trained athlete, in brief high-intensity exercise (eg, tennis, sprinting), the size of the glycogen store is not a limiting factor, provided that it is not grossly subnormal at the beginning of the exercise. On the other hand, with high-intensity exercise of long duration, glycogen stores can be a limiting factor for the endurance capacity, especially considering that, at the end of the competition, a capacity to increase the performance (spurt) may be decisive for winning. Such long-duration, high-intensity exercise includes long-distance running, cross-country skiing and possibly some team sports, such as soccer and ice hockey. The amount of glycogen stores must also be considered when athletes perform repeatedly during one day.

Bergstrom et al observed that, after the muscle glycogen stores had been depleted by previous exercise, a high-carbohydrate diet for one to three days greatly enhanced the synthesis of muscle glycogen.[34] They also showed that, when carbohydrate was given without any previous exercise, muscle glycogen stores only moderately increased.

Slovic confirmed that carbohydrate loading does improve performance, with the improvement most pronounced in the final stages of the event.[36] The available information indicates that the glycogen content of the working muscle is one of the most important factors for prolonged exercise.

The carbohydrate loading technique has been published in many forms, but essentially consists of three phases: phase I, the depletion phase, consists of days 7 to 4 before the event; phase II, the glycogen synthesis phase, days 3 to 1 before the event; phase III, the day of the event[37].

In phase I, the specific muscles to be used must be exercised to exhaustion by the same type of activity as performed during the event, to deplete them of their glycogen stores. Phase I is done about six to seven days before the day of the endurance event,. so that the muscles can be rested before the event. The diet during this phase is crucial. While depleting the muscles of glycogen, a high-fat, high-protein, low-carbohydrate diet is followed for three days. The glycogen content of the muscles is kept low during this time. One possible problem during phase I is a feeling of fatigue, irritability, nervousness, or nausea, due to the low carbohydrate intake. During this phase, many athletes will refuse all forms of dietary carbohydrate and eat only protein and fat, resulting in ketosis. Intake of carbohydrate should be kept at about 100 grams per day.

After three days on the low-carbohydrate diet, the athlete begins the high-carbohydrate diet of phase II. This diet is adequate in protein and fat but the major source of calories is carbohydrate. A minimum of 250 to 525 grams of carbohydrate is needed each day in phase II. During this period, glycogen synthesis is enhanced and is localized to the muscles that were depleted during phase I. Exercise is not recommended at this time, because it depletes the glycogen stores. Diets during phases I and II should be similar in caloric value and should be designed to meet the athlete's protein and energy needs.

Phase III is the day of the event. The athlete may eat anything he wishes. If an athlete thinks any one food will help his performance, he should eat it. The pre-event meal should be eaten three to four hours before the event, so that the stomach is empty at the time of competition. Intake of food or fluid is necessary during an endurance event, to maintain hydration and blood glucose.

A shorter method of carbohydrate loading would consist of the exhausting exercise on day 4 before the event, followed by three days of high-carbohydrate diet. Many misconceptions exist about diet for carbohydrate loading. Many equate carbohydrate with foods containing simple sugar, such as candy, soft drinks, and honey, neglecting the complex carbohydrate sources such as vegetables, breads, and cereals.

Several investigators believe that the carbohydrate loading technique should be used with caution and done at most two to three times a year[37]. In addition to glycogen, water is also deposited in muscle in amounts equal to about three times the amount of glycogen deposited. While this deposit of water may contribute to a sensation of muscular heaviness and stiffness, some believe that it partly compensates for the evaporative water losses experienced during the event. It does, however, result in increased body weight. For example, with glycogen storage of 700 grams, there is an increase in body water amounting to about 2 kilograms. In activities in which the body weight must be lifted, an excessive glycogen store should be avoided.

Carbohydrate loading should be used very selectively for high school and college athletes, and rarely, if ever, for early adolescent or pre-adolescent athletes.[38]

Athletes with diabetes or hypertriglyceridemia or who are at risk for cardiovascular disease should consult their physicians about endurance exercise or carbohydrate loading.[38]

Although carbohydrate loading appears to enhance performance, its use has been questioned. Mirkin reported ST-T wave changes and chest pain in a 40-year-old man who followed an extreme version of the carbohydrate-loading diet.[38,39] Blair et al[40] monitored possible electrocardiogram and blood lipid changes in a group of 14 well-trained runners who engaged in carbohydrate loading. Ten of these runners followed the classic carbohydrate-loading procedure and four runners followed their usual diets. No changes were noted for any variables in the nonloading runners. Runners who used the carbohydrate loading had higher triglyceride values after the race, and may have exhibited slight decreases in R–wave height after carbohydrate loading. It has also been suggested that athletes using carbohydrate loading may be destroying muscle fibers, due to the high glycogen stores or to the heavy exercise. Because no evidence supports this theory, no definitive statement can be made concerning possible muscular breakdown.

The purpose of carbohydrate loading is to supersaturate with glycogen the muscles to be used in competition. The competition should be longer than 30 to 60 minutes, to fully utilize the glycogen stores. The complete technique of carbohydrate loading should be used only for endurance events and, because of the demands on the muscles, it should be used sparingly, possibly two to three times a year. For shorter events, phase I can be omitted and phase II can be followed to fill but, not supersaturate, glycogen stores.

The effects of using the technique over a competitive lifetime are unknown. Adverse effects are suspected, but full knowledge of possible dangers is lacking at this time because of the limited duration of use. If this dietary manipulation is practiced by many athletes to enhance their endurance and achieve better performance, the nutritional adequacy of the diet should be carefully considered.

Precompetition Meals

Unfounded beliefs have probably placed greater restrictions than necessary on food choices for the precompetition meal. The rigidity of some well-known recommendations is obviously extreme and limited in the light of what is known about food and its digestion. There is no reason that an athlete should not enjoy his pre-event meal and have the privilege of selecting the customary food he enjoys at other times during training. Probably more important than the foods consumed during this meal is the psychologic significance ascribed to foods or combination of foods by the athlete.

The relative composition or size of the meal preceding an event of short duration has little influence on improving performance. The main concern is that the meal be consumed at a reasonable time, usually three hours before the competitive event, which allows for digestion and absorption but is not long enough for feelings of hunger to develop.

In long-duration events,[41] the meal should also be consumed about three hours before the event. The fat content of the meal should be kept at a minimum, however, because fat in any form slows stomach-emptying time. Protein intake should also be limited because most protein sources contain fat. The athlete will want digestion in the stomach to be complete before the competitive event begins. Protein also yields the nitrogen by-products of digestion, which can only be eliminated by urinary excretion, therefore requiring fluid loss. The carbohydrate content of the meal should be higher than normal, because it is easily digested and readily absorbed and will ensure adequate glycogen stores. The meal should exclude foods that are likely to cause flatulence and discomfort. To compensate for sweat losses, the athletes should drink 2 to 3 cups of water to insure adequate hydration. An additional cup of water should be taken 1½ hours before competition. Ingestion of bouillon, broth, or consomme at least three hours before the event will ensure adequate salt intake. Because of its potentially detrimental effect, alcohol should be avoided. Caffeine in coffee and tea should also be avoided because it has a diuretic effect, causing a depletion in body water and because it is a central nervous system stimulant that may impair the athlete's awareness of fatigue. Some athletes are more sensitive than others to the effects of caffeine. With the ingestion of 4 to 5 mg per kilogram body weight (2 cups of coffee for a 70 kg man), some claims have been made that caffeine prior to exercise stimulates the release of free fatty acid, thus sparing glycogen[42].

Costill believes that an experienced runner will generally learn when and what to eat during precompetition[43]. For a race that begins at noon, the runner generally eats his major meal about 6 o'clock the night before, followed in four hours by a snack. Breakfast should be taken about 4 hours before the race. All of these meals and snacks should be high carbohydrate, defined by Costill as being 60% to 70% of calories as carbohydrate. A study[44] analyzing the training methods and racing techniques of 12 athletes who have completed 100-mile runs was reported. A wide variation in the ways athletes prepare for and run a 100-mile race was seen. Moreover, the results suggest that an average marathoner can finish a 100-mile race without modifying his training program. Requisites for optimal performance in the 100- mile run remain ill-defined. These data show no consistent correlation between finishing times and a runner's age, sex, height, weight, running experience, weekly mileage, frequency and intensity of workouts, diet, use of vitamins and other supplements, or nourishment during the run.

To maintain energy and prevent dehydration in long-duration events, runners need to drink during competition. Excess amounts of glucose, dextrose pills, sugar cubes, honey, or hard candy should be avoided because they draw fluid into the intestinal tract and may add to the problem of dehydration. A concentrated sugar solution may also cause distension of the stomach, cramps, nausea, and diarrhea.

The American College of Sports Medicine position statement on prevention of heat injuries in distance running suggests that fluids containing less than 2.5 grams glucose per 100 ml of water and less than 10 mEq sodium and 5 mEq potassium per liter of solution be used.[45] These proportions are recommended as sufficiently dilute to allow for rapid gastric emptying. Commercial solutions are generally more concentrated than the recommended solution. The role of the electrolytes, sodium, and potassium in the recommended fluid is primarily to improve absorption; these electrolytes do not appear to need to be replaced during exercise.

The addition of glucose increases the blood glucose level and thus increases the insulin level, which may increase the utilization of glucose. The ingestion of glucose may decrease the rate of utilization of glycogen and thereby improve endurance. The position paper also states that runners should be encouraged to ingest fluids frequently during competition and to consume 400 to 500 ml of fluid 10 to 15 minutes before competition. In races of 16 km (10 mi) or more, fluid should be consumed every 3 to 4 km (2-2.5 mi).

Summary

Aside from heredity and training no single factor plays a bigger role in the quality of athletic performance than diet. Physical training by the athlete requires that appropriate adjustments in the diet be made in total calories, proportion of carbohydrates, water, salt, and iron to maintain optimal performance.

A varied diet, sufficient in amount to satisfy the energy needs of an athlete, will provide adequate vitamins and minerals. The energy cost of a sport depends on the intensity of the physical activity demanded, the length of time of intense exertion, and the total time of participation. Eating habits that promote obesity, semistarvation, dehydration, and excess vitamin supplementation are counterproductive to physical training and optimal performance.

REFERENCES

1. Mayer J, Bullen B: Nutrition and athletic performance. Physiol Rev 40:369-397, 1960.
2. Pemberton,CM, Morness, KE, German,M, et al., Mayo Clinic Diet Manual. Ed 6. Philadelphia, BC Decker Inc., 1988,P 546-547.
3. Mitchell HS, Rynbergen HJ, Anderson L, et al: Nutrition in Health and Disease. Philadelphia, JB Lippincott Company, 1976, p 121.
4. Bogert LJ, Briggs, GM, Calloway DH: Nutrition and Physical Fitness. Philadelphia, WB Saunders Co, 1973, p 39.
5. Consolazio CF, Johnson RE, Pecora LJ: Physiological Measurements of Metabolic Functions in Man. New York, McGraw-Hill Book Company, 1963, p 505.
6. Costill DL: Physiology of marathon running. JAMA 221:1024-1029, 1972.
7. Buskirk ER: Diet and athletic performance. Postgrad Med 61:229-236, 1977.
8. Costill DL, Bowers R, Kammer WF: Skinfold estimates of body fat among marathon runners. Med Sci Sports 2:93-95, 1970.
9. Cureton KJ, Sparling PB, Evans BW, et al: Effect of experimental alterations in excess weight on aerobic capacity and distance running performance. Med Sci Sports 10:194-199, 1978.
10. Serfass RC: Nutrition for the athlete. Contemporary Nutrition 2:May, 1977.
11. Consolazio CF, Johnson HL: Dietary carbohydrate and work capacity. Am J Clin Nutr 25:85-90, 1972.
12. Astrand PO: Nutrition and physical performance. World Rev Nutr Diet 16:59-79, 1973.
13. Pitts GC, Consolazio CF, Johnson RE: Dietary protein and physical fitness in temperate and hot environments. J Nutr 27:497, 1944.
14. Evans WJ, Fisher EC, Hoerr RA, Young VR: Protein metabolism and endurance exercise. The Physician and Sportsmedicine 11:63-72, 1983.
15. Keys A, Henschel AF, Mickelsen O, et al: The performance of normal men on controlled thiamine intake. J Nutr 26:399-415, 1943.
16. Bergstrom J, Hultman E, Jorfeldt L, et al: Effect of nicotinic acid on physical working capacity and on metabolism of muscle glycogen in man. J Appl Physiol 26:170-176, 1969.
17. Niacin and myocardial metabolism. Nutr Rev 31:80-81, 1973.
18. Gey GO, Cooper KH, Bottenberg RA: Effect of ascorbic acid on endurance performance and athletic injury. JAMA 211:105, 1970.
19. Rhead WJ, Schrauzer GN: Risks of long-term ascorbic acid overdose (letter to the editor). Nutr Rev 29:262-263, 1971.
20. Farrell PM, Bieri JG: Megavitamin E supplementation in man. Am J Clin Nutr 28:1386, 1975.

21. Lawrence JD, Bower RC, Riehl WP, et al: Effects of a tocopherol acetate on the swimming endurance of trained swimmers. Am J Clin Nutr 28:205-208, 1975.

22. United States Department of Health, Education and Welfare: Ten-State Nutrition Survey in the United States. DHEW Publication No. HSM 73-8704 Washington, DC, Government Printing Office, 1972.

23. Bunch TW: Blood test abnormalities in runners. Mayo Clin Proc 55:113-117, 1980.

24. Martin DE, Vroon DH, May DF, Pilbeam SP: Physiological changes in elite male distance runners training. The Physician and Sportsmedicine 14:152-171, 1986.

25. Ehn L, Carlmark B, Hoglund S: Iron status in athletes involved in intense physical activity. Med Sci Spor Exer 12:61- 64, 1980.

26. Pate RR: Sports anemia: A review of the current research literature. The Physician and Sportsmedicine 11:115-131, 1983.

27. Ehn L, Carlmark B, Hoglund S: Iron status in athletes involved in intense physical activity. Med Sci Sports Exercise 12(Spring):61-64, 1980.

28. Vellar OD: Studies on sweat losses of nutrients. Iron content of whole body sweat and its association with other sweat constituents, serum iron levels, hematological indices, body surface area, and sweat rate. Scand J Clin Invest 21:157-167, 1968.

29. Smith NJ: Food for Sport. Palo Alto, CA. Bull Publishing Company, 1976, p. 90-103.

30. Bergstrom J, Hultman E: Nutrition for maximal sports performance. JAMA 221:999-1006, 1972.

31. Nelson RA: Preventing and treating dehydration. The Physician and Sportsmedicine 13:176-178, 1985.

32. Williams MH: Nutritional faddism and athletics. Nutr and MD IV:1-2, 1977.

33. Food and Nutrition Board, Recommended Dietary Allowances, 1980, National Research Council-National Academy of Sciences, Washington, DC, 9th ed.

34. Bergstrom J. Hermansen L, Hultman E, et al: Diet, muscle glycogen and physical performance. Acta Physiol Scand 71:140-150, 1967.

35. Hermansen L, Hultman E, Saltin B: Muscle glycogen during prolonged severe exercise. Acta Physiol Scand 71:129-139, 1967.

36. Slovic P: What helps the long distance runner run? Nutr Today 10:18-21, 1975.

37. Forgac MT: Carbohydrate loading—a review. JADA 75:42- 45, 1979.

38. Amer Diet Assoc: Position paper: Nutrition and physical fitness. J Amer Diet Assoc 76:437-443, 1980.

39. Mirkin G: Carbohydrate loading: A dangerous practice (letter to the editor). JAMA 223:1511-1512, 1973.

40. Blair S, Sargent R, Davidson D, Krejci R: Blood lipid and ECG responses to carbohydrate loading. The Physician and Sportsmedicine 8:69-75, 1980.

41. Nutrition for Athletes: A Handbood for Coaches. Washington, DC American Association for Health, Physical Education, and Recreation, 1971.

42. Salvin JL, Joensen DJ: Caffeine and sports performance. The Physician and

Sportsmedicine 13:191-193, 1985.
43. Costil DL: Get a load of this. The Runner, May 1980, p. 68.
44. Fred HL: The 100-mile run: Preparation, performance, and recovery a case report. The Amer J of Sports Med 9:258-261, 1981.
45. American College of Sports Medicine: Prevention of heat injuries during distance running. Med Sci Sports 7:7-8, 1975.

Index